Exotic Animal Oncology

Editor

DAVID SANCHEZ-MIGALLON GUZMAN

VETERINARY CLINICS OF NORTH AMERICA: EXOTIC ANIMAL PRACTICE

www.vetexotic.theclinics.com

Consulting Editor
JÖRG MAYER

January 2017 • Volume 20 • Number 1

ELSEVIER

1600 John F. Kennedy Boulevard • Suite 1800 • Philadelphia, Pennsylvania, 19103-2899
http://www.vetexotic.theclinics.com

VETERINARY CLINICS OF NORTH AMERICA: EXOTIC ANIMAL PRACTICE Volume 20, Number 1
January 2017 ISSN 1094-9194, ISBN-13: 978-0-323-48273-8

Editor: Katie Pfaff
Developmental Editor: Meredith Clinton

Veterinary Clinics of North America: Exotic Animal Practice (ISSN 1094-9194) is published in January, May, and September by Elsevier, Inc., 360 Park Avenue South, New York, NY 10010-1710. Subscription prices are $265.00 per year for US individuals, $460.00 per year for US institutions, $100.00 per year for US students and residents, $311.00 per year for Canadian individuals, $554.00 per year for Canadian institutions, $347.00 per year for international individuals, $554.00 per year for international institutions and $165.00 per year for Canadian and foreign students/residents. To receive student/resident rate, orders must be accompanied by name of affiliated institution, date of term, and the *signature* of program/residency coordinator on institution letterhead. Orders will be billed at individual rate until proof of status is received. Foreign air speed delivery is included in all *Clinics* subscription prices. All prices are subject to change without notice. **POSTMASTER:** Send address changes to *Veterinary Clinics of North America: Exotic Animal Practice,* Elsevier Health Sciences Division, Subscription Customer Service, 3251 Riverport Lane, Maryland Heights, MO 63043. **Customer Service: Telephone: 1-800-654-2452** (U.S. and Canada); **1-314-447-8871** (outside U.S. and Canada). **Fax: 1-314-447-8029. E-mail: journalscustomerservice-usa@elsevier.com (for print support); journalsonlinesupport-usa@elsevier.com (for online support).**

Reprints. For copies of 100 or more of articles in this publication, please contact the Commercial Reprints Department, Elsevier Inc., 360 Park Avenue South, New York, New York 10010-1710. Tel.: 212-633-3874; Fax: 212-633-3820; E-mail: reprints@elsevier.com.

Veterinary Clinics of North America: Exotic Animal Practice is covered in *MEDLINE/PubMed (Index Medicus).*

Contributors

CONSULTING EDITOR

JÖRG MAYER, Dr.med.vet, MSc
Diplomate American Board of Veterinary Practitioners (Exotic Companion Mammals); Diplomate European College of Zoological Medicine (Small Mammals); Diplomate American College of Zoological Medicine; Associate Professor of Zoological Medicine, Department of Small Animal Medicine and Surgery, College of Veterinary Medicine, University of Georgia, Athens, Georgia

EDITOR

DAVID SANCHEZ-MIGALLON GUZMAN, LV, MS
Diplomate, European College of Zoological Medicine (Avian, Small Mammal); Diplomate, American College of Zoological Medicine; Associate Professor of Clinical Zoological Companion Animal Medicine and Surgery, Department of Veterinary Medicine and Epidemiology, School of Veterinary Medicine, University of California Davis, Davis, California

AUTHORS

MELANIE AMMERSBACH, DVM
Department of Pathobiology, Ontario Veterinary College, University of Guelph, Guelph, Ontario, Canada

JANE CHRISTMAN, DVM
Small Animal Intern, Department of Small Animal Clinical Sciences, College of Veterinary Medicine and Biomedical Sciences, Texas A&M University, College Station, Texas

MICHAEL DEVAU, DVM
Diplomate, American College of Veterinary Radiology (Radiation Oncology); Clinical Assistant Professor, Department of Small Animal Clinical Sciences, College of Veterinary Medicine and Biomedical Sciences, Texas A&M University, College Station, Texas

DAVID ESHAR, DVM
Diplomate, American Board of Veterinary Practitioners (Exotic Companion Mammals); Diplomate, European College of Zoological Medicine (Small Mammal); Assistant Professor of Companion Exotic Pets, Wildlife & Zoo Animal Medicine, Department of Clinical Sciences, Kansas State University, Manhattan, Kansas

JOSEPH M. GROFF, VMD, PhD
Associate Pathologist, William R. Pritchard Veterinary Medical Teaching Hospital, School of Veterinary Medicine, University of California, Davis, Davis, California

TARA MYERS HARRISON, DVM, MPVM
Diplomate, American College of Zoological Medicine; Diplomate, American College of
Veterinary Preventive Medicine; Clinical Assistant Professor, Department of Clinical
Sciences, North Carolina State University College of Veterinary Medicine, Raleigh,
North Carolina

J. JILL HEATLEY, DVM, MS
Diplomate, American Board of Veterinary Practitioners (Avian, Reptilian & Amphibian);
Diplomate, American College of Zoological Medicine; Associate Professor, Department of
Small Animal Clinical Sciences, College of Veterinary Medicine and Biomedical Sciences,
Texas A&M University, College Station, Texas

SAMUEL E. HOCKER, DVM
Oncology Resident, Department of Clinical Sciences, Kansas State University,
Manhattan, Kansas

SHARMAN HOPPES, DVM
Diplomate, American Board of Veterinary Practitioners (Avian); Clinical Associate
Professor, Department of Small Animal Clinical Sciences, College of Veterinary Medicine
and Biomedical Sciences, Texas A&M University, College Station, Texas

MICHAEL S. KENT, MAS, DVM
Diplomate, American College of Veterinary Internal Medicine (Oncology); Diplomate,
American College of Veterinary Radiology (Radiation Oncology); Director, Center for
Companion Animal Health; Professor, Department of Surgical and Radiological Sciences,
School of Veterinary Medicine, University of California, Davis, Davis, California

BARBARA E. KITCHELL, DVM, PhD
Diplomate, American College of Veterinary Internal Medicine (Internal Medicine and
Oncology); Staff Oncologist; Director of VCA Residency Training Programs, Department
of Oncology, VCA Veterinary Care Referral Center, Albuquerque, New Mexico

GREGORY A. LEWBART, MS, VMD
Diplomate, American College of Zoological Medicine; Raleigh, North Carolina

CHRISTOPH MANS, Dr med vet
Diplomate, American College of Zoological Medicine; Department of Surgical Sciences,
School of Veterinary Medicine, University of Wisconsin-Madison, Madison, Wisconsin

MARIE-EVE NADEAU, DVM
Diplomate, American College of Veterinary Internal Medicine (Oncology); Associate
Professor of Oncology, Centre Hospitalier Vétérinaire Universitaire, Faculté de médecine
vétérinaire, Université de Montréal, Saint-Hyacinthe, Québec, Canada

ALISA L. NEWTON, VMD
Diplomate, American College of Veterinary Pathologists; Wildlife Conservation Society,
Bronx, New York

RAQUEL RECH, DVM, MSC, PhD
Diplomate, American College of Veterinary Pathologists (Anatomic Pathology);
Department of Veterinary Pathobiology, College of Veterinary Medicine and Biomedical
Sciences, Texas A&M University, College Station, Texas

CECILIA S. ROBAT, Dr med vet
Diplomate, American College of Veterinary Internal Medicine (Subspecialty Oncology);
Veterinary Emergency Service, Veterinary Specialty Center, Middleton, Wisconsin

KAREN E. RUSSELL, DVM, PhD
Diplomate, American College of Veterinary Pathologists (ClinPath); Professor, Department of Small Animal Clinical Sciences, College of Veterinary Medicine and Biomedical Sciences, Texas A&M University, College Station, Texas

NICO J. SCHOEMAKER, DVM, PhD
Diplomate, European College of Zoological Medicine (Small Mammal & Avian); Diplomate, American Board of Veterinary Practitioners-Avian Practice; Associate Professor, Faculty of Veterinary Medicine, Division of Zoologic Medicine, Department of Clinical Sciences of Companion Animals, Utrecht University, Utrecht, The Netherlands

MICHELE A. STEFFEY, DVM
Diplomate, American College of Veterinary Surgeons; ACVS Founding Fellow, Surgical Oncology, Associate Professor of Small Animal Surgery, School of Veterinary Medicine, University of California, Davis, Davis, California

YVONNE VAN ZEELAND, DVM, MVR, PhD, CPBC
Diplomate, European College of Zoological Medicine (Avian, Small Mammal); Associate Professor, Division of Zoological Medicine, Department of Clinical Sciences of Companion Animals, Faculty of Veterinary Medicine, Utrecht University, Utrecht, The Netherlands

CLAIRE VERGNEAU-GROSSET, med vet, IPSAV
Diplomate, American College of Zoological Medicine; Clinical Instructor, Zoological Medicine Service, Centre Hospitalier Vétérinaire Universitaire, Faculté de médecine vétérinaire, Université de Montréal, Saint-Hyacinthe, Quebec, Canada; Veterinarian, Aquarium du Québec, Quebec, Canada

HEATHER WILSON-ROBLES, DVM
Diplomate, American College of Veterinary Internal Medicine (Oncology); Associate Professor, Department of Small Animal Clinical Sciences, College of Veterinary Medicine and Biomedical Sciences, Texas A&M University, College Station, Texas

RAELENE M. WOUDA, BVSc, MANZCVS (SAIM)
Diplomate, American College of Veterinary Internal Medicine (Oncology); Assistant Professor of Oncology, Department of Clinical Sciences, Kansas State University, Manhattan, Kansas

Contents

Exotic Animal Oncology

VETERINARY CLINICS OF NORTH AMERICA: EXOTIC ANIMAL PRACTICE

THE CLINICS ARE NOW AVAILABLE ONLINE!
Access your subscription at:
www.theclinics.com

Preface

Exotic Animal Oncology

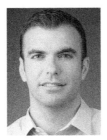

David Sanchez-Migallon Guzman, LV, MS, DECZM (Avian, Small Mammal), DACZM
Editor

With an increase in the life expectancy of our exotic patients and the increasing demand in the quality of patient care, the diagnosis and treatment of cancer in our patients have gained more importance in our daily practice. We are faced now with clients that are emotionally connected with personal experiences and more educated in the diagnosis and treatment of cancer, with higher expectations regarding prognosis for some of these diseases. While much progress has been made and we feel like we can provide advanced diagnostic and treatment options, exotic animal oncology is still in an early stage of development when compared with what is known in canine, feline, and of course, human patients.

This issue of the *Veterinary Clinics of North America: Exotic Animal Practice* covers, in separate articles, oncology in invertebrates, fish, reptiles, birds, rabbits, rodents, and ferrets as well as the principles of medical and surgical oncology and radiation therapy. The information presented here evidences the significant advances that our field has experienced in this area over the last 10 years, with numerous retrospective studies and case reports, as well as evaluation of new treatments for different types of cancer in these species.

I would like to encourage clinicians to consult with board-certified medical oncologists, surgeons, and radiation oncologists when evaluating and treating exotic patients with cancer as well as document these cases and promote research in this area. A simple way to do that is by contributing cases to the Exotic Tumor Database, a project of the Exotic Species Cancer Research Alliance (www.escra.org), where the information gained with each case reported is shared to advance the knowledge and ultimately improve the care of our patients.

Also, I would like to thank all the authors for their efforts and contribution to this issue; we hope that the reader will find the information presented here educational and clinically applicable. It was our goal to help clinicians keep up with the increasing new information in this area and present it in a clear and effective manner. Last, I would like to thank Elsevier for the opportunity given to serve as a guest editor of this issue

Vet Clin Exot Anim 20 (2017) xi–xii
http://dx.doi.org/10.1016/j.cvex.2016.10.001
1094-9194/17/© 2016 Published by Elsevier Inc.

vetexotic.theclinics.com

and for their support and guidance. It has been a great pleasure, and I look forward to contributing again to the *Veterinary Clinics of North America: Exotic Animal Practice* in the future.

David Sanchez-Migallon Guzman, LV, MS, DECZM (Avian, Small Mammal), DACZM
Department of Veterinary Medicine and Epidemiology
School of Veterinary Medicine
University of California Davis
One Shields Avenue, 2108 Tupper Hall
Davis, CA 95616, USA

E-mail address:
guzman@ucdavis.edu

Invertebrate Oncology
Diseases, Diagnostics, and Treatment

Alisa L. Newton, VMD, DACVP[a],
Gregory A. Lewbart, MS, VMD, DACZM[b],*

KEYWORDS

- Invertebrate • Neoplasia • Oncology • Surgery • Histopathology • Diagnosis
- Treatment

KEY POINTS

- Neoplasia is a documented occurrence across invertebrate taxa, but challenges remain with regard to tumor diagnosis, identification, and treatment.
- Literature reports of neoplasia are frequent in mollusks and insects, infrequent in Cnidaria and crustaceans, and are yet to be documented in Porifera and Echinodermata.
- The use of traditional methods of diagnosis in veterinary medicine is encouraged, but the unique anatomy and tissue biology of each invertebrate taxon needs to be taken into account.
- Most neoplasms described in the invertebrate literature have been benign, and many external lesions may be amenable to surgical resection.

INTRODUCTION

At the beginning of the twentieth century, it was argued that invertebrates were incapable of developing neoplasia.[1,2] This argument was based on anatomic differences in the nervous and vascular systems of invertebrates and the embryonal theory of tumor growth, which was popular at the time, believing that invertebrate cells were already in an embryonic state and therefore could not revert to a more undifferentiated state that would produce tumors.[3] After decades of study and based on the current understanding of its causes, neoplasia is a well-documented occurrence across invertebrate taxa.[4] Neoplasia is defined as the proliferation of genetically altered cells that fail to respond to the normal regulatory controls of cell growth.[5,6] The genetic alterations can be spontaneous, hereditary, or acquired as a result of exposure to mechanical (radiation), chemical (carcinogens), or infectious (oncoviruses) agents.[6] All 3 causes

---

Disclosures: The authors have nothing to disclose.
[a] Wildlife Conservation Society, Bronx, NY, USA; [b] 1060 William Moore Drive, Raleigh, NC 27607, USA
* Corresponding author.
E-mail address: greg_lewbart@ncsu.edu

have been recognized in invertebrates.[7] Importantly, the study of invertebrate neoplasms has revealed that many genes and pathways involved in neoplastic transformation and metastasis are evolutionarily conserved and invertebrate models of neoplasia, particularly in *Drosophila* spp and *Caenorhabditis elegans*, are contributing significantly to the understanding of tumorigenesis.[6]

There have been, and remain, many challenges to documenting neoplasms in invertebrates. The images and descriptions of gross and microscopic findings in the older literature, which would allow comparison or peer evaluation of the identification, are inadequate.[3] Pathologists can be inexperienced with the identification of invertebrate tissues, normal tissue reaction, inflammation, and wound repair. Invertebrate biologists are often not familiar with tumor biology, identification, and classification. Both have led to confusing diagnoses in the invertebrate neoplasia literature.[3,4,7] The classifications that exist for mammalian tumors are also difficult to apply to invertebrate neoplasms, in some cases may not be appropriate, and the tools relied on for cell identification (immunohistochemistry) are generally unavailable. The characteristics used to define neoplasms in vertebrates, particularly mammals, include (1) self-sufficiency in growth signals, (2) insensitivity to antigrowth signals, (3) evasion of apoptosis, (4) unlimited replicative potential, (5) sustained angiogenesis, and (6) tissue invasion and metastasis.[8] These characteristics may be challenging to fulfill across invertebrate taxa because the organs, organ systems, cell types, and metabolic reactions are different from their vertebrate counterparts and the anatomy of most invertebrate circulatory systems (partially open or lacking organization) makes documenting angiogenesis extremely difficult.[4] The establishment of the Registry of Tumors in Lower Animals (RTLA), a cooperative project between the National Institutes of Health (NIH) National Cancer Institute (NCI) and the Smithsonian Institution's National Museum of Natural History in 1965 greatly advanced the understanding of the occurrence, gross and microscopic pathology, and cause of invertebrate neoplasms. However, this valuable resource closed in 2007 because of a lack of funding, although the archives still exist. It is notable that, out of the 1550 invertebrate submissions made to the RTLA database and evaluated by the RTLA pathologists between 1965 and its closure in 2007, only 30% were ultimately designated to be neoplasms.[4]

This article assists veterinarians in evaluating and treating invertebrates with suspected neoplasia by (1) summarizing the major types of neoplasms that have been documented across invertebrate taxa, (2) describing the diagnostic tools available to clinicians and pathologists to identify and confirm neoplastic processes, and (3) recommending possible treatment options for invertebrates with neoplasia.

NEOPLASMS REPORTED IN INVERTEBRATES

All tumors consist of 2 major components: the parenchyma, composed of the transformed neoplastic cells; and the stroma, composed of nonneoplastic host-derived connective tissue, blood vessels, and inflammatory cells. The parenchyma largely determines a tumor's biological behavior and classification. The stroma is critical to the growth of the neoplasm by providing structure and necessary blood supply to support the growth of the parenchymal cells.[5] The fundamental characteristics used to differentiate benign from malignant neoplasms include (1) degree of cellular differentiation and anaplasia, (2) rate of growth, (3) local invasion, and (4) evidence of metastasis.[5] These features should be applied with caution because invertebrate neoplasms have rarely been studied over time, mitotic figures can be transient, cell division may be under heavy hormonal control, and evidence of local invasion and metastasis can be difficult to assess in species with open circulatory systems.[4]

The incidence of reported neoplasms across invertebrate taxa are variable both between and within phyla and subphyla. Reports of neoplasia are frequent in phylum Mollusca and subphylum Hexapoda (class Insecta), infrequent in phylum Cnidaria and subphylum Crustacea, and are not yet documented in phyla Porifera or Echinodermata. This distribution is undoubtedly biased because these reports largely reflect the extent of monitoring performed in a given taxa, which by its nature focuses on invertebrates of economic importance.[6] With notable exceptions, most neoplasms described in invertebrates have been reported to be benign, largely because of a lack of variation in cell size and shape (anaplasia), lack of mitotic figures, and a lack of organ invasion or metastatic spread.[6] A summary table of the individual invertebrate neoplasms received and documented by the RTLA between 1965 and 2007 is reproduced here with permission (**Table 1**).[4] In addition, readers are directed to several summaries of invertebrate neoplasia that have been produced over the last few decades.[3,9,10] The invertebrate neoplasms best described in the literature are discussed later and grouped by anatomic location.

Tumors of the Carapace or External Body Wall

Tumorlike lesions of the carapace have been described in crustaceans and classified as papillomas or hamartomas, a proliferation of disorganized tissue indigenous to the examined site.[4,11] Hamartomas were considered to be developmental anomalies in mammals, but recent genetic studies have documented acquired translocations in some, which suggests a neoplastic origin.[5] Carapace tumors have been described arising from the abdominal somites in brown shrimp (*Farfantepenaeus aztecus*) and an American lobster (*Homarus americanus*) with additional occurrences in lobster anecdotally reported.[11,12] Similar lesions in California brown shrimp (*Farfantepenaeus californiensis*) were reported in the RTLA archive (see **Table 1**). Affected crustaceans were adults at an intermolt stage. These tumors were broad based, firm, exophytic proliferations with a papilliform to rugose surface and increased pigmentation reported apically (**Fig. 1**). On cut section, tumors were fibrous with a convoluted cuticle of variable thickness covering the surface. On histology, the epidermis and subepidermis were continuous with the adjacent unaffected areas, but epithelial cells within the mass showed altered histomorphology, described as hypertrophic and hyperchromatic in shrimp and columnar with globose apical vacuoles in the lobster. Adnexa (tegmental glands, setal inserts and pigment cells) were locally absent in the lobster, and multifocally absent within the brown shrimp. When present in the shrimp, these glands were noted to be increased in number and in an abnormal (deep) location to the epidermis. The stroma was composed of fibrous connective tissue with scattered muscle fibers and few arterioles and small numbers of infiltrating hemocytes. Mitotic figures were not observed in either reported case but both investigators suggested that the strong hormonal control of cell division in crustaceans may limit the ability for mitoses to occur outside times of ecdysis even in neoplastic lesions. The cause of these carapace lesions remains unknown. No infectious agents have been identified within the lesions. The cause in lobster was hypothesized to be local trauma, with bleeding and wound repair to the affected somite, but the lack of adnexa suggests epidermal disruptions more complex than simply failing to unfold during ecdysis and is more consistent with a neoplasm. It is not clear whether animals affected by these lesions can survive molting because of the lack of tegmental glands (which provide lubrication during ecdysis) and the size of the lesions, which would likely adhere to the instar during molting.[11,12]

Several different benign external tumors, papillomas, polypoid tumors, or polypoid growths have been described in gastropod and bivalve mollusks. The locations and

Table 1
Invertebrate neoplasms in the RTLA collection.

Phylum Class Order	Family	Species	Common Name	Neoplasm (Number of Cases in RTLA)
Annelida				
Oligochaeta				
Haplotaxida	Lumbricidae	*Lumbricus terrestris*	Earthworm	Myoblastoma: ventral coelom (1)
Arthropoda				
Insecta				
Blattodea	Blattidae	*Leucophaea maderae*	Madeira cockroach	Neoplasm: salivary reservoir (1)
Diptera	Drosophilidae	*Drosophila melanogaster*	Fruit fly	Cystocyte neoplasm: ovary (3)
				Ganglioneuroblastoma: brain (1)
				Lethal (1) malignant blood neoplasm: systemic (1)
				Lethal (2) malignant blood neoplasm: systemic (1)
				Lethal (3) malignant blood neoplasm: systemic (1)
				Neoplasm: imaginal disk (3)
Malacostraca				
Decapoda	Lithodidae	*Paralithodes platypus*	Blue king crab	Carcinoma: antennal gland (1)
		Paralithodes camtschatica	Red king crab	Carcinoma: hindgut (1)
	Palaemonidae	*Exopalaemon (formerly Palaemon) orientis*	Oriental prawn or grass shrimp	Carcinoma: embryo (2)
	Penaeidae	*Farfantepenaeus (formerly Penaeus) aztecus*	Brown shrimp	Papilloma: epidermis (1)
		Farfantepenaeus (formerly Penaeus) californiensis	California brown shrimp	Papilloma: epidermis (1)
				Hematopoietic sarcoma: multicentric (1)
		Litopenaeus (formerly Penaeus) vannamei	Mexican white shrimp	**Papilloma: epidermis (1)**

	Family	Species	Common name	Tumor (count)
Cnidaria				
Anthozoa				
Scleractinia	Acroporidae	Acropora cervicornis	Staghorn coral	Epithelioma: calicoblastic epidermis (conjectured) (5)
		Acropora formosa	Formosan staghorn coral	Epithelioma: calicoblastic epidermis (4)
		Acropora palmata	Elkhorn coral	Epithelioma: calicoblastic epidermis (10)
		Acropora valenciennesi	Coral	Epithelioma: calicoblastic epidermis (4)
		Montipora sp	Coral	Epithelioma: calicoblastic epidermis (conjectured) (1)
Mollusca				
Bivalvia				
Myoida	Myidae	Mya arenaria	Softshell	Adenoma: kidney (4); Disseminated neoplasia: systemic (29); Germinoma: gonad (114); Germinoma: gonad; carcinoma: stomach (1); Germinoma: gonad; papilloma: epidermis (1); Germinoma: multicentric (15); Papilloma: gill (3)
		Mya truncata	Truncate softshell	Disseminated neoplasia: systemic (1); Fibrosarcoma: multicentric (1)
Mytiloida	Mytilidae	Geukensia demissa	Ribbed mussel	Teratoma: gonad (1)
		Modiolus	Northern horse mussel	Vesicular cell sarcoma: visceral mass (1)
		Mytilus edulis	Blue mussel	Carcinoma: gill (1)
		Mytilus galloprovincialis	Mediterranean mussel	Disseminated neoplasia: systemic (8)
		Mytilus sp	Mussel	Germinoma: gonad (1)
		Mytilus trossulus	Foolish mussel	Disseminated neoplasia: systemic (2)
		M trossulus (?)	Foolish mussel (?)	Fibroma: gonad (1)
		M trossulus/ galloprovincialis	Mussel	Germinoma: gonad (1); Vesicular cell sarcoma: gonad (1); Disseminated neoplasia: systemic (4); Disseminated neoplasia: systemic (2); Myxoma: multicentric (1)

(continued on next page)

Table 1
(continued)

Phylum Class Order	Family	Species	Common Name	Neoplasm (Number of Cases in RTLA)
Ostreoida	Ostreidae	*Crassostrea gigas*	Pacific oyster	Disseminated neoplasia: systemic (2)
		Crassostrea virginica	Eastern oyster	Epithelioma: mantle (1)
		Ostrea conchaphila	Olympia oyster	Ganglioneuroma: visceral mass (1)
		Ostrea edulis	Edible oyster	Gonadoblastoma: gonad (1)
		Ostrea sandvicensis	Sandwich Island oyster	Adenocarcinoma in situ: intestine (3)
		Saccostrea glomerata (formerly *commercialis*)	Sydney rock oyster	**Adenocarcinoma: gill (1)**
				Adenoma: intestine (1)
				Adenoma: kidney (1)
				Adenoma: rectum (1)
				Adenopapilloma: gill (1)
				Disseminated neoplasia: systemic (71)
				Fibroma: blood vessel wall (1)
				Fibroma: gonad (1)
				Germinoma: gonad (3)
				Gonadoblastoma: gonad (2)
				Neuroblastoma: visceral ganglion (1)
				Papilloma: gill (1)
				Sarcoma: visceral mass (1)
				Vesicular cell sarcoma: heart (1)
	Pectinidae	*Tiostrea chilensis*	Bluff oyster	Disseminated neoplasia: systemic (6)
		Argopecten irradians	Bay scallop	Disseminated neoplasia: systemic (15)
		Pecten sp	Scallop	Disseminated neoplasia: systemic (1)
				Disseminated neoplasia: systemic (4)
				Papilloma: mantle (33)
				Germinoma: gonad (21)
				Disseminated neoplasia: systemic (1)
				Germinoma: gonad (1)
				Disseminated neoplasia: systemic (1)

	Family	Genus/species	Common name	Neoplasm type
Veneroida	Cardiidae	*Cerastoderma* (formerly *Cardium*) *edule*	Edible dwarf cockle	Adenoma: digestive gland (1); Disseminated neoplasia: systemic (2)
		Cerastoderma (formerly *Cardium*) *glaucum*	Cockle	Disseminated neoplasia: systemic; germinoma: gonad (1); Germinoma: gonad (1)
	Dreissenidae	*Arctica islandica*	Ocean quahog	Disseminated neoplasia: systemic (1)
	Pharidae	***Ensis arcuatus***	**Razor clam**	Disseminated neoplasia: systemic (1)
	Mactridae	*Spisula solidissima*	Atlantic surf clam	Germinoma: gonad (1)
	Tellinidae	*Macoma balthica*	Baltic macoma	**Germinoma: gonad (1)**
		Macoma calcarea	Chalky macoma	Myoma: foot (1)
		Macoma inquinata	Stained macoma	Neurofibroma: foot (1)
		Macoma nasuta	Bent-nose macoma	Mesothelioma: heart (1)
	Veneridae	*Mercenaria*	Northern quahog	Carcinoma: gill (2); Carcinoma: gill v. disseminated neoplasia: systemic (4)
		M mercenaria/Mercenaria campechiensis	Northern southern quahog (hybrid)	Germinoma: gonad; disseminated neoplasia: systemic (1); Disseminated neoplasia: systemic (1)
		Tapes (= *Ruditapes*) *decussata*	Carpet shell clam	Germinoma: gonad (13); Germinoma: gonad (5); Disseminated neoplasia: systemic (5)
Cephalopoda				
Decabrachia	Sepiidae	*Sepia officinalis*	Common cuttlefish	Iridophoroma: dermis (1)
Octopoda	Octopodidae	*Octopus vulgaris*	Atlantic octopus	Fibropapilloma: mantle (1)
Gastropoda				
Archaeogastropoda	Haliotididae	*Haliotis* (formerly *Nordotis*) *discus*	Japanese abalone	Glioma: pleuropedal nerve cord (1)
Architaenioglossa (formerly Mesogastropoda)	Ampullariidae	*Ampullarius australis*	Applesnail	Papilloma: epidermis; adenoma: digestive gland (1)

(continued on next page)

Table 1
(continued)

Phylum Class Order	Family	Species	Common Name	Neoplasm (Number of Cases in RTLA)
Polyplacophora				
Neoloricata	Chitonidae	*Chiton tuberculatus*	West Indian green chiton	Papilloma: gastrointestinal tract (1)
Platyhelminthes				
Trematoda				
Azygiida (formerly Digenea)	Azygiidae	*Otodistomum plunketi*	Trematode	Ganglioneuroblastoma: nerve cord, parenchyma (1)
Turbellaria				
Tricladida	Dugesiidae; Planariidae	*Dugesia; Crenobia* spp	Planarians	Papilloma: epidermis (7)

Boldface indicates cases added from January 2004 through September 2007, when National Cancer Institute funding ceased.

From Peters EC, Smolowitz RM, Reynolds, TL. Neoplasia. In: Lewbart GA, editor. Invertebrate medicine. 2nd edition. Chichester: John Wiley; 2012. p. 432–4; with permission.

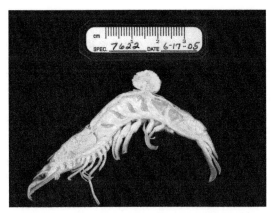

Fig. 1. An epidermal papilloma in a Pacific white shrimp (*Litopenaeus vannamei*). On hemisection, there is an approximately 1.0-cm diameter firm, papilliform mass protruding dorsally between the third and fourth abdominal segments. (*Courtesy of* Esther C. Peters, PhD, George Mason University.)

species affected include the foot of freshwater mussels (*Anodonta californiensis*), oysters (*Crassostrea virginica* and *Crassostrea gigas*) and butter clam (*Saxidomus giganteus*), and the base of the siphon of soft shell clams (*Mya arenaria*) and a horse clam (*Tresus nuttallii*).[13–17] These tumors were described as focal, exophytic, and firm with a texture and color similar to the adjacent tissue of the foot and siphon and in some cases a firm but flexible stalk.[13] On histology, the tumors were covered by normal tall columnar epithelium that was often thrown into convoluted folds. Multifocal hyperplasia of the basophilic glandular cell layer is also noted. The neoplastic portion of these growths consists of a compact, disorganized proliferation of smooth muscle cells, which form the stalk and central portion. In the butter clam, this proliferation seemed to originate from the circular layer of smooth muscle beneath the epithelium of the foot and in soft shell clam seemed to arise from the smooth muscle of the siphon.[14,15] Mitotic figures were not a feature of any of the described tumors and all were classified as benign. Inflammatory infiltrates were present in some tumors, potentially caused by trauma to the lesion.[13–15] The cause of these neoplasms is unknown. Although some investigators have suggested environmental contaminants, others have described them as spontaneous.[14,18]

Exophytic lesions similar to those described earlier have been described in apple snail (*Ampullarius australis*) and giant African snail (*Achatina fulica*), as well as Pacific oyster (*C gigas*), Sydney rock oyster (*Saccostrea glomerata*), and planarians (*Dugesia* and *Crenobia* spp). However, histologically these tumors were composed of large altered epithelial cells forming convoluted acini and covering a fibrous connective tissue stalk that contained bands of muscle. The altered epithelial cells indicated a different cell of origin and tumor type and the terms adenopapilloma, epithelioma, or epidermal papilloma were applied to these lesions.[4,7,19] All were similarly described as benign and of unknown cause.

Growth anomalies in Cnidaria have been reported in more than 40 species of scleractinian coral, 5 gorgonians, and 1 hydrozoan.[20] Despite having a similar external appearance and gross features, the histologic morphology is significantly different across species and not all growth anomalies have been classified as neoplasms.[21–24] Growth anomalies present as discrete nodular protrusions from the colony and share the gross characteristics of fewer polyps per surface area, decreased pigmentation (fewer zooxanthella per polyp), and finer (more porous) skeletal structures than normal. These foci also grow more rapidly than the adjacent normal-appearing tissues. Calicoblastic epitheliomas, tumors resulting from abnormal proliferation of the ectodermal cells that produce the aragonite skeleton, have been described in both *Acropora* spp and *Montipora* spp corals[4] (**Figs. 2** and **3**). Proliferation of gastrovascular canals and the associated calicoblastic epidermis (calicodermis) was described histologically, with a loss of normal polyp structures and decreased numbers of gastrodermal zooxanthellae, mesenteries, and gonads. Calicoblasts, instead of having a squamous morphology, were cuboidal to columnar and resembled those found near the rapidly growing regions in corals.[22] The designation of these lesions as neoplastic and specifically malignant remains controversial but is based on histologic features that suggest rapid uncoordinated growth of the tissue and skeleton and destruction of adjacent normal tissue.[20,22] Lack of anaplasia and mitotic figures have been cited as the reason for caution in considering these growth anomalies or hyperplasias rather than true neoplasms.[6,23] In areas of anomalous growth, the loss of polyps and mucous secretory cells in the affected region of the coral colony makes affected corals susceptible to sediment accumulation. This accumulation causes tissue necrosis and filamentous algae overgrowth within the coral skeleton, which can cause regional polyp or entire colony death.[4] Although the normal argonite crystalline structure is retained in areas of growth anomalies, the skeletal density is reduced, further predisposing the affected area to erosion and predation.[24] In *Montipora* spp, similar anomalies reduce fecundity of affected colonies and in some cases nearly 70% of the colony is replaced by growth anomalies.[24] The cause of these lesions is not known; viral infections and ultraviolet light exposure have been proposed but remain to be proved.[23]

Reproductive Tumors

Gonadal tumors have been described in 14 species of marine bivalve mollusks from 3 continents. Species include ocean quahog (*Arctica islandica*), bay scallop (*Argopecten irradians*), cockle (*Cerastoderma edule*), Pacific oyster (*C gigas*), Eastern oyster (*C virginica*), chalky macoma (*Macoma calcarea*), Northern quahog (*Mercenaria mercenaria*), hybrid quahog (*M mercenaria campechiensis*), soft shell clam (*M arenaria*), blue mussel (*Mytilus edulis*), bluff oyster (*Tiostrea chilensis*), and razor clam (*Ensis arcuatus*).[25–27]

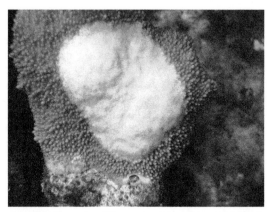

Fig. 2. A calicoblastic epithelioma in elkhorn coral (*Acropora palmata*). There is a discrete nodular protrusion from the colony with decreased regional pigmentation and decreased polyp numbers. (*Courtesy of* Esther C. Peters, PhD, George Mason University.)

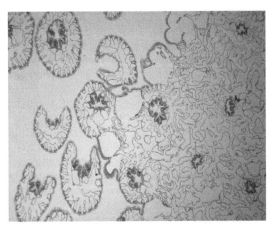

Fig. 3. Photomicrograph of a calicoblastic epithelioma in elkhorn coral (*A palmata*). There are increased numbers of gastrovascular canals evident, a regional loss of polyps and a finer (more porous) skeletal structure (hematoxylin-eosin, original magnification ×40). (*Courtesy of* Esther C. Peters, PhD, George Mason University.)

Three histologic patterns have been documented in these neoplasms: (1) tumors of germ cell origin (germinomas), (2) tumors of stromal/connective tissue origin (fibroma, myofibroma), (3) mixed tumors (gonadoblastoma) containing both components.[27] Germinomas were composed of undifferentiated germ cells that filled individual follicles, effaced the gonadal area, or spread to other adjacent tissues. Stromal tumors were composed of neoplastic cells that were myxoid to vesicular to spindle shaped and effaced the normal reproductive tissue as they grew. In mixed tumors there was a central region of the tumor mass that consisted of dense fibrous tissue, and surrounding the margins were neoplastic germ cells that showed either ovarian or spermatogenic differentiation. The mixed tumors were reported infrequently but had an aggressive pattern of growth with evidence of extension through the follicular basement membrane, invasion of the adjacent connective tissue of the gill, and mass formation along the wall of the branchial vein.[27] Small foci of isolated neoplastic cells were also identified within the gill microvasculature in soft shell clams with gonadoblastoma consistent with metastatic foci. The cause of these gonadal neoplasms has been proposed to be environmental pollutants and/or viruses but this remains to be confirmed. The cause remains undetermined at this time.[4,27] There is a single report of gonadal neoplasia in the male gonad of a gastropod, the limpet (*Patella coerulea*).[28]

A single case report of an oviductal tumor was identified in a species of orb-weaver spider (*Pachygnatha clercki*). This tumor arose from the oviductal epithelium and consisted of multiple disorganized layers of epithelial cells that filled the lumen, infiltrated the oviduct and uterine wall, and in some areas infiltrated adjacent coelomic membranes and ovary. Significant cellular and nuclear atypia were described, as were mitotic figures and central necrosis. These features were consistent with a malignant neoplasm. Although not definitively identified in the article, the morphology and origin suggested an oviductal carcinoma in this spider.[29]

Other Visceral Tumors

Epithelial and mesenchymal tumors associated with the coelomic viscera and coelomic cavity have been described in a variety of invertebrates. In pearl oyster

(*Pinctada margaritifera*), polypoid tumors attached to the visceral mass (gut loop) were reported. Described as firm, stalked, polyplike growths, these tumors were composed of a normal low columnar to cuboidal ciliated epithelium showing glandular differentiation supported by a stroma of proliferative fibrous tissue and muscle fibers that varied in thickness and showed irregular (abnormal) orientation. Blood spaces were apparent throughout the stroma with no cellular atypia or mitotic figures noted. The investigator described these neoplasms as benign fibrovascular polyps and hypothesized a developmental origin.[30]

Pericardial tumors of mesenchymal origin have been reported in *Crassostrea* spp oysters and the Olympia oyster (*Ostrea lurida*). These growths were polypoid to pedunculated masses attached to the mantle that protruded into the coelom, extended into the pericardial sinus, or compressed the pericardium and the ventricle. On histology, the masses in *Crassostrea* spp consisted of a mixture of fibrous connective tissue and Leydig cells (vesicular connective tissue) with multifocal inflammatory infiltrates present. These tumors were considered to be benign tumors of Leydig cell origin.[31] In *O lurida* the neoplasm was histologically different, consisting of a superficial cuboidal layer of mesothelial cells supported by a fibrous connective tissue stroma containing pigmented cells, collagen, reticular fibers, and striated muscle fibers. In this animal, a developmental anomaly was the favored diagnosis, but the mass was similarly described as benign.[32]

Pulmonary tumors have been described in multiple different research colonies of ghost snails (*Biomphalaria glabrata*). These tumors were evident in young snails soon after they emerged from the egg capsule, and grew proportionally with the rest of the body. They occurred along the parietal wall and histologically were composed of a loose stroma of connective tissue with intervening pigment cells. These proliferations completely occluded the pulmonary cavity in some cases, inhibited respiratory function, prevented retraction of the snail into the shell, and prevented the use of the pulmonary cavity to regulate buoyancy. The cause seems to be genetic and heritable. In one colony the disease could be traced back along breeding lines to a single snail. A designation for these pulmonary tumors was not offered by the investigator. Similar descriptions of benign proliferative lesions of the pseudobranch and mantle in this species favored a diagnosis of a choristoma (proliferative normal tissue in an abnormal location).[33,34]

A malignant epithelial tumor (carcinoma) of the hindgut was identified in an adult female red king crab (*Paralithodes camtschatica*). Grossly the lesion presented as a large (20 × 12 mm) white mass on the ventral aspect of the anterior hindgut. On histology it was composed of an unencapsulated proliferation of large pleomorphic epithelioid cells, smaller hypertrophied cells, and an inflammatory cell infiltrate. Cells had large nuclei that were pleomorphic to fissured with beaded, marginated chromatin and basophilic cytoplasm. A single eccentric nucleolus was present and mitotic figures were present in low numbers. Uniquely, this tumor showed signs of malignancy, including local tissue infiltration. Neoplastic cells were most histologically consistent with midgut epithelial cells, although the investigators thought that the cell of origin remained unclear.[35]

Hemic Tumors

Disseminated neoplasm of presumed hematogenous (hemic) origin is one of the most commonly described neoplastic conditions of invertebrates. A similar condition has been described in 15 species of bivalve mollusks as well as the white shrimp (*Penaeus vannamei*), and mutant strains of *Drosophila*.[36–39] The cytologic and histologic features described were similar across species and included the presence of large, round, anaplastic cells in the connective tissue, blood vessels, and sinuses of the visceral mass, muscle, and mantle tissue (**Fig. 4**). These cells were 2 to 4 times the diameter of a normal hemocyte, had a nuclear to cytoplasmic volume ratio of 1:1, contained 1 or more prominent nucleoli, and had 1 to several vesicles containing neutral triglycerides and lipids. Mitotic figures were common. Infiltrating cells caused displacement, compression, and necrosis of the gill, gonad, and connective tissue; arrest of gametogenesis; with gonad atrophy and degeneration. Death was the ultimate outcome of this tumor caused by both the effects of organ disruption and dysfunction of the immune system. A clear consensus has not been reached regarding the exact cell of origin beyond a sarcoma (derived from mesenchymal cells). Most investigators favor a hemic origin because of similarities between the neoplastic cells and granular or hyaline hemocytes, and their detection first within the circulatory system, although a gonadal origin has also been proposed.[39,40] Clinical signs in affected individuals are challenging and nonspecific, including emaciation, pallor of the digestive gland, and mantle recession, all considered general signs of poor health in bivalves.[40,41] A single cause for the disease has not been identified in bivalves or crustaceans. A relationship between the prevalence of disseminated neoplasia and environmental carcinogens, biotoxins, stress, and genetics has not been proved.[40,42,43] There is some support for an infectious cause, but the nature is unclear, although a virus is suggested as a primary candidate. There is a variation in the occurrence of disseminated neoplasia between species, locations, and time of year, suggesting that this is likely a complex multifactorial process.[42] In the single case report of disseminated neoplasia of shrimp, lesions consistent with penaeid shrimp virus (Infectious Hypodermal Haematopoietic Necrosis [IHHN]) were present in the neoplastic hematopoietic tissue, suggesting a possible role for viral infection.[36]

The disseminated (hemic) neoplasia of *Drosophila* is genetic in origin and can be caused by 4 different gene mutations that result in malignant transformation of the plasmatocyte cell lineage. Transformation of proplasmatocytes causes increased blood cell counts in hematopoietic organs and hemolymph and ultimately death before puparium formation. Grossly, larvae appear enlarged and bloated because of a failure of release of maturing hemocytes to the hemolymph and enlargement of

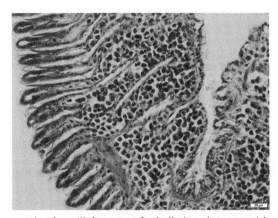

Fig. 4. Photomicrograph of a gill from a soft shell clam (*M arenaria*) with disseminated neoplasia. Vascular spaces are filled with neoplastic cells showing anisocytosis, anisokaryosis, and increased nucleus/cytoplasm ratio compared with adjacent normal hemocytes (hematoxylin-eosin, original magnification ×400). (*Courtesy of* Roxanna Smolowitz, Roger Williams University.)

the hematopoietic organs by 30 to 40 times wild type. The cells that are released into the hemolymph invade larval organs and form pigmented (melanotic) masses throughout the posterior fat body, ultimately resulting in death.[37]

ONCOGENES

It is important to recognize that, even in the absence of reports of neoplasms, pro-oncogenes and oncogenes similar to those that are important in human cancers (eg, *ras*, *src*, and *ets*) have been identified in nearly all invertebrate species investigated, which suggests that oncogenic transformation is possible.[6] Genes and pathways of malignancy exist in cnidarians and include the p53 tumor suppressor–like protein nvp63 in the starlet sea anemone (*Nematostella vectensis*).[44] In mollusks, mutations in the ras oncogene and deregulated expression of p53 tumor suppressor are supported as important causes of disseminated neoplasia.[6] *C elegans* has been a model organism to study the genes and pathways affected during tumorigenesis, such as apoptosis and *Ras* signaling. A homologue of the retinoblastoma susceptibility gene (Rb) that is functionally inactivated in most human solid tumors has been characterized and plays a role in cell proliferation and differentiation in *Drosophila*.[6] Hyperactivation of the JAK/STAT pathway results in the development of epithelial and hematopoietic tumors in *Drosophila*.[7,45] The potential for metastasis of *Drosophila melanogaster* tumors is supported by conservation of molecular control of cell migration (SAP97, TGF) pathways, which plays a role in mammalian cancer cell metastasis. Large numbers of mammalian tumor suppressor genes and other genes controlling proliferation and migration (serine/threonine-protein kinase LATS 1, Ras signaling, Raf/MAPK pathway) have been characterized in *D melanogaster*, which supports that spontaneous neoplasia and malignancies are possible.[6]

DIAGNOSTIC TESTING

The diagnosis of neoplasia in invertebrates can be challenging, and although external neoplasms can be grossly recognized, internal or systemic neoplasms are generally not detected.[40] Clinical pathology and flow cytometry have been recognized as important methods for identifying hemic neoplasia in bivalve mollusks. Hemolymph samples (0.1–0.5 mL), collected through the posterior adductor muscle and diluted with filtered seawater, can be placed on a glass slide coated in poly-L-lysine for differential evaluation. Samples show increased cellularity (opacity) and can be examined by phase contrast or can be stained with regular histochemical stains (Romanowsky) for bright-field evaluation.[46] Immunohistochemical stains (indirect peroxidase staining method) for neoplastic hemocytes have also been developed for marine bivalves.[47] The neoplastic cells also contain more DNA than normal cells and therefore can be separated from normal hemocytes in hemolymph samples using flow cytometry.[48]

No radiographic diagnoses of internal neoplasms are described in the literature but radiography is still a useful tool in invertebrate medicine. Diagnostic imaging of invertebrates is challenged because of the lack of a mineralized internal skeleton or fat bodies to provide contrast. Successful radiographic techniques have been described in terrestrial and aquatic invertebrates with and without the use of gastrointestinal contrast media and radiology is encouraged during the work-up of any invertebrate with suspected neoplasia.[49–52] Davis and colleagues[52] found that plain film radiography in a variety of common terrestrial invertebrate taxa (tarantulas, scorpions, hissing cockroaches, and millipedes) provided fair body cavity detail but limited visceral detail in all but cockroaches because of the lack of a fat body. Gastrointestinal contrast (Hypaque and barium) does provide enhanced detail of the gastrointestinal tract in these species and could be useful for detecting mass effect or luminal masses within the intestinal tract. Advanced imaging techniques, including computed tomography and MRI, have proved useful in describing the internal anatomy of several terrestrial and aquatic invertebrate species. Exceptionally detailed anatomic images were created in urchin using MRI and freshwater crayfish using manganese-enhanced MRI.[53,54]

Histopathology remains a critical tool for further documenting and understanding neoplastic disease in invertebrate patients. Ten percent neutral buffered formalin is an adequate fixative for all samples, although zinc-based formalin fixatives (Z-fix), seawater buffered formalin, and Davidson solution have advantages in some invertebrate species because of an ability to better preserve fine cellular detail and harden at times very soft amorphous tissues. Pathologists should be contacted in advance to determine their preference for case materials. Further, pathologists with both knowledge of tumor biology and knowledge of invertebrate biology should be sought for the most reliable identification. Histopathology laboratories need to understand the special tissue processing and handling necessary to prepare and section invertebrate tissues. Regular hematoxylin-eosin sections have proved useful for the basic structure of various neoplasms, but additional histochemical stains can be useful in characterizing the content of the cytoplasm. Immunohistochemical stains may be used to attempt to identify cells of origin but, as in other exotic species, they are often unsuccessful because such antibodies are developed for species-specific and tissue-specific antigens.

TREATMENT

Descriptions of treatments for invertebrate neoplasms are lacking, even descriptions as simple as mass removal, and whether this results in normal tissue repair.[4] There is 1 research reference to the use of chemotherapy in soft shell clams (*M arenaria*) with disseminated neoplasia, which shows mortalin-based cytoplasmic sequestration of p53 similar to human colorectal cancer and glioblastoma.[42,43] Treatment of normal and neoplastic clam hemocytes in vivo and in vitro with genotoxic topoisomerase II toxins (effective against human leukemia and lymphoma), etoposide, or a combination of etoposide and mitoxantrone, resulted in increased wild-type p53 production in neoplastic cells and apoptosis. Treatment of neoplastic cells with the chemotherapeutic rhodocyanin dye MKT-077 resulted in nontranscriptional induction of p53-mediated apoptosis.[55,56] For other invertebrate neoplasms, the potential exists to identify chemotherapeutic agents from the human and veterinary literature if a better understanding of the nature of these tumors and their pathogenesis were available.

Based on the gross and histologic descriptions of the neoplasms identified to date, it is likely that many of the external lesions described in invertebrates could be amenable to surgical resection. As with any animal patient, adequate chemical immobilization and analgesia should be provided during surgical procedures. Although many procedures described in the literature do not indicate the use anesthesia, sufficient reviews on the topic are available in the veterinary literature and should be consulted.[57] An appropriate review with the normal anatomy and physiology of the species is highly recommended before embarking on any surgical procedure.

Controlled fracturing (fragging) of hard and soft corals is a common practice used in coral propagation, as is field sampling for disease investigations. Both processes use rongeurs, pliers, chisels, or sharp cylindrical cores and mallets in the case of hard corals, or scissors in the case of soft corals, to bluntly dissect polyps and the underlying skeleton from the parent colony.[58] These defects can be left open or can be filled with marine epoxy following sampling to prevent endolithic fungal, algal, and Porifera infections. In soft corals, resection sites are not often treated or closed, but monofilament suture or fishing line have been used to tether and transplant fragments and could be used to reseal the exposed coral skeleton following tissue removal. A single case report describes the surgical removal of growth anomalies from *Acropora* spp and *Montipora* spp corals with mixed success. Although the treated *Acropora acuminata* remained growth anomaly free for 9 months following the procedure, *Montipora efflorescens* showed 100% recurrence.[59] This finding highlights the need to better understand invertebrate neoplasms, their cause, and their pathogenesis in order to better effect treatment.

With local tissue dissection papilliform tumors of the body wall and carapace of invertebrates could likely be removed. Care should be used if removing soft tissue tumors in the region of the free edge of the mantle in mollusks because damage to these sensitive tissues may disrupt shell formation. Surgical treatment of carapace lesions in crustaceans, arthropods, hexapods, myriapods, and decapods must always take into consideration the impact that carapace disruption and healing may have on the ability of the animal to molt. Avoidance of the underlying hemolymph sinuses is also important. Within the gastropod mollusk research literature there are descriptions of amputations of eyes and tentacles.[60–63] None used a method of wound closure following tissue resection. Studies of wound healing in sea hares (*Aplysia californica*) successfully used a variety of suture materials for wound closure, including monofilament nylon, monofilament poliglecaprone polydioxanone, and polyglactin 910 with similar histologic evidence of successful healing. For cephalopod mollusks the only mass removal described in the veterinary literature is the removal of fungal granulomas from the mantle of a cuttlefish. Anesthesia, surgical preparation, and wound closure are described and could be extrapolated to address neoplastic lesions in these species.[64]

REFERENCES

1. Teutschlaender O. Beiträge zur vergleichenden Onkologie mit Berücksichtigung der Identitätsfrage. Ztschr f Krebsforsch 1920;17:285–407.
2. Engel CS. Warum erkranken wirbellose Tiere nicht an Krebs? Ztschr f Krebsforsch 1930;32:531–43.
3. Scharrer B, Szabó-Lochhead L. Tumors in the invertebrates: a review. Cancer Res 1950;10(7):403–19.
4. Peters EC, Smolowitz RM, Reynolds TL. Neoplasia. In: Lewbart GA, editor. Invertebrate medicine. 2nd edition. Chichester: John Wiley; 2012. p. 448–525.
5. Kumar V, Abbas AK, Aster AC. Neoplasia. In: Kumar V, Abbas AK, Aster AC, editors. Robbins and Cotran, pathologic basis of disease. 9th edition. Philadelphia: Elsevier; 2015. p. 265–340.
6. Robert J. Comparative study of tumorigenesis and tumor immunity in invertebrates and non-mammalian vertebrates. Dev Comp Immunol 2010;34(9):915–25.
7. Tascedda F, Ottaviani E. Tumors in invertebrates. Invertebrate Surviv J 2014;11:197–203.
8. Hanahan D, Weinberg RA. The hallmarks of cancer. Cell 2000;100(1):57–70.
9. Sparks AK. Review of tumors and tumor-like conditions in protozoa, coelenterata, platyhelminthes, annelida, sipunculida, and arthropoda, excluding insects. Natl Cancer Inst Monogr 1969;31:671–82.

10. Sparks AK. Tumors and tumor-like conditions in invertebrates. In: Sparks AK, editor. Invertebrate pathology noncommunicable diseases. New York: Academic Press; 1972. p. 271–371.
11. Shields JD, Small HS. An unusual cuticular tumor-like growth on the abdomen of a lobster, *Homarus americanus*. J Invertebr Pathol 2013;114:245–9.
12. Sparks AK, Lightener DV. A tumorlike papilliform growth in the brown shrimp (*Penaeus aztecus*). J Invertebr Pathol 1973;22:203–12.
13. Pauley GB. Four freshwater mussels (*Anodonta californiensis*) with pedunculated adenomas arising from the foot. J Invertebr Pathol 1966;9:459–66.
14. Pauley GB. A butter clam (*Saxidomus giganteus*) with a polypoid tumor of the foot. J Invertebr Pathol 1967;9(4):577–9.
15. Pauley GB, Cheng TC. A tumor on the siphons of a soft shell clam *Mya arenaria*. J Invertebr Pathol 1968;11(3):504–6.
16. Potter M, Kuff E. A developmental anomaly of the siphon of the soft-shell clam, *Mya arenaria*, from the Chesapeake Bay. In: Harshbarger JC, Cantwell GE, editors. Activities report of the Registry of Tumors in Lower Animals from the period Sept. 1, 1967 to March 31, 1967. Washington, DC: Smithsonian Institute; 1967. p. 11.
17. DesVoigne DM, Mix MC, Pauley GB. A papillomalike growth on the siphon of the horse clam, *Tresus nuttalli*. J Invertebr Pathol 1970;15:262–7.
18. Odintsova NA, Usheva LN, Yakovlev KV, et al. Naturally occurring and artificially induced tumor-like formations in invertebrates: a search for permanent cell lines. J Exp Mar Bio Ecol 2011;407:241–9.
19. Michelson EH. A neoplasm in the giant African snail *Achatina fulica*. J Invertebr Pathol 1972;20:264–7.
20. Doumart-Coulon IJ, Traylor-Knowles N, Peters E, et al. Comprehensive characterization of skeletal tissue growth anomalies of the finger coral *Porites compressa*. Coral Reefs 2006;25:531–43.
21. Loya Y, Bull G, Pichon M. Tumor formations in scleractinian corals. Helgol Merrsunters 1984;37:99–112.
22. Peters EC, Halas JC, McCarty HB. Calicoblastic neoplasms in *Acropora palmata*, with a review of reports on anomalies and form in corals. J Natl Cancer Inst 1986; 76(5):895–912.
23. Work TM, Aeby GS, Coles SL. Distribution and morphology of growth anomalies in Acropora from the Indo-pacific. Dis Aquat Org 2008;78:255–64.
24. Burns JHR, Takabayashi M. Histopathology of growth anomaly affecting the coral, *Montipora capitata*: implications on biological functions and population viability. PLoS One 2011;6(12):e28854.
25. Hessleman DM, Blake NJ, Peters EC. Gonadal neoplasms in hard shell clams *Mercenaria* spp., from the Indian River, Florida: occurrence, prevalence and histopathology. J Invertebr Pathol 1988;52:436–46.
26. Darriba S, Iglesias D, Harshbarger JC, et al. Germinoma in razor clam *Ensis arcuatus* (Jeffreys, 1865) in Galicia (NW Spain). J Invertebr Pathol 2006;93: 140–2.
27. Peters EC, Yevish PP, Harshbarger JC, et al. Comparative histopathology of gonadal neoplasms in marine bivalve molluscs. Dis Aquat Org 1994;20:59–76.
28. Carella F, Restucci B, Maiolino P, et al. A case of germinoma in a limpet (*Patella coerulea*). J Invertebr Pathol 2009;101:154–6.
29. Lopez A. Tumoral pathology of spiders. J Invertebr Pathol 1979;34:224–30.
30. Dix TG. Two mesenchymal tumors in a pearl oyster (*Pinctada margaritifera*). J Invertebr Pathol 1972;20:317–20.

31. Dinamani P, Wolf PH. Multiple tumors in the pericardial cavity of an Australian rock oyster, *Crassostrea commercialis* (Iredale and Roughley). Int J Cancer 1973;11: 293–9.
32. Mix MC, Riley RT. A pericardial tumor in a native (Olympia) oyster, *Ostrea lurida*, from Yaquina Bay, Oregon. J Invertebr Pathol 1977;30:104–7.
33. Richards CS. Tumors in the pulmonary cavity of *Biomphalaria glabarata*: genetic studies. J Invertebr Pathol 1973;22:283–9.
34. Richards CS. Inherited abnormal growths on the mantle of *Biomphalaria glabrata*. J Invertebr Pathol 1980;35:119–23.
35. Sparks AK, Morado JF. A putative carcinoma-like neoplasm in the hindgut of a red king crab, *Paralithodes camtschatica*. J Invertebr Pathol 1987;50:45–52.
36. Lightener DV, Brock JA. A lymphoma-like neoplasm arising from hematopoietic tissue in the white shrimp, *Penaeus vannamei* Boone (Crustacea: Decapoda). J Invertebr Pathol 1987;49(2):188–93.
37. Shrestha R, Gateff E. Ultrastructure and cytochemistry of the tumorous blood cells in the mutant lethal (3) malignant blood neoplasm of *Drosophila melanogaster*. J Invertebr Pathol 1986;48:1–12.
38. Farley CA. Probable neoplastic disease of the hematopoietic system in oysters *Crassostrea virginica* and *Crassostrea gigas*. Natl Cancer Inst Monogr 1969; 31:541–55.
39. Farley CA. Sarcomatoid proliferative disease in a wild population of blue mussels (*Mytilus edulis*). J Natl Cancer Inst 1969;43:509–16.
40. Barber BJ. Neoplastic diseases of commercially important marine bivalves. Aquat Living Resour 2004;17:449–66.
41. Elston RA, Moore JD, Brooks K. Disseminated neoplasia of bivalve molluscs. Rev Aquat Sci 1992;6:405–66.
42. Walker CW, Van Veneden RJ, Muttray AF, et al. P53 superfamily proteins in marine bivalve cancer and stress biology. In: Lesser MA, editor. Advances in marine biology, vol. 59. London: Academic Press; 2011. p. 1–36.
43. Böttger A, Amarosa EJ, Geoghegan P, et al. Chronic natural occurrence of disseminated neoplasia in select populations of soft-shell clam, *Mya arenaria*, in New England. Northeast Nat (Steuben) 2013;20(3):430–40.
44. Pankow S, Bamberger C. The p53 tumor suppressor-like protein nvp63 mediates selective germ cell death in the sea anemone *Nematostella vectensis*. PLoS One 2007;2(9):e782.
45. Amoyel M, Anderson AM, Bach EA. JAK/STAT pathway dysregulation in tumors: A drosophila perspective. Semin Cell Dev Biol 2014;28:96–103.
46. Howard DW, Lewis EJ, Keller BJ, et al. Histological techniques for marine bivalves and crustaceans. 2nd edition. NOAA technical memorandum NOS NCCOS 2004;5:218.
47. Smolowitz RM, Reinisch CL. Indirect peroxidase staining using monoclonal antibodies for *Mya arenaria* neoplastic cells. J Invertebr Pathol 1986;48:139–45.
48. Vassilenko E, Baldwin SA. Using flow cytometry to detect haemic neoplasia in mussels (*Mytilus trossulus*) from the Pacific Coast of southern British Columbia, Canada. J Invertebr Pathol 2014;117:68–72.
49. Bock C, Frederich M, Wittig RM, et al. Simultaneous observations of hemolymph flow and ventilation in marine spider crabs at different temperatures: a flow weighted MRI study. Magn Reson Imaging 2001;19:1113–24.
50. Nollens HH, Schofield JC, Keogh JA, et al. Evaluation of radiography, ultrasonography and endoscopy for detection of shell lesions in live abalone *Haliotis iris* (Mollusca: Gastropoda). Dis Aquat Organ 2002;50:145–52.

51. Wecker S, Hornschemeyer T, Hoehn M. Investigation of insect morphology by MRI: assessment of spatial and temporal resolution. Magn Reson Imaging 2002;20:105–11.
52. Davis MR, Gamble KC, Matheson JS. Diagnostic imaging in terrestrial invertebrates: Madagascar hissing cockroach (*Gromphadorhina portentosa*), desert millipede (*Orthoporus* sp.), emperor scorpion (*Pandinus imperator*), Chilean rosehair tarantula (*Grammostola spatulata*), Mexican fireleg tarantula (*Brachypelma boehmei*) and redknee tarantula (*Brachypelma smithi*). Zoo Biol 2008; 27:109–25.
53. Herberholz J, Mims CJ, Zhang X, et al. Anatomy of a live invertebrate revealed by manganese enhanced magnetic resonance imaging. J Exp Biol 2004;207: 4542–50.
54. Ziegler A, Faber C, Mueller S, et al. Systematic comparison and reconstruction of sea urchin (Echinoidea) internal anatomy: a novel approach using magnetic resonance imaging. BMC Biol 2008;6(33):1–15.
55. Walker CW, Böttger SA. A naturally occurring cancer with molecular connectivity to human diseases. Cell Cycle 2008;7(15):1–4.
56. Böttger S, Jerszyk E, Low B, et al. Genotoxic stress induced expression of P53 and apoptosis in leukemic clam hemocytes with cytoplasmically sequestered P53. Cancer Res 2008;68:777–82.
57. Gunkel C, Lewbart GA. Invertebrates. In: West G, Heard D, Caulkett N, editors. Zoo animal and wildlife immobilization and anesthesia. Ames (IA): Blackwell Publishing; 2007. p. 147–58.
58. Work T. Collecting corals for histopathology: a practical guide. National Wildlife Health Center, Honolulu Field Station, USGS; 2013. Available at: https://www.nwhc. usgs.gov/hfs/Globals/Products/Collecting%20corals%20for%20histopathology.pdf.
59. Williams GJ. Contrasting recovery following removal of growth anomalies in corals *Acropora* and *Montipora*. Dis Aquat Org 2013;106:181–5.
60. Matsuo R, Kobayashi S, Murakami J, et al. Spontaneous recover of the injured higher olfactory center in the terrestrial slug *Limax*. PLoS One 2010;5(2):e9054.
61. Matsuo R, Kobayashi S, Tanaka Y, et al. Effects of tentacle amputation and regeneration on the morphology and activity of the olfactory center of the terrestrial slug *Limax valentianus*. J Exp Biol 2010;213:3144–9.
62. Moffett SB. Regeneration as an application of gastropod neural plasticity. Microsc Res Tech 2000;49:579–88.
63. Tartakovskaya OS, Borisenko SL, Zhukov VV. Role of the age factor in eye regeneration in the gastropod *Achatina fulica*. Biol Bull Acad Sci USSR 2003;30(3): 228–35.
64. Harms CA, Lewbart GA, McAlarney R, et al. Surgical excision of mycotic (*Cladosporium* sp.) granulomas from the mantle of a cuttlefish (*Sepia officinalis*). J Zoo Wildl Med 2006;37(4):524–30.

Fish Oncology

Diseases, Diagnostics, and Therapeutics

Claire Vergneau-Grosset, med vet, IPSAV, DACZM[a,b,]*,
Marie-Eve Nadeau, DVM, DACVIM (Oncology)[a], Joseph M. Groff, VMD, PhD[c]

KEYWORDS

• Fish • Oncology • Chemotherapy • Cancer • Neoplasm

KEY POINTS

• Fish neoplasms have frequently been reported in fish.
• Advanced imaging is helpful to plan surgical interventions but requires knowledge of normal specific anatomy.
• Fish oncologic treatment plans should integrate water residue management to avoid exposure to conspecific fish and caretakers.
• Additional studies are required to establish the best course of action for the treatment of neoplasms in ornamental fish, especially when taking into consideration the decline of wild fish populations and the increasing educational and conservation value of captive fish in public aquaria.

INTRODUCTION

Piscine species are the most numerous and diverse group among vertebrates, with more than 27,000 species.[1,2] The scientific literature contains a wealth of information concerning spontaneous fish tumors,[1,3] although ornamental fish oncology is still in its infancy. Certain neoplasms affecting fishes have been associated with oncogenic viruses, parasites, and environmental contaminants, whereas association between environmental contaminants and fish neoplasms can be used as sentinels for environmental degradation. In addition, because fish are often an important source of protein, especially for developing countries, an investigation of piscine neoplasms may have implication for human consumers.[4]

Malignant neoplasms[5] with or without metastasis are reported rarely in fish compared with mammals.[1,3,6] This could be due to a different antitumor immunity in

The authors have nothing to disclose.
[a] Centre Hospitalier Vétérinaire Universitaire, Faculté de médecine vétérinaire, Université de Montréal, 3200 rue Sicotte, Saint-Hyacinthe J2S 2M2, Quebec, Canada; [b] Aquarium du Québec, 1675 Avenue des Hôtels, Ville de Québec, QC G1W 4S3, Canada; [c] William R. Pritchard Veterinary Medical Teaching Hospital, School of Veterinary Medicine, University of California, Davis, Shields Avenue, Davis, CA 95616, USA
* Corresponding author.
E-mail address: claire.grosset@umontreal.ca

Vet Clin Exot Anim 20 (2017) 21–56
http://dx.doi.org/10.1016/j.cvex.2016.07.002
vetexotic.theclinics.com

fish versus mammals.[7] Malignant cells in nonmammalian vertebrates may also be more susceptible to apoptosis than in mammals.[8] Additional explanations for the rarity of metastasis in fishes include the absence of frequent metastatic sites that are present in mammals, including lung, lymph nodes, and bone marrow[2,3,9]; differences in the lymphatic system in fishes versus mammals[3]; lower body temperatures in fishes[3]; and the more common differentiation of neoplasms in fishes versus mammals.[3] In this context, the tumor, node, metastasis (TNM) staging system in mammals, which is a classic evaluation of the initial neoplastic lesion, lymph node involvement, and the occurrence of metastasis, is not applicable to fishes. Examples of malignant neoplasms have previously been reviewed,[3,10,11] and metastasis may be detected in fish hematopoietic organs, such as the spleen, kidney, and thymus.[12] Differential diagnoses for tumoral lesions in fish include non-neoplastic masses commonly encountered, such as xanthomas,[13] granulomas, and masses associated with parasites or fungi, such as microsporidia.[14,15]

FISH NEOPLASMS
Commonly Encountered Neoplasms in Fish

Spontaneous neoplasms have been commonly reported in fishes, but an average incidence is unknown,[1] although the incidence of neoplasms in fishes is considered less common than the incidence in higher vertebrates, for the reasons discussed previously.[3,7,8] On revision of a pathology database, including 883 fish necropsies from a public aquarium over a 5-year period, 6% of the cases presented with spontaneous neoplasms (Stéphane Lair, DVM, DACZM, personal communication, 2016). Captive display fish may have a longer life span than wild ones and, as a consequence, spontaneous neoplasms may be detected more commonly in this population. Various models of human cancers, however, have been developed in genetically modified fish,[16,17] including zebrafish (Brachydanio rerio) that are easily kept in captivity, because zebrafish develop tumors that resemble human tumors both histologically and at the genetic level of expression.[18] Studies using these fish have revealed a low propensity for spontaneous tumors; rather, they require exposure to carcinogens and mutagens to induce tumor formation.[3,12,19-21] Information concerning the etiologies of neoplasms in wild and production fishes may, therefore, provide information applicable or relevant to ornamental and hobby fish seen by the veterinary practitioner. For example, up to 10% of salmon (Salmo salar) from a commercial aquaculture facility fed commercial pellets without any known potential carcinogens in the feed developed intestinal adenocarcinomas and other types of tumors.[12] Carcinogenesis was attributed to chronic intestinal inflammation caused by the ingestion of omega-6 and other vegetable compounds in this carnivorous species.[12] Neoplasms in elasmobranchs have been reported as rare, although recent reports suggest that neoplasms in this taxonomic group may be more common than once believed.[22-24]

Examples of tumors reported in fish are included in **Table 1**. Generally, ectoderm-derived and endoderm-derived epithelial neoplasms are the most common neoplasms in fishes, whereas the integument is the most common organ for the manifestation of neoplasms in fishes.[1,50,57-62] Cutaneous neoplasms are generally benign with few exceptions, although recurrence is common in cases of incomplete surgical excision.[1] The histologic classification of cutaneous neoplasms in fishes, however, is often confused due to the common shared features of the lesions.

Papillomas are the most common cutaneous neoplasms in fishes,[57] especially because various raised, cutaneous lesions are often classified as papillomatous lesions regardless of size, appearance, and histogenesis. The distribution of papillomas

Table 1
Examples of spontaneous neoplasms reported in fish

	Neoplasm	Location	Example of Reports and Corresponding Fish Species
Round cell tumors	Melanoma	Skin	Thornback skate[22]
	Lymphosarcoma		Pike,[25] bonnethead shark[26]
Epithelial tumors	Papilloma	Skin	Koi[27]
	Carcinoma	Choroid plexus	Spiny dogfish[28]
	Squamous cell carcinoma		Koi[27], Blue shark[22]
	Adenoma	Hepatic	Salmon[12]
	Adenocarcinoma	intestine	Coho salmons[29]
	Spindle cell tumors or neoplasms		Bicolor damselfish[30], Spiny dogfish[22]
	Peripheral nerve sheath tumor (Schwannoma, Neurofibroma, Neurilemmoma)		
	Neuroblastoma	Olfactory tissue	Koi,[31] goldfish,[32] medaka,[33] gilt-head bream,[34] bloater[35]
Mesenchymal tumors	Leiomyoma		Indian catfish,[36] goldfish[37]
	Leiomyosarcoma		Largemouth bass[38]
	Fibroma	Skin	Salmon[39]
	Fibrosarcoma		Hooknose[40]
	Myxoma		Goldfish,[41] lined seahorse[42]
	Chromatophoroma		European eel[43]
	Sertoli cell tumor	Gonad	Koi,[44] goldfish,[45] croaker,[46] corydoras[47]
	Seminoma	Swim bladder	Cyprinidae[48]
	Teratoma	Coelom	Black sea bass[49]
	Chondroma		Guppy, platyfish[50]
	chondrosarcoma		Mediterranean dogfish[51]
	Osteochondroma		Paddlefish[52]
	Osteoma		Gilthead sea bream[53]
	Osteosarcoma		Mediterranean dogfish[51]
	Odontoma		Barbel[54]
	Hemangioma	Spleen	Mediterranean dogfish[55]
	Hemangiosarcoma		Salmon,[12] starry skate[22]
	Nephroblastoma		Mangrove killifish[56], Salmon[12]
	Branchioblastoma		Salmon[50]

is random and often multicentric. The lesions may be ulcerated due to continual trauma,[57] and the development of papillomas in captive fishes is often associated with chronic cutaneous trauma or irritation. Histologically, papillomas may have a primary squamous (epidermal) or connective tissue (dermal) component due to desmoplasia or a mixture of both components. Papillomas have previously been described in koi carp (*Cyprinus carpio*) and may progress to squamous cell carcinoma.[27]

Squamous cell carcinoma is rare in fishes but has been reported in various wild populations and may occur spontaneously in individual captive fishes.[3,50,63,64] A squamous cell carcinoma with hepatic metastasis has been reported in a hybrid sunfish.[65] Cutaneous distribution is random, although the cranial integument is a common site of involvement. Squamous cell carcinomas may grossly resemble papillomas or originate from papillomatous lesions[27,34–64,66] or may be a diffuse, infiltrative neoplasm that results in erosion and ulceration of the integument with subsequent involvement of the subcutaneous tissue.[50]

Neoplasms that have generally been classified as spindle cell tumors are also common, spontaneous, cutaneous lesions in fishes. The general classification is due to the fusiform to elongated microscopic appearance of the neoplastic cells, although the cells may also have oval or spherical profiles. Due to the common features of these neoplasms, a more definitive diagnosis requires ultrastructural examination of the neoplastic cells. Regardless, the general category of spindle cell tumors includes mesenchymal tumors, such as fibromas and fibrosarcomas, pigment cell tumors or chromatophoromas, and tumors of the peripheral nerves, such as schwannomas, neurofibromas, and neurilemmomas.

Cutaneous fibromas are not uncommon in fishes.[50,57,58] Myxomatous fibromas, or myxomas, are a variation of the typical fibroma with a loose, soft, mucinous texture due to the glycosaminoglycan matrix with an abundance of hyaluronic acid. Fibrosarcomas are less common, locally invasive neoplasms that grossly resemble fibromas.[50] Fibromas and fibrosarcomas have previously been described in wild and laboratory fishes exposed to chemical agents,[3] and fibrosarcomas have also been reported in goldfish (*Carassius auratus*),[41,67] although these neoplasms may be confused with pigment cell neoplasms or erythrophoromas of goldfish or may be characterized as papillomas. Additional neoplasms of mesenchymal origin, including neoplasms that originate from smooth and striated muscle or cartilaginous and osseous tissue, may also involve the integument but are rare in fishes.[50,61]

Neoplasms of the peripheral nerves may be the most common neoplasms in fishes according to some investigators[57,68] and include neurofibromas that are derived from endoneurial and epineurial connective tissue and neurilemmomas that are derived from Schwann cells.[57] As discussed previously, these tumors are often difficult to differentiate from other spindle cell tumors, such as nonpigmented chromatophoromas and fibromas without ultrastructural examination. Multiple neurofibromas and schwannomas have been described in various fishes,[50,69] including the bicolor damselfish (*Pomacentrus partitus*)[70] and goldfish.[71,72] These tumors may be confused with fibromas or fibrosarcomas.[67,73] Rarely, metastasized malignant nerve sheath tumors have been described.[29,72,74]

Pigment cells are derived from the neural crest, and pigment cell neoplasms or chromatophoromas in fishes are more specifically classified according to the pigment cell origin of the neoplasm and include erythrophoromas, melanophoromas (**Fig. 1**), xanthophoromas, guanophoromas, and iridophoromas. Pigment cell tumors are commonly confused with connective tissue tumors, such as fibromas and peripheral nerve tumors. Regardless, pigment cell neoplasms are common in fishes[50,57,58,75,76] and may be the primary type of neoplastic disease in certain fishes.[68] For example,

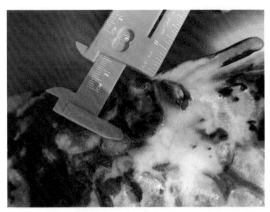

Fig. 1. A nonpigmented melanophoroma in a koi, a rare chromatophoroma. (*Courtesy of Companion Exotic Animal Medicine and Surgery Service, University of California, Davis, Davis, California.*)

aquatic animal practitioners may be familiar with goldfish that present with focal or multifocal, discrete, raised, tan to light brown or yellow to orange, nodular, or papillomatous lesions.[44,68] The neoplasms are generally benign but may be locally invasive and may recur with or without complete surgical excision. In contrast, melanomas may be the most common pigment cell tumor in various other fishes.[50,57] The most well-known example of melanoma in fishes occurs in platyfish crossed with swordtail hybrids (*Xiphophorus* sp),[77,78] whereas similar melanomas also occur spontaneously in nonhybrid strains of *Xiphophorus* species.[79]

Neoplasms of the gills in fishes are rare lesions, which is surprising considering the large epithelial surface area of the gills and the consequent exposure of the gills to various environmental agents, including chemicals and infectious agents.[58] Nasal adenocarcinomas can be encountered (**Fig. 2**). Neoplasms of the alimentary tract are also rare in fishes and, therefore, are not significant in ornamental or display fishes. Aggressive carcinomas and mixed malignant neoplasms of the intestine in the zebrafish, however, have been associated with the nematode *Pseudocapillaria tomentosa*.[80] Gastric adenopapillomas have been reported in rainbow trout (*Oncorhynchus mykiss*) exposed to chemicals,[20] whereas esophageal and gastric adenomas and invasive adenomas and adenocarcinomas of the intestine have also been induced in laboratory fish exposed to chemical agents.[3]

Hepatobiliary neoplasms are the most common visceral neoplasms of fishes, although an accurate determination of the prevalence of these neoplasms is difficult to establish in nonlaboratory fishes, because internal neoplasms are obviously less apparent than external neoplasms. These neoplasms include hepatomas, hepatocellular carcinomas, cholangiomas, cholangiocarcinomas, and mixed neoplasms that contain hepatic and biliary components. Metastasis of hepatobiliary carcinomas to the kidney and spleen is not uncommon, as described for hepatocellular carcinomas in rainbow trout exposed to aflatoxins.[11,81,82] Hepatic neoplasms are uncommonly reported, however, in ornamental species.

Lymphohematopoietic neoplasms in fishes that are often referred to as round cell tumors have generally been characterized as lymphosarcomas.[83] Lymphosarcomas have been reported in various species, including zebrafish,[84] Japanese medaka (*Oryzias latipes*),[83] African tilapia (*Sarotherodon spiluris spiluris*),[85] astyanax (*Astyanax* spp),[86] rainbow trout,[87,88] coho salmon (*Oncorhynchus kisutch*),[89] and esocids,

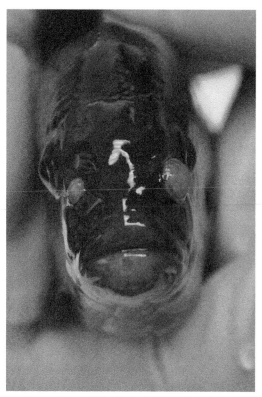

Fig. 2. Nasal adenocarcinoma in a *Labidochromis* sp.

such as northern pike *(Esox lucius)* and muskellunge *(Esox masquinongy)*.[90–92] The lymphosarcomas in Japanese medaka are cutaneous neoplasms that may also infiltrate the subcutaneous skeletal muscle or result in thymic, splenic, or renal metastases.[83] Likewise, lymphosarcomas in adult northern pike and muskellunge are large, irregular, proliferative, cutaneous neoplasms that may invade the subcutaneous skeletal muscle and metastasize to the liver, spleen, and kidney.[91,92] Affected fish may also have internal neoplasms that originate in the kidney without cutaneous involvement and are frequently associated with a leukemic condition.[86,91–93] Lymphosarcoma in salmonids and zebrafish often have a thymic origin[84,88,89] and may also be associated with a leukemic condition in salmonids.[58,87]

The most significant gonadal neoplasms in ornamental fishes are the gonadal neoplasms of ornamental koi carp,[94] which are similar to the gonadal neoplasms of wild hybrids of goldfish and carp.[95,96] The neoplasms are common in sexually mature female koi and apparently originate from the ovary, although the cellular origin of these neoplasms is often difficult to determine.[97] Regardless, affected fish generally present with coelomic distension (**Fig. 3**); ascites; subcutaneous edema with lepidorthosis, the scientific term for pine-coning, which is a condition when fish present with raised scales due to edema (**Fig. 4**); and an inability to maintain normal equilibrium in severe cases. Affected fish generally present with advanced, aggressive neoplasms with local invasion that involves and often replaces the liver, intestine, and other visceral organs (**Fig. 5**). Rupture of the body wall at the posterioventral midline is not uncommon in fish with advanced neoplasms and severe coelomic distension that results in exposure of the viscera and subsequent coelomic herniation.

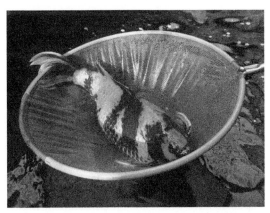

Fig. 3. Marked coelomic distension in a male koi with a seminoma.

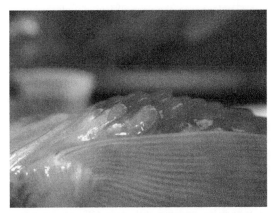

Fig. 4. Close-up view of the skin of a koi presented with lepidorthosis: the scales appear raised instead of being flat, due to cutaneous edema.

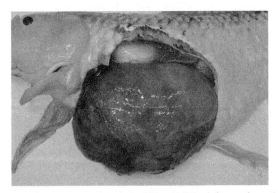

Fig. 5. Gross necropsy picture: large invasive cavitary gonadal neoplasm in a koi presented with buoyancy problems. (*Courtesy of* Joe Groff, VMD, PhD, Pathology Service, University of California, Davis, Davis, California.)

Neoplasms of mesenchymal origin with the exception of fibromas and fibrosarcomas are generally rare in fishes but have been reported in laboratory fishes (osteosarcoma, rhabdomyosarcoma, and leiomyosarcoma) exposed to chemical agents.[3] Leiomyomas are often difficult to differentiate from other neoplasms and may be confused with neurilemmomas in the goldfish.[50,98] Occasional spontaneous neoplasms of cartilage and bone have been reported as previously reviewed.[1]

Possible Causes and Predisposing Factors

Neoplasia is the result of a genetic mutation that may be acquired as an inherited characteristic and/or may occur as a result of exposure to an environmental agent, such as various chemicals,[3] radiation, or infectious agents, especially oncogenic viruses,[99] although the cause of most neoplasms in fishes has not been definitively determined.

UV radiation has been shown to play a role in the oncogenesis of certain fish tumors.[100] Many fish species have evolved in an environment with very low UV exposure, due to the attenuation of radiation by the depth of water and dissolved organic matter.[101] Fishes living in shallow water have also developed adaptations to high UV-B exposure, such as effective DNA repair systems,[101] UV-screening mucus in the saddle wrasse (*Thalassoma duperrey*)[102] or development of photoprotective substances, such as melanin, when exposed to radiation.[101,103] Melanomas have been shown to occur or be induced in free-ranging and captive (laboratory) fish, respectively, exposed to UV radiation.[100,104] *Xiphophorus* spp hybrids have been used as a model for human melanophoroma[104,105] and, more recently, zebrafish models have also been developed.[106] The manifestation of melanophoromas in these fish is linked to a spontaneous duplication of the epidermal growth factor receptor gene, also called the XMRK oncogene.[104,105] Cutaneous melanophoromas have also been reported in wild-caught nonhybrid *Xiphophorus* and in *Plectropomus* spp[100]; 15% of coral trout (*Plectropomus leopardus*) from a wild population exhibited cutaneous melanoma and a genetic predisposition was suspected in addition to a suspected induction by UV radiation; however, no pathogenic agent or toxin could be detected in these cases.[100] Fish possess cutaneous biochemical pathways to synthesize vitamin D, but only in small quantities due to the low concentration of cutaneous provitamin D, which is approximately only 10% of the quantity present in the integument of humans.[107]

Oncogenic viruses in fish include retroviruses, such as the walleye dermal sarcoma retrovirus, salmon swimbladder sarcoma virus[39,99] and the esocid lymphoma virus (ie, pike and muskellunge),[25] and herpesviruses in salmonids and smelt that result in papillomatous lesions.[2] Other suspected retroviral-induced tumors include odontomas/fibromas in angelfish (*Pterophyllum* spp) (**Fig. 6**),[2,108] schwannomas/neurofibromas in the bicolor damselfish detected concurrently with a virus-like agent,[108] papillomas in the common dab,[109] and leukemia in red sea bream were detected concurrently with an adenovirus,[110] but causality has not been established in these cases.[99]

It has been well documented that chemical compounds can induce or promote neoplasia in fish.[3] For example, aflatoxins have been shown to induce hepatobiliary neoplasms in rainbow trout, which is particularly susceptible to this toxin among vertebrates.[19,20] Cottonseed meal incorporated in pelleted diets can become infected by toxin-producing *Aspergillus* spp and the cyclopropenoid fatty acids of cottonseeds enhance the carcinogenic effect of aflatoxins.[19] Feeds that contain an increased amount of lipids associated have been shown to result in steatohepatitis and hepatocellular carcinomas in medaka exposed to carcinogenic agents.[17] The medaka has also been used as a model of hepatocellular carcinomas to study nonalcoholic

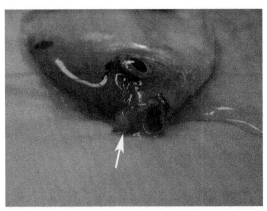

Fig. 6. Labial mass (*white arrow*) in an angelfish: histologic analysis was compatible with a fibroma. (*Courtesy of* Companion Exotic Animal Medicine and Surgery Service, University of California, Davis, Davis, California.)

hepatosteatitis in humans, which is a condition that can progress toward hepatic cirrhosis and hepatocellular carcinoma.[17] Halogenates have been suspected to promote some neurogenic tumors in salmons,[29] and N-methyl-N'-nitro-N-nitrosoguanidine has been used to experimentally induce branchial blastomas in medaka.[21] Also, free-ranging fish living in close contact to humans are exposed to multiple pharmaceutical residues,[111] although the effects of multiple and combined pharmaceutical residues in wastewater are still unknown and require more attention.[111,112] For instance, an up-regulation of oncogenes in fish has been demonstrated after exposure to endocrine disruptors, such as 17β-estradiol found in contraceptives.[113] Papillomas have also been induced in laboratory fishes exposed to chemical agents or been described in wild fishes from contaminated environments.[3] Hepatobiliary neoplasms have also been detected in wild fishes, especially fishes that inhabit polluted or contaminated environments,[3,114–116] and laboratory species that are experimentally exposed to various carcinogenic chemicals.[3]

Genetic predispositions for neoplasia in fish have been hypothesized, but not demonstrated, in epizootic cases of tumors.[29] As discussed previously, hybrids of swordtail and platyfish have been studied for their susceptibility to UV-induced melanomas due to a sex-linked oncogene.[104,105]

Complications

Malignant neoplasms may become locally invasive (**Figs. 7** and **8**),[1] which can result in organ displacement, such as exophthalmos (**Fig. 9**) or intracoelomic organ compression, as frequently observed with gonadal tumors in koi (see **Fig. 5**). Metastases have also been reported in fish with malignant tumors.[11,29,57,58,65,72,74,81–83,91,92]

DIAGNOSING FISH NEOPLASMS
Patient Evaluation

In addition to usual information collected for mammalian species, history should include water quality, exposure to toxins, and food storage in aquatic patients. Life support system assessment is also an important part of the evaluation.[117] This may include the filter, frequency of water changes, disinfection, and connections between the various parts of the system. Water source and water quality should be assessed

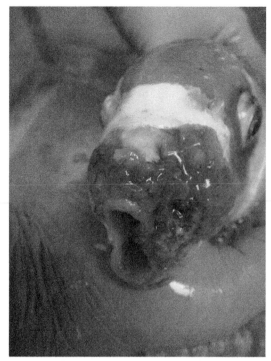

Fig. 7. Invasive and extensive squamous cell carcinoma in a koi preventing food prehension. (*Courtesy of* Companion Exotic Animal Medicine and Surgery Service, University of California, Davis, Davis, California.)

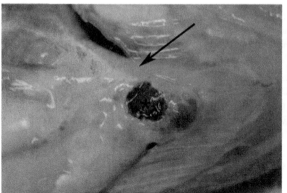
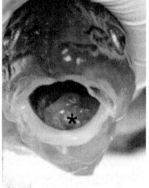

Fig. 8. Invasive thyroid adenocarcinoma (*asterisk*) in an Atlantic tomcod (*Microgadus tomcod*) causing dyspnea due to invasion of the branchial arches. Left part of the figure: ventral view: the mass is visible ventrally to the operculum (*arrow*): the head of the fish is toward the right. Right part of the figure: rostral view showing invasion of the oral cavity by the mass. (*Courtesy of* Aquarium du Québec, Université de Montréal, Québec.)

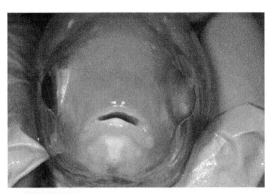

Fig. 9. Exophthalmos of the left eye due to an intraocular spindle cell sarcoma in a goldfish. (*Courtesy of* Companion Exotic Animal Medicine and Surgery Service, University of California, Davis, Davis, California.)

because water-borne toxins have been linked to neoplasm development. Cold-water fish are able to fast for months and it is not uncommon for owners to report prolonged anorexia associated with neoplastic disease conditions, although anorexia is a nonspecific sign of various disease conditions and has been reported as a manifestation of pain in some fish species[117]; therefore, anorexia should not be overinterpreted.

Physical examination

Fish are examined from a distance to evaluate buoyancy, swimming ability, and general level of activity. After this first assessment, a complete physical examination may be performed under general anesthesia unless the patient is deemed too unstable. The physical examination of fishes has previously been described.[118] Clinical signs associated with neoplasms are variable and include anorexia in cases of oral mass (**Figs. 10** and **11**); goiter (**Fig. 12**); exophthalmos in cases of retro-orbital masses; external lesions, including cutaneous (**Fig. 13**) and vent masses (**Fig. 14**); coelomic distension; and negative buoyancy in cases of intracoelomic mass (see **Fig. 3**). Complementary examinations typically performed under anesthesia include a skin scrape and gill biopsy. Water-borne anesthetic agents used in fish include buffered tricaine methanesulfonate (MS-222), clove oil (eugenol and isoeugenol),[119] isoeugenol,[120] propofol,[121] alfaxalone,[122] xylazin, ketamine,[123] and phenoxyethanol[124] among others. The quantity of buffer that should be added to MS-222 depends on the alkalinity of the water and ranges between a ratio of 1:2 and 1:1 MS-222:sodium bicarbonate.[125]

Currently, the only FDA-approved anesthetic agent in fish is MS-222, while metomidate (Aquacalm®, Syndel Laboratories Ltd., Nanaimo, Canada) is indexed for sedation during fish transportation[126] and isoeugenol and benzocaine are under an Investigational New Animal Drug program for ornamental fish.[120] Gill irrigation is required throughout anesthesia regardless of the anesthetic agent selected.[125] When using an injectable anesthetic agent, clinicians should be aware that the pharmacokinetics of the agent may vary depending on the site of muscular injection: drugs injected in red versus white muscles may have a different pharmacokinetic profile and many fish have a renal and/or hepatic portal system[9] that may affect the excretion of drugs injected in the caudal part of the body. In addition, some commonly used injectable anesthetic agents, like alfaxalone should not be used intramuscularly in koi.[127] For more information, the reader can refer to more in-depth reviews regarding fish anesthesia.[128,129]

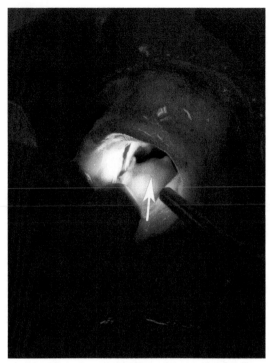

Fig. 10. Oral examination of an anesthetized koi with a transilluminator: a large mass is detected (*white arrow*). (*Courtesy of* Companion Exotic Animal Medicine and Surgery Service, University of California, Davis, Davis, California.)

Life support system assessment is also an important part of the evaluation.[118] This may include the filter, frequency of water changes, disinfection, and connections between the various parts of the system. Water source and water quality should be assessed as water-borne toxins have been linked to neoplasm development.[29]

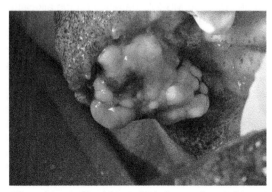

Fig. 11. Palatal papilloma in a wolf eel (*Anarrhichthys ocellatus*). (*Courtesy of* Aquarium du Québec, Université de Montréal, Québec.)

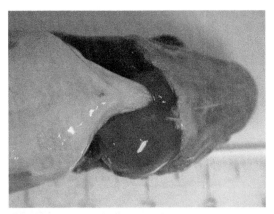

Fig. 12. Goiter in a mummichog (*Fundulus heteroclitus*). (*Courtesy of* Aquarium du Québec, Université de Montréal, Québec.)

Population evaluation

Occurrence of tumors in numerous specimens of the same species in a tank or exhibit should prompt additional diagnostic tests. In particular, the environment should be carefully examined for factors, such as the presence of toxins, or excessive exposure to UV radiation or other types of lights.[130] In addition, infection by oncogenic viruses may be suspected and investigated by electron microscopy, viral cell culture, and molecular diagnostic tests for a more definitive determination of the neoplastic etiology.

Diagnostic Modalities

Imaging

Similar to mammals, fish neoplasms can be identified and characterized via imaging techniques. The limited literature available, however, regarding advanced imaging poses a challenge to the use of these modalities in fish oncology. Furthermore, surgical planning may be challenging when description of the normal anatomy is not readily

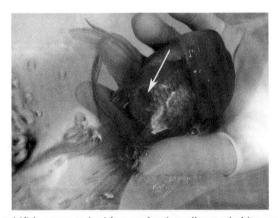

Fig. 13. Oranda goldfish presented with a coelomic wall mass (*white arrow*). (*Courtesy of* Companion Exotic Animal Medicine and Surgery Service, University of California, Davis, Davis, California.)

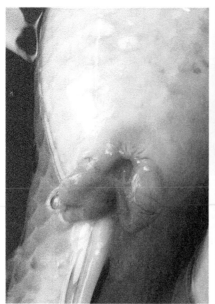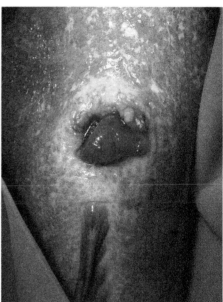

Fig. 14. Two fish presented with vent masses: a koi presented with a leiomyoma (*left*) and a kelp greenling (*Hexagrammos decagrammus*) presented with a vent adenocarcinoma (*right*). (*Courtesy of* Companion Exotic Animal Medicine and Surgery Service, University of California, Davis, Davis, California.; and Aquarium du Québec, Université de Montréal, Québec.)

available for the species. Regardless, clinicians should thoroughly review the literature whenever planning a surgical tumor excision. The anatomy for certain species of fish is available,[9,131] and an increasing number of articles describing normal and abnormal images obtained with ultrasonography,[23,132–134] radiography,[135–137] CT,[138,139] and MRI[140] have recently been published. In some cases, ultrasound, CT, and MRI may be obtained with the fish remaining in water.[138]

Coelomic contrast is limited on fish radiographs, with the exception of the swim bladder, which is radiotransparent and may be used to investigate a mass effect or to detect a swim bladder lesion (**Fig. 15**). For instance, the swim bladder is displaced ventrally in cases of renal neoplasm and displaced dorsally or compressed in cases of gonadal or caudal digestive tract neoplasm (**Fig. 16**). A dilated pneumatic duct may also be visualized in physostomous fish, that is, fish having a connection between the digestive tract and the swim bladder. Mineralized neoplasms are sometimes detected and should not be confused with digestive foreign bodies associated with substrate ingestion (**Fig. 17**). To improve digestive tract visualization, digestive contrast studies may be performed with oral and/or rectal administration of barium via a red rubber tube. Some fishes, like cyprinidae, do not have a stomach and the barium is administered in the esophagus. Knowledge of the normal digestive anatomy allows detection of mass effects associated with coelomic neoplasms. If normal anatomy is unknown, it is wise to image a healthy conspecific for comparison because some anatomic features of fish, such as pyloric ceca, can be misleading for clinicians used to domestic animal anatomy (**Fig. 18**).

Conversely, ultrasonography enables to investigate most coelomic masses more easily than with radiographs (**Fig. 19**), because the only air-filled structure is the

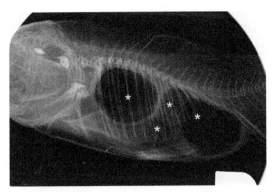

Fig. 15. Coelomic radiograph obtained with a dentistry radiology equipment in a goldfish presented with cystic lesions of the swim bladder: the multiple air-filled cavities are indicated by asterisks; only 2 chambers are usually present in the goldfish swim bladder. (*Courtesy of* Companion Exotic Animal Medicine and Surgery Service, University of California, Davis, Davis, California.)

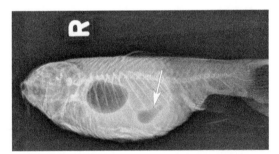

Fig. 16. Coelomic radiographs of a goldfish: a ventral displacement of the caudal chamber of the swim bladder (*arrow*) is associated with a renal mass. (*Courtesy of* Companion Exotic Animal Medicine and Surgery Service, University of California, Davis, Davis, California.)

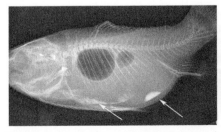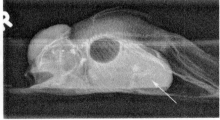

Fig. 17. Coelomic mineral opacities (*arrows*) associated with respectively, digestive mineral foreign bodies in a comet goldfish (*left*) and mineralized ovarian lesions in a ranshu goldfish (*right*). (*Courtesy of* Companion Exotic Animal Medicine and Surgery Service, University of California, Davis, Davis, California; and Davis and Zoologic medicine service, Université de Montréal, Quebec)

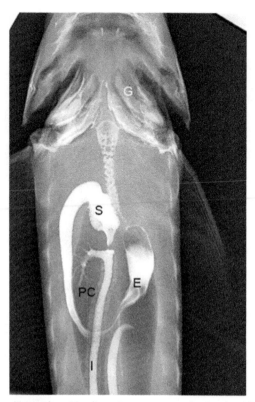

Fig. 18. Coelomic radiograph with digestive contrast obtained with administration of barium with a soft oroesophageal feeding tube in a healthy yellow sturgeon (*Acipenser fulvescens*). E, esophagus; G, gills; I, intestine; PC, pyloric ceca; S, stomach. (*Courtesy of* Aquarium du Québec, Université de Montréal, Québec.)

swim bladder in teleosts. Renal masses may be imaged with a dorsal approach due to the dorsal location of the kidney relative to the swim bladder. The ultrasound probe may be protected by a plastic sheath filled with acoustic gel to ultrasound the fish in water. When working with saltwater fishes, particular care should be taken to avoid contact between the water and electric connectors, even for impermeable ultrasound machines, because repeated salt exposure can damage the equipment. Most fish have a gallbladder, with the notable exception of some sharks. The gallbladder should not be confused with a cystic lesion. Ultrasound enables to differentiate mineralized masses from intraluminal foreign bodies (**Fig. 20**). A diffuse hepatopancreas is present in many fishes. Gonadal development may take impressive proportions during the reproductive season, to the point where other coelomic organs are difficult to locate. Developed ovaries prior to spawning should not be confused with ovarian neoplasms (**Fig. 21**). Ocular ultrasounds may allow detection of retro-orbital masses (**Fig. 22**). Ultrasound-guided aspirates may be performed to investigate masses and effusion.

Pathology
Similar to mammals, some fish neoplasms may be diagnosed by fine-needle aspiration followed by cytologic examination.[141] Diagnostic cytology of fish has been

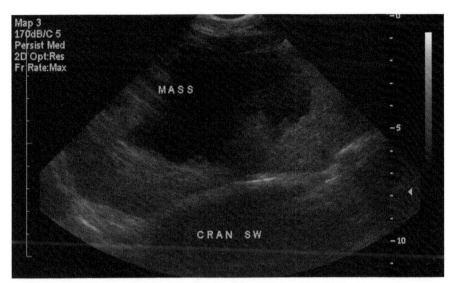

Fig. 19. Coelomic ultrasound of a koi presented with a cystic seminoma (*mass*). The cranial chamber of the swim bladder is visible dorsally to the gonadal mass (*cran sw*). (*Courtesy of* Companion Exotic Animal Medicine and Surgery Service, University of California, Davis, Davis, California.)

described previously.[142] Familiarity with fish cytology is paramount to obtaining an accurate diagnosis, which may complicate interpretation. For instance, it is expected to find diatomaceous algae on seahorse integument and normal fish flora should not be confused with cutaneous lesions (**Fig. 23**). Alarm cells, which are giant cells, are normally found in the depth of the epithelium. Mitotic figures are also commonly found in circulation, among other surprising features for mammalian pathologists. Due to the peculiarities of piscine cytology, pathologists should carefully assess apparent abnormalities. Cutaneous biopsies may be obtained from fish skin for histopathology or

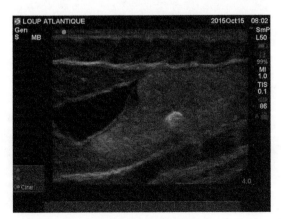

Fig. 20. Ultrasonographic image of tissular mineralizations in a hepatic xanthoma visualized in an Atlantic wolffish (*Anarhichas lupus*). (*Courtesy of* Aquarium du Québec, Université de Montréal, Québec.)

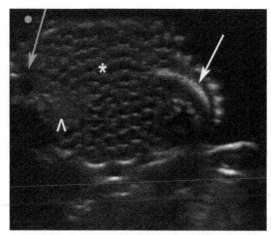

Fig. 21. Coelomic ultrasound in a reproductive Pacific spiny lumpsucker (*Eumicrotremus orbis*): the cranial part of the fish is on the left and the caudal fin is visible in the right (*white arrow*): ovarian tissue occupies the majority of the coelomic space (*asterisk*), the liver is visible cranially (*arrowhead*), near the opercular cavities (*gray arrow*). This appearance is physiologic and should not be confused with a gonadal neoplasm. (*Courtesy of* Aquarium du Québec, Université de Montréal, Québec.)

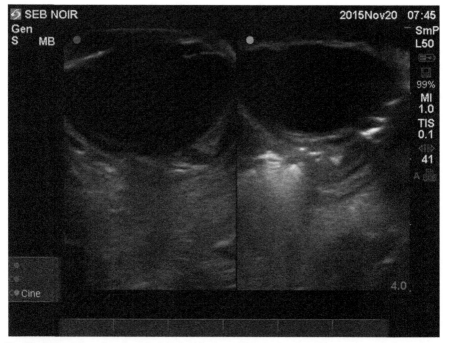

Fig. 22. Bilateral ocular ultrasound of a black rockfish (*Sebastes melanops*) presented with a unilateral retro-orbital mass (*right* part of the image). (*Courtesy of* Aquarium du Québec, Université de Montréal, Québec.)

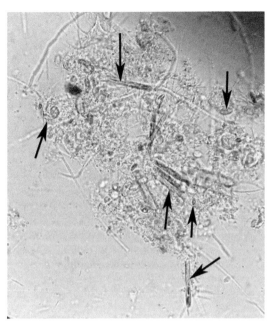

Fig. 23. Skin scrape from a big-belly seahorse (*Hippocampus abdominalis*): black arrows indicate diatomaceous algae. (*Courtesy of* Aquarium du Québec, Université de Montréal, Québec.)

microbial cultures; a biopsy punch or a scalpel blade may be used. Hemostasis is obtained by compression or the use of a handheld cautery. Compared with mammals, fish skin has a very low elasticity due to the dermal scales[143] and biopsy sites may be left open for second intention healing.

Incisional or excisional biopsies of external lesions in fish are accomplished similarly to the procedure in mammals. Local anesthesia with lidocaine, 2 mg/kg, is commonly used and anecdotally seems to allow for the use of lower general anesthetic concentrations in the authors experience. Differential diagnoses for external masses include neoplasms; bacterial, fungal, and parasitic granulomas; abscesses; cysts[144]; hyperplasia[145]; microsporidial xenomas; and traumatic hematomas; among others. Wedge biopsies may also be performed: 1 sample is placed in formalin, impression smears may be obtained, and the rest of the mass can be frozen for future diagnostic investigations. Because the body wall of fishes is usually thin compared with aquatic mammals that display a thick blubber layer, however, the surgical margins are rarely obtained following the excision of coelomic wall neoplastic lesions. Therefore, body wall reconstruction should be planned carefully prior to removal of the lesion due to the low elasticity of the tissues.[143]

Histopathology In addition to routine histologic staining of tissues using hematoxylin-eosin, special histochemical stains used in mammals are also useful in fish, such as Masson trichrome stain to highlight connective tissue,[39,98] phosphotungstic acid–hematoxylin to highlight striated muscle, alcian blue to stain mucinic substances,[12] and Sudan stain for lipids, among others.

Additional diagnostic tests Transmission electron microscopy may be required for a definitive pathologic diagnosis[141] and/or the detection of intralesional viral agents. The presence of intralesional viral particles may be incidental and Koch postulates should be verified to determine causality.

The use of immunochemical methods for the diagnosis of neoplastic lesions based on the expression of cytoskeletal proteins, including intermediate filaments and other cellular markers, such as the CD antigens, are not reliable and should be avoided or used with caution for fishes. Specifically, the expression and tissue distribution patterns of intermediate filaments in fishes is more diverse and less specific than in mammals.[146–150] In this context, interpretation of results using immunochemical techniques for the determination of the histogenesis of neoplasms in fishes should be based on prior studies of normal tissue distribution in the relevant species rather than the patterns known to occur in mammals. In this context, there are numerous peer-reviewed publications that describe the use of antibodies directed against mammalian antigens for the diagnosis of neoplasms in fishes,[151,152] although these investigations failed to perform normal distribution and expression studies and should be interpreted with skepticism. Furthermore, it is surprising that not only the investigators of these reports but also the reviewers and editors did not consider the possible differences that may occur in such distant taxons. As highlighted in some case reports,[97,153,154] clinicians should remain careful regarding interpretation of tissue staining with antibodies validated in mammalian species. The use of control tissue of piscine origin is recommended whenever immunohistochemistry is attempted,[141] and more extensive studies are needed to validate the use of immunohistochemistry in piscine species.

TREATING FISH NEOPLASMS
General Principles

Fish oncology is still in its infancy and most treatment attempts have been extrapolated from domestic animal medicine. Similar to other vertebrates, treatment of fish neoplasms may be attempted using surgery, radiation therapy, chemotherapy, or a combination of these treatments. An additional pitfall in fish medicine is the omnipresence of water and the risks associated with waterborne residues. As with other exotic species, there is a need to better understand fish nociception to take into account the welfare and attempt to minimize the discomfort and pain experienced by aquatic patients. In large groups of fish, such as populations maintained in aquaculture facilities and public aquaria, a prophylactic approach as practiced in population medicine may be favored, whereas the treatment of individual ornamental fish may be pursued for valued animals. Isolating fish patients may be preferable to favor treatment observance and appetite monitoring and avoid conspecific aggression. Social behavior of the species should be taken into account, however, because reintroducing an individual into a population may be difficult in some cases. In addition, some fish may be stressed when kept individually, whereas keeping patients in their group may be preferred.

Surgical Treatment Options

Tumor excision may be performed under general anesthesia. Preanesthetic patient evaluation may be challenging in fish due to the lack of hematological and biochemical reference intervals available in most species and due to the numerous environmental factors affecting these reference values.[155] An increasing number of reference intervals pertaining to fish species are, however, available.[156–159] It has been suggested that evaluation of acute-phase proteins and serum proteins by electrophoresis may be more relevant as part of a preanesthetic evaluation in fishes.[160–163]

Anesthetic monitoring is particularly challenging in fish, because a fish that expires under anesthesia may retain cardiac activity for hours, decreasing the value of electrocardiography and ultrasonographic Doppler monitoring. In addition, pulse oxymetry does not reliably monitor hemoglobin saturation in fish.[125] Monitoring the respiratory rate remains, albeit crude, a method to monitor anesthetic depth, because it varies with oxygenation[125] and nociception. Because of these difficulties, anesthesia should be kept to a minimal duration. Furthermore, because the pharmacokinetics of anesthetic agents is affected by environmental parameters, such as pH and temperature,[164] similar to other poikilothermic species, the water quality, including temperature, dissolved oxygen, and pH, should be kept stable throughout the procedure.

Intraoperative hemostasis may be achieved by compression or the use of handheld cautery. Cryotherapy has also been used to excise locally invasive masses (**Fig. 24**); in cases of cryotherapy used, a biopsy should be obtained first for histologic diagnosis. Surgical sites are ideally sutured with monofilament sutures[165] to avoid osmolar disorders postoperatively. Freshwater fish are especially prone to hyperhydration, whereas nonosmoconformer marine fish are prone to dehydration when cutaneous integrity is damaged.[166]

Fish wound healing has been studied extensively in zebrafish.[167] Fish have exceptional regeneration capability[168] and possess the ability to regenerate fins[169] and the caudal peduncle when amputated repeatedly.[170] Healing time, however, depends on environmental parameters, such as water temperature.[169] Because cutaneous healing may require months in cold-water species, keeping patients at higher temperature decreases healing time.[169,171] Conversely, immersion of fish in a 20-mg/L dexamethasone continuous bath has been shown to slow wound healing.[168] This should be taken into consideration if corticosteroids are elected as part of a palliative therapy regimen after tumor excision.

The excision of intraocular and retro-orbital neoplasms may require enucleation (**Fig. 25**).[172,173] In public aquaria, a prosthetic eye has been placed successfully for aesthetic purposes,[174] but long-term retention may be problematic.[175] More complete reviews of surgical techniques in fish are available.[143,176]

Surgical excision of koi gonadal neoplasms is generally only successful in the early stages of the disease condition without involvement of the other visceral organs.[97]

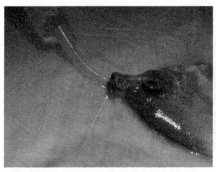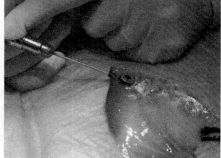

Fig. 24. Cryotherapy applied on an angelfish fibroma (*arrow*). Irrigation of the gills through the oral cavity with MS-222-containing water to prevent any movement from the fish during the procedure (*left*). Cryotherapy being applied to the mass (*right*). (*Courtesy of* Companion Exotic Animal Medicine and Surgery Service, University of California, Davis, Davis, California.)

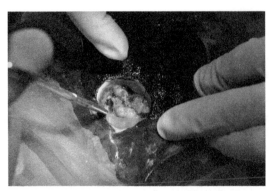

Fig. 25. Dissection of a retro-orbital mass during enucleation of a black rockfish. (*Courtesy of* Aquarium du Québec, Université de Montréal, Québec.)

Surgical intervention in a majority of advances cases is unsuccessful and, therefore, is a questionable procedure that is generally not indicated.

Chemotherapeutic Treatment Options

Few clinical reports are available regarding use of chemotherapy in fish. Some chemotherapeutics have been investigated, however, in fish to assess environmental contamination because fish may concentrate exogenous pollutants, including chemotherapeutic agents that have been experimentally administered to evaluate their effect on hematologic parameters, and further enable screening of free-ranging fish. Agents studied include mitomycin C,[177] 5-fluorouracil, bleomycin,[178] cyclophosphamide, and vinblastine among others.[179,180] In addition, cholesterol-lowering agents, such as ezetimibe, have been investigated in medaka because of their prophylactic effect on hepatocellular carcinomas.[181]

Challenges encountered when using chemotherapeutic agents in fishes is the lack of available pharmacokinetic studies and the risk of potential residues in the water. Because metabolism of these drugs is mostly unknown in fish, it is also unknown whether active metabolites are excreted in the water and subsequently recycled through the filtration system, potentially resulting in owner and conspecific exposure. Therefore, studies are needed to assess residues after fish treatment.

Bleomycin and cisplatin have been used empirically as intralesional treatments for fish neoplasms. More specifically, they were used for the treatment of an undifferentiated sarcoma of the body wall in a goldfish,[135] leiomyoma of the periventiductal area of a koi,[98] and a facial myxoma in an oranda goldfish.[182] Intralesional injections can be administered using a grid pattern in anesthetized patients (**Fig. 26**). Involved personal should wear appropriate personal protective equipment and residues should be handled following established guidelines for chemotherapeutics usage and disposal.

Concerning efficacy, there was recurrence of the undifferentiated sarcoma of the body wall in the goldfish, discussed previously, despite 2 cisplatin injections administered a month apart and the fish was subsequently euthanized 2 months after surgery.[135] Status of the surgical margins was not specified in this case report. The fish was hospitalized for a month, however, due to concerns of cisplatin residues in the environment.[135] The koi that presented with a periventiductal leiomyoma underwent a debulking surgery with incomplete margins, followed by an intralesional injection of bleomycin. A bleomycin dose of 10 IU/m^2 to 20 IU/m^2 was used and

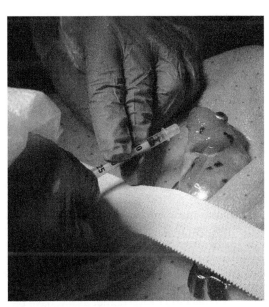

Fig. 26. Intralesional administration of bleomycin into a facial myxoma in a goldfish. Water containing the anesthetic agent (buffered MS-222) is administered in a retrograde fashion over the gills to facilitate intraoral access as some injections are performed from the labial aspect of the mass. (*Courtesy of* Companion Exotic Animal Medicine and Surgery Service, University of California, Davis, Davis, California.)

extrapolated from the dosages used in dogs and no recurrence of the mass was noted after 5 months.[183]

Bleomycin has been used in another case by one of the authors.[182] A 4.5-year, 36-g, male calico ranchu goldfish presented for exophthalmos and abnormal food prehension associated with a facial mass. A diagnosis of myxoma was achieved by incisional biopsy representing approximately 10% of the volume of the mass. A dose of 0.09 IU or 2,5 IU/kg of bleomycine, extrapolated from rat dosages, was administered into the facial myxoma in a grid pattern under general anesthesia (see **Fig. 26**). The mass volume decreased by approximately 60%. This resulted in improved food prehension and improved the exophthalmos in the patient. After 3 months, a second identical dose of bleomycin was administered due to tumor progression. The owner reported a 20% to 30% reduction in tumor size after this injection, but tumor expansion recurred at 8 to 9 weeks postadministration. Regardless, intralesional bleomycin may have utility as a potential local treatment of some neoplasms in ornamental fishes. Bleomycin is rapidly metabolized by tissue hydrolases after intratumoral injection,[184] and bleomycin hydrolase has been demonstrated in koi leukocytes.[185] In addition, clinical preparations of bleomycin contain multiple glycoproteins, which would be rapidly denatured in the environment in the event of leakage from the injection site.[184] Therefore, using this drug may limit the risk of potential exposure of the owner and counterparts to therapeutic metabolites. Further studies are needed, however, to evaluate and define optimal treatment protocols and toxicity and to assess metabolism and environmental residues. Electrochemotherapy may enhance cisplatin and bleomycin action, but this technique has not been investigated in fish to the authors' knowledge.[186,187]

Radiation Treatment Options

Radiation therapy results in cellular damage by ionization, which is the ejection of an electron from a cellular component resulting in the formation of highly reactive free-radical species.[188] In mammals, hematopoietic neoplasms are generally more radio-sensitive followed by epithelial neoplasms, whereas mesenchymal neoplasms are typically more radioresistant,[188] although it is unknown whether this also applies to fish. Ionizing radiations can be classified in 2 categories: photon radiation (x-rays and megavoltage gamma rays produced by cobalt) and particle radiation (electrons produced by linear accelerators, protons, carbon ions, and alpha and beta particles, as produced by strontium-90, for instance).[189] The energy associated with each type of radiation determines the depth of action.[189]

Effects of radiations on fish species have been mostly investigated to assess environmental risks associated with nuclear-power incidents and radioactive contaminants.[180] In addition, radiation therapy has also been investigated in zebrafish used as models for human neoplasms.[190] Zebrafish irradiated with 45 Gy or higher delivered in a single fraction at 13 Gy/min in the caudal part of their body developed muscle fibrosis 30 days later, which is a late adverse effect of radiation therapy.[190] In contrast, only 25% of zebrafish receiving 30 Gy during a single irradiation session developed fibrosis.[190] Gamma radiation effects on fish erythrocytes, including micronuclei formation and DNA strand breaks detected by the comet assay, have been documented in koi,[191] goldfish,[192] and zebrafish,[193] among others.[180] To the authors' knowledge, peer-reviewed reports documenting the clinical applications of radiation therapy in fish are still lacking with the exception of a single case report describing the use of monthly megavoltage radiation therapy at 8 Gy in a goldfish affected with a recurring myxoma of the face.[182] No clinical effect was observed and the fish was ultimately euthanized. Protocols for irradiation of soft tissue masses still need to be developed and evaluated in piscine patients, although irradiation would be technically feasible.

Supportive Treatment

Options in fish include attempts to use antinociceptive drugs and anti-inflammatories. In addition, various devices are created by fish hobbyists to compensate for buoyancy disorders and avoid exposure of the fish to air, which causes complications, such as cutaneous infections. Typically, weights or floaters are fixed to the fish to compensate. Tumors involving the coelomic cavity or the swim bladder are more commonly associated with buoyancy issues.

Recent studies have investigated fish nociception.[117] Nociception is defined as the transmission of noxious stimuli and subsequent processing of the stimulus in the brain, whereby the pain experience, if present, is mediated.[194] Fish do not have a neocortex and, therefore, the occurrence of pain, as opposed to nociception, is controversial.[196] Regardless of the proper terminology, veterinary practitioners should take measures to alleviate potential pain, because nociceptive receptors are present in fish.[195]

Clinical signs of the nociception in fish are also controversial[196] and decreased appetite has been shown associated with postoperation discomfort in koi,[117] although abnormal position in the water column as an indication of nociception is debatable.[117,197] Various models have been used to investigate fish pain,[195] including the minimum anesthetic concentration (MAC) reduction model that has been questioned because experiments have shown that MS-222 MAC increased overtime when goldfish are repeatedly anesthetized with MS-222.[198,199] That is, the duration of anesthesia had more impact than the dosage of MS-222 concentration.[199] In these experiments, however, MS-222 was not been buffered and it is unknown whether an effect of pH or a degradation of MS-222 potency overtime in an open container could have affected the results of the study.[199] More independent studies are needed to confirm this finding. In addition, the up-down method of sequential population sampling has been used to evaluate MAC reduction in fish that uses multiple individuals to adjust anesthetic bath concentration.[198] In other species, however, it is well known that nociception may vary among individuals.[200]

Opioid drugs are recommended for preemptive analgesia, but data regarding long-term administration in fish are still lacking, although the use of morphine, 5 mg/kg intramuscularly (IM), has been suggested in koi.[117] In contrast, koi administered butorphanol, at 10 mg/kg IM, after gonadectomy did not show an improved appetite compared with control fish receiving saline, and buoyancy disorders and respiratory depression were noticed after administration of 10 mg/kg IM.[118] Another experiment resulted, however, in improved appetite after a butorphanol injection of 0.4 mg/kg IM in the same species.[197] Therefore, it could be questioned whether adverse effects associated with butorphanol may be due to high dosages. Butorphanol may still be an appropriate antinociceptive agent in fish at a lower dose, although further studies are needed to determine dosage and efficiency. A study in goldfish has shown an MAC reduction when using low doses but not high doses of butorphanol.[198] IM administration of tramadol was shown to increase the electrical stimulation threshold in koi.[201] Regardless, further evaluation of noncontrolled antinociceptive drugs in fish is needed.

Anti-inflammatory drugs may be used in fish with neoplastic lesions as a component of a multimodal antinociceptive protocol. Ketoprofen,[197,202] carprofen,[203] and meloxicam[204] have been evaluated in a limited number of fish. Meloxicam safety has been evaluated in goldfish after a single injection of 5 mg/kg,[204] whereas ketoprofen has been shown to reduce the MAC in goldfish[198] and to decrease postoperative creatine kinase in koi.[197] Adverse effects of some nonsteroidal anti-inflammatory drugs (NSAIDs), however, have been previously reported in fish and empirical use at high doses is, therefore, discouraged.[205,206] Toxicity of NSAIDs in aglomerular fish species, such as seahorses and other syngnathids,[9] has not been evaluated to the authors' knowledge.

Steroidal anti-inflammatory drugs have shown to result in similar adverse in vitro effects[207] that occur in mammals, including immunosuppression[208] and osteoporosis associated with prolonged scale regeneration.[209] More studies are needed to evaluate whether glucocorticoids may improve fish comfort and appetite as part of the palliative care of patients with neoplasms.

Evaluation of Outcome and Long-Term Recommendations

Little information is available regarding the duration of survival in fishes with neoplastic lesions. It is, therefore, important to document long-term monitoring of patients receiving treatments that will progressively expand the knowledge regarding fish oncology.

ACKNOWLEDGMENTS

The authors thank Dr Stéphane Lair, DVM, Dipl. ACZM, for his contribution to the cases included in this article as illustrations.

REFERENCES

1. Groff JM. Neoplasia in fishes. Vet Clin North Am Exot Anim Pract 2004;7:705–56.
2. Claver JA, AIE Q. Comparative morphology, development and function of blood cells in non-mammalian vertebrates. J Exotic Pet Med 2009;18:87–97.

3. Grizzle J, Goodwin A. Neoplasms and related lesions. In: Leatherland A, Woo P, editors. Fish diseases and disorders. Wallingford (CT): CABI Publishing; 1998. p. 37–104.

4. Lee HK, Jeong Y, Lee S, et al. Persistent organochlorines in 13 shark species from offshore and coastal waters of Korea: Species-specific accumulation and contributing factors. Ecotoxicol Environ Saf 2015;115:195–202.

5. Cooper GM. Cancer - the development and causes of cancer. Chapter 15. In: Cooper G, editor. The cell: a molecular approach. 2nd edition. Sunderland (MA): Sinauer Associates; 2000.

6. D. M, H.W. F. Neoplasia. In: H.W. F, editor. Systemic pathology of fish. 2nd edition. London: Scotian Press; 2006. p. 313–35.

7. Bubanovic I, Najman S. Comparative oncology and comparative tumor immunology. J Biol Sci 2005;5:114–8.

8. Laurens N. Cancer resistance in amphibia. Dev Comp Immunol 1997;21:102–6.

9. Stoskopf M. Anatomy. Chapter 1. In: MK S, editor. Fish medicine. Apex (NC): Saunders; 1993. p. 2–30.

10. Machotka S, McCain B, Myers M. Metastases in fish. In: Kaiser H, editor. Comparative aspects of tumor development. Dordrecht (The Netherlands): Kluwer; 1989. p. 48–54.

11. Ashley L, Halver J. Multiple metastasis of rainbow trout hepatoma. Trans Am Fish Soc 1963;92:365–71.

12. Dale OB, Torud B, Kvellestad A, et al. From chronic feed-induced intestinal inflammation to adenocarcinoma with metastases in salmonid fish. Cancer Res 2009;69:4355–62.

13. Santamaria-Bouvier A, Lair S. Xanthomatous lesions in captibe Atlantic wolffish (Anarhichas lupus). Proceedings of the 45th International Association for Aquatic Animal Medicine annual conference 2014.

14. Lom J, Dykova I. Microsporidian xenomas in fish seen in wider perspective. Folia Parasitol (Praha) 2005;52:69–81.

15. Vergneau-Grosset C, LS. Microsporidiosis in vertebrate companion exotic animals. Journal of Fungi 2016;2:1–20.

16. Etchin J, Kanki JP, Look AT. Zebrafish as a model for the study of human cancer. Methods Cell Biol 2011;105:309–37.

17. Asaoka Y, Terai S, Sakaida I, et al. The expanding role of fish models in understanding non-alcoholic fatty liver disease. Dis Model Mech 2013;6:905–14.

18. White R, Rose K, Zon L. Zebrafish cancer: the state of the art and the path forward. Nat Rev Cancer 2013;13:624–36.

19. Lee D, Wales J, Ayres JL, et al. Synergism between cyclopropenoid fatty acids and chemical carcinogens in rainbow trout (Salmo gairdneri). Cancer Res 1991; 28:2312–8.

20. Bailey GS, Williams DE, Hendricks JD. Fish models for environmental carcinogenesis: the rainbow trout. Environ Health Perspect 1996;104:5–21.

21. Brittelli MR, Chen HH, Muska CF. Induction of branchial (gill) neoplasms in the medaka fish (Oryzias latipes) by N-methyl-N'-nitro-N-nitrosoguanidine. Cancer Res 1985;45:3209–14.

22. Stoskopf M. Neoplasia in sharks. Chapter 101. In: MK S, editor. Fish Medicine. Apex (NC): Saunders; 1993. p. 808–9.

23. Jafarey YS, Berlinski RA, Hanley CS, et al. Presumptive dysgerminoma in an orange-spot freshwater stingray (Potamotrygon Motoro). J Zoo Wildl Med 2015; 46:382–5.

24. Borucinska J, Harshbarger J, Bogicevic T. Hepatic cholangiocarcinoma and testicular mesothelioma in a wild-caught blue shark, Prionace glauca (L.). J Fish Dis 2003;26:43–9.
25. Papas T, Dahlberg JE, Sonstegard R. Type C virus in lymphosarcoma in northern pike (Esox lucius). Nature 1976;261:506–8.
26. Manire C. Lymphosarcoma in a captive bonnethead shark, Sphyrna tiburo (L.). J Fish Dis 2013;36:437–40.
27. Wildgoose W. Papilloma and squamous cell carcinoma in koi carp (Cyprinus carpio). Vet Rec 1992;130:153–7.
28. Prieur D, Fenstermacher J, Guarino A. A choroid plexus papilloma in an elasmobranch (Squalus acanthias). J Natl Cancer Inst 1976;56:1207–9.
29. Masahito P, Ishikawa T, Yanagisawa A, et al. Neurogenic tumors in coho salmon (Oncorhynchus kisutch) reared in well water in Japan. J Natl Cancer Inst 1985; 75:779–90.
30. Schmale MC, Gill KA, Cacal SM, et al. Characterization of Schwann cells from normal nerves and from neurofibromas in the bicolour damselfish. J Neurocytol 1994;23:668–81.
31. Ishikawa T, Masahito P, Takayama S. Olfactory neuroepithelioma in a domestic carp (Cyprinus carpio). Cancer Res 1978;38:3954–9.
32. Vigliano FA, Marcaccini AJ, Sarradell J, et al. First description of an olfactory neuroblastoma in goldfish Carassius auratus: a case report. Dis Aquat Organ 2011;96:61–8.
33. Torikata C, Mukai M, Kageyama K. Spontaneous olfactory neuroepithelioma in a domestic medaka (Oryzias latipes). Cancer Res 1989;49:2994–8.
34. Thomas L. Sur un cas de stiboneuroépithélioblastome chez une daurade. Bullerin de l'Association française pour l'étude du cancer 1932;21:385–96.
35. Dawe CJ, Harshbarger JC. Neoplasms in feral fishes: their significance to cancer research. In: Ribelin WE, Migaki G, editors. The pathology of fishes. Madison (WI): University of Wisconsin Press; 1975. p. 871–94.
36. Sarkar HL, Kapoor BG, Duttachaudhuri R. A study of leiomyoma, a mesenchymal tumour on the fins of an Indian catfish, Mystus Osteobagrus seenghala Sykes. Growth 1955;19:257–61.
37. Schlumberger HG. Cutaneous leiomyoma of goldfish; morphology and growth in tissue culture. Am J Pathol 1949;25:287–99.
38. Herman RL, Landolt M. A testicular leiomyoma in a largemouth bass, Micropterus salmoides. J Wildl Dis 1975;11:128–9.
39. Bowser PR, Casey JW, Casey RN, et al. Swimbladder Leiomyosarcoma in Atlantic salmon (Salmo salar) in North America. J Wildl Dis 2012;48:795–8.
40. K. A, Hilger I, Möller H. Lentivirus-like particles in connective tissue tumours of fish from German coastal waters. Dis Aquat Organ 1991;11:151–4.
41. Probasco D, Noga E, Marcellin D, et al. Dermal fibrosarcoma in a goldfish: case report. J Small An Med 1994;2:173–5.
42. Willens S, Dunn JL, Frasca S. Fibrosarcoma of the brood pouch in an aquarium-reared lined seahorse (Hippocampus erectus). J Zoo Wildl Med 2004;35:107–9.
43. Gjurčević E, Kužir S, Sfacteria A, et al. Spontaneous multicentric myxoma of the dermal nerve sheaths in farmed European eels Anguilla anguilla. Dis Aquat Organ 2014;111:173–6.
44. Murchelano R, RL. E. An erythrophoroma in ornamental carp, Cyprinus carpio L. J Fish Dis 1981;4:265–8.

45. Ishikawa T, Masahito P, Matsumoto J, et al. Morphologic and biochemical characterization of erythrophoromas in goldfish (Carassius auratus). J Natl Cancer Inst 1978;61:1461–70.
46. Kimura I, Taniguchi N, Kumai H, et al. Correlation of epizootiological observations with experimental data: chemical induction of chromatophoromas in the croaker, Nibea mitsukurii. Natl Cancer Inst Monogr 1984;65:139–54.
47. Noga E. Fish disease: diagnosis and treatment. 2nd edition. Ames (IA): Wiley-Blackwell; 2010.
48. Leatherland J, Sonstegard R. Structure of normal testis and testicular tumours in cyprinids from Lake Ontario. Cancer Res 1978;38:3164–73.
49. Weisse C, Weber ES, Matzkin Z, et al. Surgical removal of a seminoma from a black sea bass. J Am Vet Med Assoc 2002;221:240–1.
50. Roberts R. Neoplasia of teleosts. In: RJ R, editor. Fish pathology. London: WB Saunders; 2001. p. 151–68.
51. Thomas L. Sur deux cas de tumeurs testiculaires chez la roussette. Bullerin de l'Association française pour l'étude du cancer 1933;22:306–15.
52. Bean-Knuden D, Uhazy L, Wagner J. Cranial chondrosarcoma in a paddlefish Polyodon spathula (Walbaum). J Fish Dis 1987;10:363–70.
53. Nash G, Porter C. Branchial osteochrondoma in a gilthead sea bream, Sparus aurata L. cultured in the Gulf of Aqaba. J Fish Dis 1985;8:333–6.
54. Manera M, Biavati S. Branchial osteogenetic neoplasm in a barbel Barbus barbus plebejus. Dis Aquat Organ 1999;37:231–6.
55. Ladreyt F. Sur un odontome cutané chez un Scyllium catulus. Bull Inst Oceanogr Monaco 1929;539:1–4.
56. Couch JA. Invading and metastasizing cardiac hemangioendothelial neoplasms in a cohort of the fish Rivulus marmoratus: unusually high prevalence, histopathology and possible etiologies. Cancer Res 1995;55:2438–47.
57. Harshbarger J, Spero P, Wolcott N. Neoplasms in wild fish from marine ecosystems emphasizing environmental interactions. In: Couch J, Fournie J, editor. Pathobiology of marine and estuarine organisms. Boca Raton (FL): CRC Press; 1993. p. 157–76.
58. Hayes M, Ferguson H. Neoplasia in fish. In: Ferguson H, editor. Systemic pathology of fish. Ames (IA): Iowa State University Press; 1989. p. 230–47.
59. Mawdesley-Thomas L. Neoplasia in fish: a review. Curr Top Comp Pathobiol 1971;1:87–170.
60. Peters N. Diseases caused by neoplasia. In: O K, editor. Diseases of marine animals. Hamburg (Germany): Biologische Anstalt Helgoland; 1984. p. 400–23.
61. Wellings S. Neoplasia and primitive vertebrate phylogeny: echinoderms, prevertebrates and fishes. A review. Natl Cancer Inst Monogr 1969;31:59–128.
62. Wolf K. Fish viruses and fish viral diseases. Ithaca (NY): Cornell University Press; 1988.
63. Poulet F, Wolfe M, Spitsbergen J. Naturally occurring orocutaneous papillomas and carcinomas of brown bullheads (Ictalurus nebulosus) in New York State. Vet Pathol 1994;31:8–18.
64. Roberts R. Oral carcinomata in a salmon (Salmo salar L.). Vet Rec 1972;91:199.
65. Fitzgerald S, Carlton W, Sandusky G. Metastatic squamous cell carcinoma in a hybrid sunfish. J Fish Dis 1991;14:481–8.
66. Wolke R, Murchelano R. A case report of an epidermal papilloma in Mustelus canis. J Wildl Dis 1976;12:167–71.
67. Ahmed ATA, ES-. Dermal fibrosarcoma in goldfish Carassius auratus (L.). J Fish Dis 1980;3:249–54.

68. Masahito P, Ishikawa T, Sugano H. Pigment cells and pigment cell tumors in fish. J Invest Dermatol 1989;92:266–70.

69. Overstreet R. Aquatic pollution problems, Southern U.S. coasts: histopathological indicators. Aquat Toxicol 1988;11:213–39.

70. Schmale MC, Hensley G, Udey LR. Neurofibromatosis, von Recklinghausen's disease, multiple schwannomas, malignant schwannomas. Multiple schwannomas in the bicolor damselfish, Pomacentrus partitus (pisces, pomacentridae). Am J Pathol 1983;112:238–41.

71. Grizzle J, Bunkley-Williams L, Harshbarger J. Renal adenocarcinoma in Mozambique tilapia, neurofibromas in goldfish, and osteosarcoma in channel catfish from a Puerto Rican hatchery. J Aquat Anim Health 1995;7:178–83.

72. Schlumberger HG. Nerve sheath tumors in an isolated goldfish population. Cancer Res 1952;12:890–9.

73. Duncan T, Harkin J. Ultrastructure of goldfish tumours previously classified as neurofibromas. Am J Pathol 1968;52:33.

74. Johnston CJ, Deveney MR, Bayly T, et al. Gross and histopathological characteristics of two lipomas and a neurofibrosarcoma detected in aquacultured southern bluefin tuna, Thunnus maccoyii (Castelnau), in South Australia. J Fish Dis 2008;31:241–7.

75. Okihiro M. Chromatophoromas in two species of Hawaiian butterflyfish, *Chaetodon multicinctus* and C. miliaris. Vet Pathol 1988;25:422–31.

76. Okihiro M, JA W, Groff JM, et al. Chromatophoromas and related hyperplastic lesions in Pacific rockfish (*Sebastes* spp.). Mar Environ Res 1992;34:53–7.

77. Ozato K, Wakamatsu Y. Multi-step genetic regulation of oncogene expression in fish hereditary melanoma. Differentiation 1983;24:181–90.

78. Sobel H, Marquet E, KK, et al. Melanomas in platy/swordtail hybrids. In: Ribelin W, Migaki G, editors. The pathology of fishes. Madison (WI): University of Wisconsin Press; 1975. p. 945–81.

79. Schartl A, Malitschek B, Kazianis S. Spontaneous melanoma formation in nonhybrid Xiphophorus. Cancer Res 1995;55:159–65.

80. Kent M, Bishop-Stewart JK, Matthews JL, et al. *Pseudocapillaria tomentosa*, a nematode pathogen, and associated neoplasms of zebrafish (*Danio rerio*) kept in research colonies. Comp Med 2002;52:354–8.

81. Majeed S, Jolly D, Gopinath C. An outbreak of liver cell carcinoma in rainbow trout, Salmo gairdneri Richardson, in the U. K. J Fish Dis 1984;7:165–8.

82. Núñez O, Hendricks J, Arbogast D, et al. Promotion of aflatoxin B1 hepatocarcinogenesis in rainbow trout by 17b-estradiol. Aquat Toxicol 1989;15:289–302.

83. Harada T, Hatanaka J, Kubota SS, et al. Lymphoblastic lymphoma in medaka (*Oryzias latipes*) (Temminck et Schlegel). J Fish Dis 1990;13:169–73

84. Kuiper R, Kimpfler S, Grinwis G. Case report: epitheliotropic lymphoma in a zebrafish (*Danio rerio*). Tijdschr Diergeneeskd 2009;134:1018–20.

85. Haller R, Roberts R. Dual neoplasia in a specimen of *Sarotherodon spiluris spiluris* (Gunther) (=*Tilapia spiluris*). J Fish Dis 1980;3:63–6.

86. Nigrelli R. Spontaneous neoplasms in fishes; Lymphosarcoma in Astyanax and Esox. Zool Sci Contrib N Y Zool Soc 1947;32:101–8.

87. JW. B. Leukaemic lymphosarcoma in a hatchery-reared rainbow trout *Salmo gairdneri* Richardson. J Fish Dis 1984;7:83–6.

88. Warr G, Griffin B, DPA. A lymphosarcoma of thymic origin in the rainbow trout *Salmo gairdneri* Richardson. J Fish Dis 1984;7:73–82.

89. Kieser D, Kent M, JM G, et al. An epizootic of epitheliotrophic lymphoblastic lymphoma of thymic origin in coho salmon Oncorhynchus kisutch. Dis Aquat Org 1991;11:1–8.

90. Ljungberg O. Epizootiological and experimental studies of skin tumours of northern pike (Esox lucius L.) in the Baltic Sea. Prog Exp Tumor Res 1976;20: 156–65.

91. Mulcahy M, Winqvist G, Dawe C. The neoplastic cell type in lymphoreticular neoplasms of the northern pike, *Esox lucius* L. Cancer Res 1970;30:2712–7.

92. Sonstegard R. Lymphosarcoma in muskellunge. In: Ribelin WE, MG, editors. The Pathology of fishes. Madison (WI): University of Wisconsin Press; 1975. p. 907–24.

93. Nigrelli RF. Virus and tumors in fishes. Ann N Y Acad Sci 1952;54:1076–92.

94. Ishikawa T, Takayama S. Ovarian neoplasia in ornamental hybrid carp (nishiki-goi) in Japan. Ann N Y Acad Sci 1977;298:330–41.

95. Down N, Leatherland J. Histopathology of gonadal neoplasms in cyprinid fish from the lower Great Lakes of North America. J Fish Dis 1989;12:415–37.

96. Sonstegard R. Environmental carcinogenesis studies in fishes of the Great Lakes of North America. Ann N Y Acad Sci 1978;298:261–9.

97. Lewisch E, Reifinger M, Schmidt P, et al. Ovarian tumor in a koi carp (*Cyprinus carpio*): diagnosis, surgery, postoperative care and tumour classification. Tierarztl Prax Ausg K Kleintiere Heimtiere 2014;42:257–62.

98. Grosset CSN, Rodriguez CO Jr, Cenani A, et al.Excision and subsequent treatment of a leiomyoma from the periventiduct of a Koi (*Cyprinus carpio koi*). Journal of Exotic Pet Medicine, in press.

99. Coffee L, Casey JW, PR. B. Pathology of tumors in fish associated with retroviruses: a review. Vet Pathol 2013;50:390–403.

100. Sweet M, Kirkham N, Bendall M, et al. Evidence of melanoma in wild marine fish populations. PLoS One 2012;7:e41989.

101. Hader DP, Helbling EW, Williamson CE, et al. Effects of UV radiation on aquatic ecosystems and interactions with climate change. Photochem Photobiol Sci 2011;10:242–60.

102. Harborne AR. The ecology, behaviour and physiology of fishes on coral reef flats, and the potential impacts of climate change. J Fish Biol 2013;83:417–47.

103. Lowe C, Goodman-Lowe G. Suntanning in hammerhead sharks. Nature 1996; 383:677.

104. Nairn RS, Morizot DC, Kazianis S, et al. Nonmammalian models for sunlight carcinogenesis: genetic analysis of melanoma formation in Xiphophorus hybrid fish. Photochem Photobiol 1996;64:440–8.

105. Butler AP, Trono D, Beard R, et al. Melanoma susceptibility and cell cycle genes in *Xiphophorus* hybrids. Mol Carcinog 2007;46:685–91.

106. van der Weyden L, Patton EE, Wood GA, et al. Cross-species models of human melanoma. J Pathol 2016;238:152–65.

107. Pang PKT, MP S. Regulation of calcium and phosphate. In: P.K.T. P, editor. Vertebrate Endocrinology. London: Academic Press Limited; 1989. p. 501–27.

108. Rahn J, Gibbs P, Schmale M. Patterns of transcription of a virus-like agent in tumor and non-tumor tissues in bicolor damselfish. Comp Biochem Physiol C Toxicol Pharmacol 2004;138:401–9.

109. Bloch B, Mellergaard S, Nielsen E. Adenovirus-like particles associated with epithelial hyperplasia in dab, *Limanda limanda (L.)*. J Fish Dis 1986;9:281–5.

110. Miyazaka T, Asai Y, Kobayashi T, et al. Lympholeukemia in madai *Pagrus major* in Japan. Dis Aquat Organ 2000;40:147–55.

111. Kostich M, Lazorchak J. Risks to aquatic organisms posed by human pharmaceutical use. Sci Total Environ 2008;389:329–39.

112. Jobling S, Williams R, Johnson A, et al. Predicted exposures to steroid estrogens in U.K. rivers correlate with widespread sexual disruption in wild fish populations. Environ Health Perspect 2006;114(Suppl 1):32–9.

113. Rhee JS, Lee YM, Raisuddin S, et al. Expression of R-ras oncogenes in the hermaphroditic fish Kryptolebias marmoratus, exposed to endocrine disrupting chemicals. Comp Biochem Physiol C Toxicol Pharmacol 2009;149:433–9.

114. Falkner S, Emdin S, Ostberg Y. Tumour pathology of the hagfish (Myxine glutinosa) and the river lamprey (Lampretra fluviatilis). A light microscopy study with special reference to primary liver carcinoma, islet cell tumors, and epidermoid cysts of the skin. Prog Exp Tumor Res 1976;20:217–50.

115. S. K, LD. C, Morizot DC. Overexpression of a fish CDKN2 gene in a hereditary melanoma model. Carcinogenesis 2000;21:599–605.

116. Manier JF, Raibaut A, Lopez A, et al. A calcified fibroma in the common carp, Cyprinus carpio L. J Fish Dis 1984;7:283–92.

117. Baker TR, Baker BB, Johnson SM, et al. Comparative analgesic efficacy of morphine sulfate and butorphanol tartrate in koi (Cyprinus carpio) undergoing unilateral gonadectomy. J Am Vet Med Assoc 2013;243:882–90.

118. Hadfield CA, Whitaker BR, Clayton LA. Emergency and critical care of fish. Vet Clin North Am Exot Anim Pract 2007;10:647–75.

119. Javahery S, Nekoubin H, Moradlu AH. Effect of anaesthesia with clove oil in fish (review). Fish Physiol Biochem 2012;38:1545–52.

120. Gladden JN, Brainard BM, Shelton JL, et al. Evaluation of isoeugenol for anesthesia in koi carp (Cyprinus carpio). Am J Vet Res 2010;71:859–66.

121. Oda A, Bailey KM, Lewbart GA, et al. Physiologic and biochemical assessments of koi (Cyprinus carpio) following immersion in propofol. J Am Vet Med Assoc 2014;245:1286–91.

122. Minter LJ, Bailey KM, Harms CA, et al. The efficacy of alfaxalone for immersion anesthesia in koi carp (Cyprinus carpio). Vet Anaesth Analg 2014;41:398–405.

123. Al-Hamdani AH, Ebrahim SK, Mohammad FK. Experimental xylazine-ketamine anesthesia in the common carp (Cyprinus carpio). J Wildl Dis 2010;46:596–8.

124. Witeska M, Dudyk J, Jarkiewicz N. Haematological effects of 2-phenoxyethanol and etomidate in carp (Cyprinus carpio L.). Vet Anaesth Analg 2015;42:537–46.

125. Mylniczenko N, Neiffer D, Clauss. Bony fish (lungfish, surgeon, and teleosts). In: West G, Heard D, Caulkett N, editors. Zoo animal and wildlife immobilization and anesthesia. 2nd edition. Ames (IA): Wiley Blackwell; 2014. p. 209–60.

126. Kilgore KH, Hill JE, Powell JF, et al. Investigational use of metomidate hydrochloride as a shipping additive for two ornamental fishes. J Aquat Anim Health 2009; 21:133–9.

127. Bailey KM, Minter LJ, Lewbart GA, et al. Alfaxalone as an intramuscular injectable anesthetic in koi carp (Cyprinus carpio). J Zoo Wildl Med 2014;45:852–8.

128. Stoskopf M, Posner LP. Anesthesia and restraint of laboratory fish. Chapter 21. In: Fish RE, Danneman P, Brown M, et al, editors. Anesthesia and analgesia in laboratory animals. San Diego (CA): American College of Laboratory Animal Medicine Series; 2014. p. 519–34.

129. Whiteside D. Analgesia. In: West G, Heard D, Caulkett N, editors. Zoo animal and wildlife immobilization and anesthesia. 2nd edition. Ames (IA): Wiley Blackwell; 2014. p. 83–108.

130. Scala C, Lair S. Clusters of retinal neoplasms in aquarium-housed Atlantic striped basses (Morone saxatilis) and Pajama cardinalfish (Sphaeramia

nematoptera). Proceedings of the International Association for Aquatic Animal Medicine 2016.

131. Harder W. Anatomie der Fische. Stuttgart (Germany): Schweizerbart'sch Verlagsbuchhandlung; 1975.

132. Walsh MT, F.S. P, Brendemuehl CA, et al. Ultrasonography as a diagnostic tool in shark species. Vet Radiol Ultrasound 1993;34:213–8.

133. Raidal SR, Shearer PL, Stephens F, et al. Surgical removal of an ovarian tumour in a koi carp (Cyprinus carpio). Aust Vet J 2006;84:178–81.

134. Grant KR, Campbell TW, Silver TI, et al. Validation of an ultrasound-guided technique to establish a liver-to-coelom ratio and a comparative analysis of the ratios among acclimated and recently wild-caught southern stingrays, Dasyatis americana. Zoo Biol 2013;32:104–11.

135. Love NE, Lewbart GA. Pet fish radiography: technique and case history reports. Vet Radiol Ultrasound 1997;38:24–9.

136. Bakal RS, Love NE, Lewbart GA, et al. Imaging a spinal fracture in a Kohaku Koi (Cyprinus carpio): techniques and case history report. Vet Radiol Ultrasound 1998;39:318–21.

137. Govett PD, Olby NJ, Marcellin-Little DJ, et al. Stabilisation of scoliosis in two koi (Cyprinus carpio). Vet Rec 2004;155:115–9.

138. Pees M, Pees K, Kiefer I. The use of computed tomography for assessment of the swim bladder in koi carp (Cyprinus carpio). Vet Radiol Ultrasound 2010;51:294–8.

139. Carr A, Weber EP 3rd, Murphy CJ, et al. Computed tomographic and cross-sectional anatomy of the normal pacu (Colossoma macroponum). J Zoo Wildl Med 2014;45:184–9.

140. Chanet B, Fusellier M, Baudet J, et al. No need to open the jar: a comparative study of Magnetic Resonance Imaging results on fresh and alcohol preserved common carps (Cyprinus carpio (L. 1758), Cyprinidae, Teleostei). C R Biol 2009;332:413–9.

141. Sirri R, Diana A, Scarpa F, et al. Ultrasonographic and pathologic study of schwannoma in a Goldfish (Carassius auratus). Vet Clin Pathol 2015.

142. Reavill D, Roberts H. Diagnostic cytology of fish. Vet Clin North Am Exot Anim Pract 2007;10:207–34.

143. Wildgoose W. Fish surgery: an overview. Fish Veterinary Journal 2000;5:22–36.

144. Shin SP, Jee H, Han JE, et al. Surgical removal of an anal cyst caused by a protozoan parasite (Thelohanellus kitauei) from a koi (Cyprinus carpio). J Am Vet Med Assoc 2011;238:784–6.

145. Petty BD, Fraser WA. Viruses of pet fish. Vet Clin North Am Exot Anim Pract 2005;8:67–84.

146. Groff JM, Naydan DK, Higgins RJ, et al. Cytokeratin-filament expression in epithelial and non-epithelial cells of the common carp (Cyprinus carpio). Cell Tissue Res 1997;287:375–84.

147. Groff J, Naydan D, Zinkl J, et al. Immunological cross-reactivity of type I-III intermediate filaments in the common carp: in situ localization using heterologous antibodies. Trans Am Fish Soc 1997;126:948–60.

148. Markl J. Cytokeratins in mesenchymal cells: impact on functional concepts of the diversity of intermediate filament proteins. J Cell Sci 1991;98:261–4.

149. Markl J, Franke WW. Localization of cytokeratins in tissues of the rainbow trout: fundamental differences in expression pattern between the fish and higher vertebrates. Differentiation 1988;39:97–122.

150. Markl J, Winter S, Franke W. The catalog and the expression complexity of cytokeratins in a lower vertebrate: biochemical identification of cytokeratins in a teleost fish, the rainbow trout. Eur J Cell Biol 1989;50:1–16.

151. Marino F, Germana A, Bambir S, et al. Calretinin and S-100 expression in goldfish, Carassius auratus (L.), schwannoma. J Fish Dis 2007;30:251–3.

152. Lubojemska A, Borejko M, Czapiewski P, et al. Of mice and men; olfactory neuroblastoma among animals and humans. Vet Comp Oncol 2016;14:e70–82.

153. Lewbart GA, Spodnick G, Barlow N, et al. Surgical removal of an undifferentiated abdominal sarcoma from a koi carp (Cyprinus carpio). Vet Rec 1998; 143:556–8.

154. Magi GE, Renzoni G, Piccionello AP, et al. Primary ocular chondrosarcoma in a discus (Symphisodon aequifasciatus). J Zoo Wildl Med 2013;44:225–31.

155. Clauss TM, Dove AD, Arnold JE. Hematologic disorders of fish. Vet Clin North Am Exot Anim Pract 2008;11:445–62, v.

156. Groff JM, Zinkl JG. Hematology and clinical chemistry of cyprinid fish. Common carp and goldfish. Vet Clin North Am Exot Anim Pract 1999;2:741–76.

157. Tripathi NK, Latimer KS, Burnley VV. Hematologic reference intervals for koi (Cyprinus carpio), including blood cell morphology, cytochemistry, and ultrastructure. Vet Clin Pathol 2004;33:74–83.

158. Palmeiro BS, Rosenthal KL, Lewbart GA, et al. Plasma biochemical reference intervals for koi. J Am Vet Med Assoc 2007;230:708–12.

159. Innis C, Davis D, Mandelman J, et al. Hematologic values of captive Acadian redfish (Sebastes fasciatus). J Zoo Wildl Med 2010;41:432–7.

160. Pionnier N, Adamek M, Miest JJ, et al. C-reactive protein and complement as acute phase reactants in common carp Cyprinus carpio during CyHV-3 infection. Dis Aquat Organ 2014;109:187–99.

161. Krol L, Allender M, Cray C, et al. Plasma proteins and selected acute-phase proteins in the whitespotted bamboo shark (*Chiloscyllium plagiosum*). J Zoo Wildl Med 2014;45:782–6.

162. Christiansen EF, C. C, Lewbart G, et al. Plasma protein electrophoresis and acute phase proteins in koi carp (Cyprinus carpio) following exploratory coeliotomy. Journal of Exotic Pet Med 2015;24:76–83.

163. Manera M, Britti D. Assessment of serum protein fractions in rainbow trout using automated electrophoresis and densitometry. Vet Clin Pathol 2008;37:452–6.

164. E.D.Stevens, Balahura RJ. Aspects of morphine chemistry important to persons working with cold-blooded animals, especially fish. Comp Med 2007;57:161–6.

165. Hurty CA, Brazik DC, Law JM, et al. Evaluation of the tissue reactions in the skin and body wall of koi (Cyprinus carpio) to five suture materials. Vet Rec 2002; 151:324–8.

166. Stoskopf M. Physiology. Chapter 3. In: MK S, editor. Fish medicine. Apex (NC): Saunders; 1993. p. 48–52.

167. Rapanan JL, Pascual AS, Uppalapati CK, et al. Zebrafish keratocyte explants to study collective cell migration and reepithelialization in cutaneous wound healing. J Vis Exp 2015;(96).

168. Ochandio B, Bechara I, Parise-Maltempi P. Dexamethasone action on caudal fin regeneration of carp Cyprinus carpio (Linnaeus, 1758). Braz J Biol 2015;75: 442–50.

169. Andrews M, Stormoen M, Schmidt-Posthaus H, et al. Rapid temperature-dependent wound closure following adipose fin clipping of Atlantic salmon Salmo salar L. J Fish Dis 2015;38:523–31.

170. Azevedo AS, Grotek B, Jacinto A, et al. The regenerative capacity of the zebrafish caudal fin is not affected by repeated amputations. PLoS One 2011;6: e22820.
171. Jensen LB, Wahli T, McGurk C, et al. Effect of temperature and diet on wound healing in Atlantic salmon (Salmo salar L.). Fish Physiol Biochem 2015.
172. da Silva EG, Gionfriddo JR, Powell CC, et al. Iridociliary melanoma with secondary lens luxation: distinctive findings in a long-horned cowfish (Lactoria cornuta). Vet Ophthalmol 2010;13(Suppl):123–7.
173. Lair S, Santamaria-Bouvier A, Marvin J. Clusters of retinoblastoma-like neoplasms in a group of aquarium-housed striped basses (*Morone saxatilis*). Proceedings of the 45th International Association for Aquatic Animal Medicine annual conference 2014.
174. Nadelstein B, Bakal R, Lewbart GA. Orbital exenteration and placement of a prosthesis in fish. J Am Vet Med Assoc 1997;211:603–6.
175. Harms CA, Wildgoose W. Surgery. Chapter 31. In: Wildgoose W, editor. BSAVA manual of ornamental fish. 2nd edition. Quedgeley (England): British Small Animal Veterinary Association; 2001. p. 159–266.
176. Vergneau-Grosset C III, WE. Fish Surgery In: Bennett RA, GW P. Exotic animal surgery. Wiley, in press.
177. CK G. A comparison between mouse and fish micronucleus test using cyclophosphamide, mitomycin C and various pesticides. Mutat Res 2002;518: 145–50.
178. Grisolia C, Cordeiro C. Variability in micronucleus induction with different mutagens applied to several species of fish. Genet Mol Biol 2000;23:235–9.
179. Matsumoto F, Colus I. Micronucleus frequencies in *Astyanax bimaculatus* (Characidae) treated with cyclophosphamide or vinblastine sulfate. Genet Mol Biol 2000;23:489–92.
180. Kumar P, Soorambail KS, Bhagatsingh Harisingh S, et al. The effect of gamma radiation on the Common carp (Cyprinus carpio): In vivo genotoxicity assessment with the micronucleus and comet assays. Mutat Res Genet Toxicol Environ Mutagen 2015;792:19–25.
181. Oishi T, Terai S, Kuwashiro S, et al. Ezetimibe reduces fatty acid quantity in liver and decreased inflammatory cell infiltration and improved NASH in medaka model. Biochem Biophys Res Commun 2012;422:22–7.
182. Stevens B, Vergneau-Grosset C, Rodriguez C, et al. Treatment of a facial myxoma in a goldfish (*Carassius auratus*) with intralesional bleomycin chemotherapy and radiation therapy. Proceedings of the International Association for Aquatic Animal Medicine 2016.
183. Kelly JM, Belding BA, Schaefer AK. Acanthomatous ameloblastoma in dogs treated with intralesional bleomycin. Vet Comp Oncol 2010;8:81–6.
184. Chabner B. Bleomycin and other antitumor antibiotics. In: Chabner B, Longo D, editors. Cancer chemotherapy and biotherapy: principles and practice. Philadelphia: Wolters Kluwer, Lippincott Williams & Wilkins; 2014. p. 323–41.
185. Yin Z, He JY, Gong Z, et al. Identification of differentially expressed genes in Con A-activated carp (Cyprinus carpio L.) leucocytes. Comp Biochem Physiol B Biochem Mol Biol 1999;124:41–50.
186. Brunner CH, Dutra G, Silva CB, et al. Electrochemotherapy for the treatment of fibropapillomas in Chelonia mydas. J Zoo Wildl Med 2014;45:213–8.
187. Lanza A, Baldi A, Spugnini EP. Surgery and electrochemotherapy for the treatment of cutaneous squamous cell carcinoma in a yellow-bellied slider (Trachemys scripta scripta). J Am Vet Med Assoc 2015;246:455–7.

188. Mauldin GN, Shiomitsy K. Principles and practice of radiation therapy in exotic and avian species. Seminars in Avian and Exotic Pet Medicine 2005;14:168–74.

189. Society. AC. The Science behind radiation, 2014.

190. Epperly MW, Bahary N, Quader M, et al. The zebrafish- Danio rerio - is a useful model for measuring the effects of small-molecule mitigators of late effects of ionizing irradiation. In Vivo 2012;26:889–97.

191. Driver C. Ecotoxicity literature review of selected Hanford site contaminants. Richland (WA): Pacific Northwest Lab; 1994. PNL-9394.

192. Cavaş T, S. K. Detection of cytogenetic and DNA damage in peripheral erythrocytes of goldfish (*Carassius auratus*) exposed to a glyphosate formulation using the micronucleus test and the comet assay. Mutagenesis 2007;22:263–8.

193. Jarvis RB, JF K. DNA damage in zebrafish larvae induced by exposure to low-dose rate gamma-radiation: detection by the alkaline comet assay. Mutat Res 2003;541:63–9.

194. Stevens CW. Analgesia in amphibians: preclinical studies and clinical applications. Vet Clin North Am Exot Anim Pract 2011;14:33–44.

195. Weber ES 3rd. Fish analgesia: pain, stress, fear aversion, or nociception? Vet Clin North Am Exot Anim Pract 2011;14:21–32.

196. Braithwaite B. Pain in fish: the evidence and ethical implications. A review of do fish feel pain. Oxford University Press; 2010.

197. Harms CA, Lewbart GA, Swanson CR, et al. Behavioral and clinical pathology changes in koi carp (Cyprinus carpio) subjected to anesthesia and surgery with and without intra-operative analgesics. Comp Med 2005;55:221–6.

198. Ward J, McCartney S, Chinnadurai S, et al. Development of a minimum-anesthetic-concentration depression model to study the effects of various analgesics in goldfish (Carassius auratus). J Zoo Wildl Med 2012;43:214–22.

199. Posner L, Scott GN, JM. L. Repeated exposure of goldfish (Carassius auratus) to tricaine methanesulfonate (MS-222). J Zoo Wildl Med 2013;44:340–7.

200. Pecina M, Love T, Stohler CS, et al. Effects of the Mu opioid receptor polymorphism (OPRM1 A118G) on pain regulation, placebo effects and associated personality trait measures. Neuropsychopharmacology 2015;40:957–65.

201. Chervova LS, Lapshin DN. Opioid modulation of pain threshold in fish. Dokl Biol Sci 2000;375:590–1.

202. Davis MR, Mylniczenko N, Storms T, et al. Evaluation of intramuscular ketoprofen and butorphanol as analgesics in chain dogfish (*Scyliorhinus retifer*). Zoo Biol 2006;25:491–500.

203. Mettam J, Oulton L, McCrohan C, et al. The efficacy of three types of analgesic drugs in reducing pain in the rainbow trout, Oncorhynchus mykiss. Appl Anim Behav Sci 2011;133:265–74.

204. Larouche C. Evaluation of toxic effets of meloxicam intramuscular injection in goldfish (*Carassius auratus auratus*). 47th Annual Conference of the American Association of Zoo Veterinarians. 2015;58.

205. Schwaiger J, Ferling H, Mallow U, et al. Toxic effects of the non-steroidal anti-inflammatory drug diclofenac. Part I: histopathological alterations and bioaccumulation in rainbow trout. Aquat Toxicol 2004;68:141–50.

206. Lovy J, Speare DJ, Wright GM. Pathological effects caused by chronic treatment of rainbow trout with indomethacin. J Aquat Anim Health 2007;19:94–8.

207. Lee LE, NC. B. The corticosteroid receptor and the action of various steroids in rainbow trout fibroblasts. Gen Comp Endocrinol 1989;74:85–95.

208. Mikriakov D, Mikriakov VR, MA. S. Influence of stress hormones (adrenalin and glucocorticoids) on the infestation rate of the carp Cyprinus carpio L. by Dactylogyrus sp. (Monogenoidea). Parazitologiia 2009;43:90–6.

209. Pasqualetti S, Congiu T, Banfi G, et al. Alendronate rescued osteoporotic phenotype in a model of glucocorticoid-induced osteoporosis in adult zebrafish scale. Int J Exp Pathol 2015;96:11–20.

Avian Oncology
Diseases, Diagnostics, and Therapeutics

Cecilia S. Robat, Dr med vet, DACVIM (Oncology)[a],*, Melanie Ammersbach, DVM[b],
Christoph Mans, Dr med vet, DACZM[c],*

KEYWORDS

- Neoplasia • Tumor • Neoplastic • Bird • Psittacine • Cancer

KEY POINTS

- Cytologic examination of fine-needle aspirates of neoplastic lesions should be performed whenever feasible, because it has a potential to provide a rapid diagnosis with low morbidity and costs associated.
- Surgical excision of a neoplastic lesion should only be formed after staging to evaluate extend of disease and optimize the surgical planning.
- Safe and effective chemotherapy dosages and frequency of administration in companion birds are yet to be established and although many published drug protocols seem safe, they are also largely ineffective, likely due to subtherapeutic drug concentrations reached.
- Radiation therapy seems to be well tolerated in birds; however, the need for general anesthesia and lack of established radiation protocols limit its use in companion birds.

INTRODUCTION

Birds kept as companion animals are increasingly living longer due to improved husbandry, nutrition, and veterinary care provided. As a consequence, a growing number of geriatric disease conditions, such as degenerative and neoplastic diseases, are diagnosed and managed by veterinarians. The increasing awareness of bird owners of diagnostic and treatment options for neoplastic diseases in humans and domestic animals has led to an increasing demand to provide advanced diagnostic and treatment modalities for companion birds diagnosed with neoplasia.

Among companion birds, Psittaciformes are most frequently diagnosed with neoplasia, with budgerigars the most commonly affected species (17%–24% overall incidence).[1] Passeriformes have the lowest reported incidence of neoplasia among

The authors have nothing to disclose.
[a] Veterinary Emergency Service, Veterinary Specialty Center, 1612 North High Point Road, Middleton, WI 53562, USA; [b] Department of Pathobiology, Ontario Veterinary College, University of Guelph, Building 89, 50 Stone Road East, Guelph, Ontario N1G 2W1, Canada; [c] Department of Surgical Sciences, School of Veterinary Medicine, University of Wisconsin-Madison, 2015 Linden Drive, Madison, WI 53706, USA
* Corresponding author
E-mail addresses: ceciliarobat@hotmail.com; christoph.mans@wisc.edu

companion birds. Cutaneous neoplasia, followed by urogenital neoplasia, is the most frequently diagnosed in companion birds.

Diagnostic and treatment attempts remain challenging in many companion birds due to the often small patient size, difficulty to gain repeated intravascular access, increased anesthetic risks compared with other domestic animals and lack of information regarding prognosis and efficacy of antineoplastic treatments in companion bird species. Although several reviews of avian neoplasia exist, reported numbers of clinical cases are low, and there is no established standard of care for most neoplasias in companion birds. Collaboration among veterinarians and multi-institutional studies are needed to increase understanding of cancer behavior in the companion birds.

DIAGNOSIS

As in any other species, a definitive diagnosis should always be obtained prior to determining the prognosis and treatment options. A definitive diagnosis can usually be obtained either by cytology or, if the obtained samples are nondiagnostic, by histopathology of a biopsy specimen.

BODY MAP

A body map, which documents the location and size of the neoplastic masses, should be performed anytime a new mass is found in a patient (**Fig. 1**). Calipers should be used to measure the longest diameter of a mass, and this value should be recorded on the body map form, with the visit date. This allows for close monitoring of the changes in mass size. If owners have declined further diagnostics, or if the mass was diagnosed as benign but is growing, repeated discussion with the clients about benefits of therapeutic intervention could be pursued.

BLOOD WORK

Blood work should be performed to assess overall health as well as to look for abnormal blood counts, which could be linked to the presence of neoplasia. A complete blood cell count may reveal cytopenias, which may result from the presence of hematopoietic malignancies in which the neoplastic cells may crowd the bone marrow (myelophthisis). Anemia may occur in patients with cancer for a variety of reasons, including bleeding from a tumor or bone marrow infiltration by hematopoietic tumors. Leukocytosis, consisting of a mature lymphocytosis (chronic lymphocytic leukemia)[2,3] or a population of large immature blasts (acute leukemia), may be seen in patients with leukemia.

An abnormal biochemistry profile may be the sign of organ involvement by the tumor or organ dysfunction related to age or other diseases and may preclude the use of certain therapies. Paraneoplastic syndromes, such as hypercalcemia and hyperglobulinemia, are commonly described in canine patients with hematopoietic malignancies. Hypercalcemia was present in 2 Amazon parrots with malignant lymphoma and believed to be paraneoplastic.[4] Ionized calcium should be determined if hypercalcemia of malignancy is suspected.

Diagnostic Imaging

Many malignant tumors have the propensity to spread to other organs, commonly to lungs but also to coelomic organs or bones.[5–8] Radiographs allow for visualization of bone lesions (**Fig. 2**) and soft tissue masses; however, whole-body CT, preferably contrast enhanced, is becoming the mainstay in diagnostic imaging of avian patients,

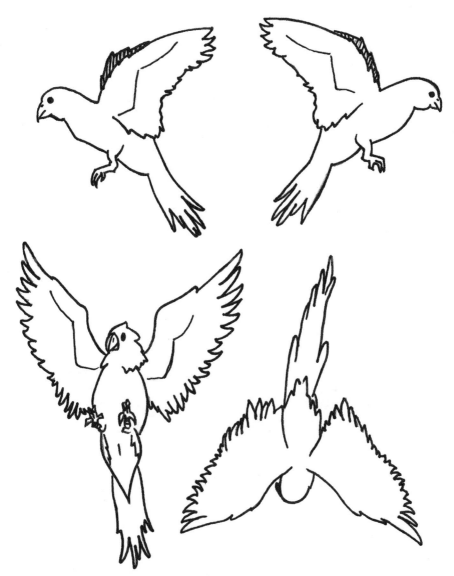

Fig. 1. Avian body map. (*Courtesy of* Ruth Houseright, DVM, DACVP, Madison, WI.)

because it allows for 3-D visualization and better assessment of internal organs for the presence of primary or metastatic lesions (**Fig. 3**A, B). CT images also allow for better surgical planning. CT can be performed in sedated avian patients in most instances, therefore eliminating anesthetic risks (**Fig. 4**) Noniodinated contrast material (eg, iohexol) can be administered either intravenously (IV) or intraosseously (IO) after catheter placement.

Ultrasound is a valuable diagnostic tool in avian patients, in particular for large coelomic masses; however, the presence of air sacs may reduce its suitability in some instances. Ultrasound-guided fine-needle aspirates should be performed whenever possible to increase the chance of obtaining a diagnostic sample and to reduce

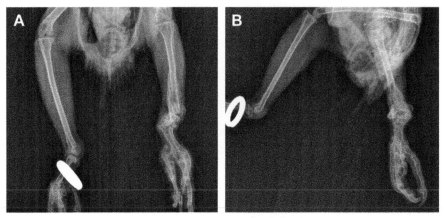

Fig. 2. Ventrodoral (*A*) and lateral radiographs of a 33-year-old blue-fronted Amazon parrot (*Amazona aestiva*), which presented with left leg lameness. Radiographs show expansion of left distal tibiotarsus and tarsometatarsus and abnormal angulation, consistent with chronic osteomyelitis or neoplasia. Fine-needle aspiration did not reveal a diagnostic sample. Postmortem diagnosis was a well-differentiated chondrosarcoma affecting the left tibiotarsus and metatarsus. (*Courtesy of* Christoph Mans, Madison, WI.)

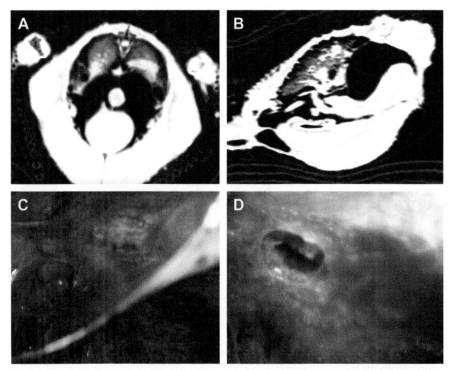

Fig. 3. CT and laparoscopy in a 35-year-old Congo African gray parrot (*P erithacus*) diagnosed with primary lung neoplasia. (*A*) Cross-sectional and (*B*) sagittal CT views. Note the bilateral asymmetric soft tissue attenuation in the lungs. (*C*) Laparoscopic examination of the lung was performed and (*D*) biopsies for histopathologic examination collected using 5F biopsy forceps. The biopsy samples did not reveal a neoplastic or infectious underlying cause. Necropsy revealed a primary pulmonary carcinoma. (*Courtesy of* Christoph Mans, Madison, WI.)

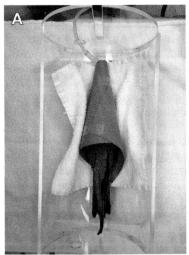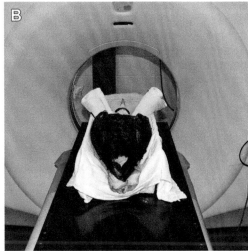

Fig. 4. CT in sedated avian patients. (*A*) Cockatiel (*N hollandicus*); note the supplemental oxygen provided and the cardboard cone, which facilitates to keep the patient in a sternal body position without restraint. (*B*) Bald eagle (*Haliaeetus leucocephalus*) hooded and sedated for whole-body CT scan in dorsal recumbence. (*Courtesy of* Christoph Mans, Madison, WI.)

associated morbidity. A 3-D ultrasound has been successfully used to identify the origin of a coelomic mass in a mynah, by providing better spatial perspective of the internal organs.[9]

Cytology

Cytology is a readily available tool, which is inexpensive and associated with low patient morbidity. The turnaround time for results is also faster than for histopathology. Cytology can often be used to differentiate between an inflammatory process (eg, septic heterophilic inflammation, or granuloma) and neoplasia and, depending on the type of tumor, can lead to the differentiation between a benign and malign tumor. Most masses can be sampled with little concern for complications. Patients may need to be sedated for a fine-needle aspirate. If deeper-seated tumors are to be sampled, ultrasound guidance may be helpful.

Fluid aspirates (effusions) can also be evaluated, either as a direct smear (if cell count is high) or after cytocentrifugation (if low cellularity). Some neoplasias tend to exfoliate well, such as hematopoietic tumors (eg, lymphoma) and carcinomas. Many sarcomas exfoliate poorly, however, because they contain more connective tissue, which holds cells together. Bone lesions and bone marrow can readily be sampled although patients need to be under a short general anesthesia.

When sampling a mass, a small-gauge needle should be used first (eg, 25G or 23G). Larger needles are rarely helpful, because blood contamination is a common complication. Nonaspiration techniques are preferred for cytologic sample collection, because blood contamination and cell lysis are common with the aspiration techniques. If the nonaspiration technique does not yield an adequately cellular sample, the aspiration technique can be attempted. This technique uses a syringe attached to the needle. Once a needle has been introduced into the mass, negative pressure is applied by quickly pulling on the plunger and releasing. This increases the chance of obtaining a sufficient number of cells to obtain a diagnostic sample. If a mass easily bleeds during aspiration, putting a finger on the hub of the needle (**Fig. 5**) and introducing the needle into the mass once or twice only may be helpful to obtain an adequate sample. Several slides should be prepared, quickly spread to avoid clotting and quickly air dried to avoid drying artifact. A representative slide should be stained and evaluated under the microscope to ensure that a sample of sufficient quality and quantity has been obtained, prior to submitting remaining slides to a clinical pathologist. Nonstained slides are preferred for assessment, because in-house stain is usually Diff-Quik, but clinical pathologists prefer alcohol-based modified Romanowsky-type stains (eg, Wright-Giemsa) for their increased ability to evaluate cellular structures. A common complaint from clinical pathologists is that they receive inadequate samples, either because they are poorly cellular, composed of ruptured cells, hemodiluted, too thick, understained, or not representative tissue (**Fig. 6**). Certain types of tumors, however, result in virtually acellular slides (eg, lipomas) or slides containing only blood (eg, vascular tumors) despite appropriate sampling techniques.

Histopathology

Although cytology sampling is easy, quick, inexpensive, and associated with low morbidity, a definitive diagnosis more readily is obtained by histopathology of a biopsy sample. Biopsy samples allow for evaluation of a larger specimen and provide information on architecture (important for staging) and surgical margins. Additional immunohistochemical (IHC) testing may be necessary in some cases where cell morphology alone is insufficient to yield a definitive diagnosis; however, the antibodies used for immunohistochemistry in cats and dogs may not cross-react with avian tissues and should be evaluated independently in each bird species. In addition, the lack of established positive controls in birds further complicates interpretation of IHC staining. IHC has been used successfully to diagnose various tumors in birds such as, an intestinal leiomyosarcoma in a zebra rinch (*Taeniopygia guttata*),[10] a rhabdomyosarcoma in a budgerigar (*Melopsittacus undulatus*)[11] and in a yellow-headed caracara (*Milvago chimachima*),[12] a hemangiosarcoma in a Java sparrow (*Padda oryzivora*),[7] and various cases of lymphoid malignancy in birds.[2,13–15]

Several techniques may be used to obtain a biopsy sample. Under sedation and local anesthesia, a punch biopsy or core needle (Tru Cut TM) biopsy of cutaneous or subcutaneous masses can be performed. Punch biopsies are a good choice for superficial lesions. Tru-cut biopsies are commonly used for larger, cutaneous or

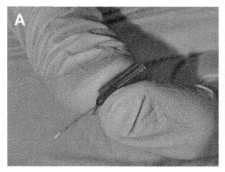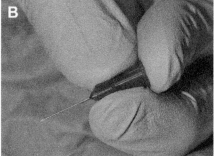

Fig. 5. (*A*) Fine-needle aspiration technique using a 25-G needle. (*B*) Occlusion of the needle hub should using the index finger reduces the risk of blood contamination of the sample. (*Courtesy of* Christoph Mans, Madison, WI.)

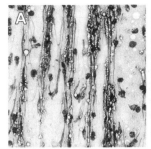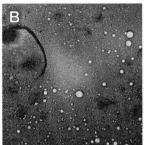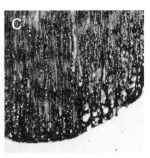

Fig. 6. Cytologic artifacts. (*A*) Most of the nucleated cells are lysed. Bare nuclei are present and nuclear streaming (spread chromatin) is evident. Cell lysis can occur after excessive suction during sample collection, use of a needle that is too small, or excessive pressure during spreading of the sample with a glass slide. (*B*) This sample is poorly spread therefore individual cell morphology cannot be assessed. Cytology samples that are too thick are also often poorly stained unless stained more than once. (*C*) Edge of the sample shows poor cell spread and cell lysis. (*Courtesy of* Melanie Ammersbach, Guelph, Ontario.)

subcutaneous masses and sampling of internal organs using ultrasound guidance. General anesthesia may be necessary for deeper-seated lesions or sampling of bone lesions. Once a biopsy sample has been obtained, impression smears can be performed and may yield a preliminary diagnosis.

Biopsies of internal organs in birds are often obtainable by laparoscopy. Using standard laparoscopic equipment suitable for companion birds (eg, 2.7-mm telescope with operating sheath and 5 French [F] biopsy forceps), biopsies can be obtained from many internal organs, including the lungs, air sacs, liver, spleen, kidney, and gonads (**Fig. 3**C, D). Owing to the small size of the laparoscopic biopsy specimens obtained, however, a sample may be nondiagnostic or not representative of the pathologic process (see **Fig. 3**C, D).

In other species, grading of malignancy is performed on biopsy samples. Most grading systems consist of low (grade 1), intermediate (grade 2), or high (grade 3) grade. Grades are obtained by a veterinary pathologist by assessing the sample for various criteria, such as number of mitotic figures, degree of pleomorphism, anisocytosis and anisokaryosis, percent necrosis, and so forth. Grade helps predict behavior and dictates how aggressively a tumor should be treated. Grading schemes have not been established in avian medicine. Further evaluation of avian tumors is warranted for establishment of a grading system for common tumors.

STAGING

Staging should be performed in all patients diagnosed with cancer, to determine whether or not the neoplastic disease has spread to other parts of the body and, if so, how extensively. In other species, such as cats and dogs, there is a plethora of information on the metastatic behavior of most tumor types, and this helps dictate which staging tests are necessary. In avian medicine, the behavior of most tumors is poorly described, and clinicians are encouraged to perform full staging in these patients to gather and report further information on tumor behavior. With this information, appropriate therapy can be recommended and prognosis can be discussed with clients. A thorough history, including information on diet, past diseases and trauma, current medications, and reproductive history, should be obtained and a complete physical examination performed.

Treatment

Surgery

When possible, surgical excision of a tumor, with adequate margins, will always result in a better outcome. Prior to any surgical intervention, careful planning should be performed to increase chances of the first surgery being successful. This includes making every effort to obtain a presurgical diagnosis with cytology or histopathology as well as, if necessary, using imaging techniques to assess the extent of disease and help plan the optimal approach. Full staging should be performed, and benefits and risks of surgical intervention discussed with the owners. The goal is to remove the tumor with adequate margins to avoid recurrence. Recurrent tumors are harder to manage surgically, because tissues have been disrupted and the resulting surgical field is much larger, making a second excision exceedingly difficult. Recurrent tumors carry a poorer prognosis, and many avian patients are euthanized due to local tumor progression.[16,17] Surgery can sometimes be performed in a purely palliative setting, to relieve discomfort associated with the size and/or location of the tumor. If margins are incomplete, adjuvant treatment options should be discussed with the owners, such as a second surgery, radiation therapy, or chemotherapy. Most benign tumors are cured with adequate surgical excision. Recurrence is still possible, however, and has been reported in cases of a surgically removed lipoma in an orange-winged Amazon parrot (*Amazona amazonica*).[18]

Radiation therapy

Radiation therapy is a form of local therapy, used either in a gross disease setting to provide palliation of clinical signs and attempt to shrink the tumor (palliative, coarse-fractionation radiation therapy) or in a microscopic disease setting to kill cells remaining after surgical excision and extend survival time (curative/definitive radiation therapy). The tumor is irradiated as well as a margin of normal surrounding tissue to account for microscopic tumor extension.

Several reports of radiation therapy in birds exist and show mixed results in terms of success and side effects. Major problems include the lack of information on adequate fractionation and schedule in avian patients, knowledge of radiosensitivity of avian tumors, and tolerance of normal tissues. Some of this information can be extrapolated from other species, in which hematopoietic tumors are exquisitely sensitive to radiation therapy, whereas carcinomas are moderately sensitive and sarcomas much less so.[19]

The tolerance of skin and mucosal tissues to radiation therapy has been evaluated in ring-necked parakeets.[20] Each bird was treated with cobalt-60 teletherapy and received 4-Gy fractions to a total of 48 Gy, 60 Gy, or 72 Gy. Minimal epidermal changes were noted in all birds, including in the high-dose group, and no chronic side effects were present 9 months post-therapy. This suggests that birds may have higher tissue tolerance to radiation and may require higher radiation dosages to treat sensitive tumors.

Radiotherapy has been used after surgery to treat a squamous cell carcinoma (SCC) of the mandibular beak in a Buffon macaw (*Ara ambigua*).[21] The bird was treated on a Monday-Wednesday-Friday schedule with 5.6 Gy per fraction to a total of 48 Gy and an additional 8-Gy boost, with cobalt-60, with no effect on the tumor and no side effects. Possible explanations for lack of response include a high number of hypoxic cells (presence of infection/necrosis), lack of radiosensitivity of the tumor (as in other species, such as felines, where best responses are mostly stable or partial, with only modest improvements in survival time compared with untreated patients[22]), or inadequate radiation dose.

Partial response to radiation therapy has been reported in a few cases. A stage 4 mandibular beak melanoma in a thick-billed parrot was treated with 20 daily fractions (Monday through Friday) of 2.5 Gy (total 50 Gy), using a linear accelerator, yielding a partial response at the primary tumor site; however, the bird died of metastatic disease 11.5 weeks postdiagnosis.[23] A hemangiosarcoma on the wing of a budgerigar resolved without complications after radiotherapy with [137]cesium teletherapy (10 fractions of 4 Gy, Monday-Wednesday-Friday) but recurred 1 month later, and the bird was subsequently euthanized 2 months postdiagnosis due to disseminated hemangiosarcoma.[24]

Orthovoltage was used to treat an intraocular osteosarcoma after exenteration and mass removal in an umbrella cockatoo (*Cacatua alba*) using a Monday-Wednesday-Friday schedule to a total dose of 68 Gy over 6 weeks.[25] The bird died of neurologic signs 3 months later and no necropsy was performed. Although the treatment was administered without complications, response could not be evaluated due to the rapid death of the bird.[26] A malignant lymphoma involving the periorbital area in an African gray parrot (*Psittacus erithacus*) was treated with orthovoltage teletherapy for 10 fractions of 4 Gy on a Monday-Wednesday-Friday schedule. By the third treatment, the mass had markedly shrunk but at a 2-month recheck had grown back to at least 50% of its original size.[27]

Combination therapies have been evaluated using intralesional chemotherapy and radiation. A fibrosarcoma of the wing in a blue-and-yellow macaw (*Ara ararauna*) was treated with 4 Gy per fraction on a Monday-Wednesday-Friday schedule to a total of 40 Gy with a cobalt-60 unit, with concurrent administration of intratumoral cisplatin. Complete tumor response was noted 2 months postcompletion of therapy.[28] There was no evidence of reoccurrence 15 months post-treatment. Intralesional cisplatin was also used in a treatment protocol using surgery and orthovoltage radiation (before the 8th and 11th radiation treatments) to treat a fibrosarcoma on the face of a blue-and-yellow macaw.[29] The tumor had been increasing in size at the 6th radiation treatment, so intralesional cisplatin was added. The patient remained in remission for 29 months.

In general, avian patients seem to tolerate radiation better than other species. Protocols using 4-Gy fractions, administered 3 times a week (10–12 total fractions), for a cumulative dose of 40 Gy to 48 Gy seem most commonly reported. Side effects are either absent or mild and include erythema, feather loss in the radiation field, pigmentary changes, and, rarely, necrosis, fibrosis, and leukopenia. A recent study of radiation of the head in birds concluded that the unique anatomy of this species, with the presence of an elaborate set of sinuses, resulted in inhomogeneity of dose distribution and that the intended amount of radiation delivered did not reach intended levels.[30]

Chemotherapy

When considering the use of chemotherapy in companion birds, several precautions must be taken. Every effort should be made to include a board-certified oncologist in the decision-making process. There is no established standard of care for the treatment of avian cancer; dosages are mostly unknown and side effects difficult to predict. This should be discussed with clients so that expectations are realistic. Reports of avian species with various neoplasms treated with chemotherapy (mostly hematopoietic diseases) have been published[2,3,13,15,28,31–36]; however, responses and outcome remain anecdotal.

Dosages of chemotherapy are extrapolated from those used in canine and feline species; however, they may not be appropriate for use in avian patients. Most chemotherapy agents are dosed based on body surface area (BSA); however, concerns have been raised that BSA does not adequately correlate with the physiologic/pharmacologic factors that influence drug exposure.[37] Another commonly used formula is based on weight (milligrams per kilogram). Pharmacokinetics of several chemotherapy agents have been studied in healthy sulphur-crested cockatoos and other avian species in an attempt to improve dosage of chemotherapy agents in birds.[38–42]

Chemotherapy kills rapidly dividing cells (neoplastic cells) but may cause collateral damage on normal rapidly dividing cells, such as cells in the hair follicles, gastrointestinal tract, and bone marrow. Gastrointestinal side effects usually occur 3 to 5 days post-therapy and are readily managed with supportive medications. Bone marrow suppression and resulting heteropenia happen most commonly at approximately 1 week after chemotherapy and close monitoring of blood cell counts is, therefore, necessary. In canine and feline patients, treatment is administered if the neutrophil count is greater than 1500/μL. Antibiotic therapy is initiated if the neutrophil count is less than 1000/μL, and a febrile and neutropenic patient is considered a medical emergency and should be hospitalized on IV antibiotics.

Side effects of chemotherapy in avian species have been reported (**Table 1**). Cisplatin, if given at the dog dosage, can cause severe nephrotoxicity, but it seems safe at a dose of 1 mg/kg IV.[25] Carboplatin has been used at 5 mg to 27 mg/kg IV or IO, every 3 to 4 weeks with minimal toxicity.[35,36,43] Both carboplatin and cisplatin have been used intralesionally, in an oil-based emulsion.[21,28,29,34,44] Cyclophosphamide causes marked heteropenia in birds, in experimental settings[45,46] and causes feather lesions in chicken.[47] Lomustine (CCNU) causes hepatotoxicity in humans and dogs but this has not yet been reported in birds. Topical 5-fluorouracil has successfully been used for the treatment of cutaneous SCC.[1] Vincristine and doxorubicin are vesicants in humans, dogs, and cats. Doxorubicin has been used at 2 times the typical dog dose with no side effects observed.[48] L-Asparaginase has been used by the authors at both the canine/feline dosage (400 U/kg) and 4 times that dose, with no effect and no toxicity in a finch with lymphoma. Metronomic chemotherapy (low dose, daily oral chemotherapy, and using cyclophosphamide and meloxicam) has been used successfully to delay recurrence in a kori bustard (Ardeotis kori) with an incompletely excised myxosarcoma.[31] No side effects were reported. In dogs, metronomic chemotherapy has also been shown to slow down recurrence of soft tissue sarcomas.[49] Although maximum tolerated dose chemotherapy targets the DNA of rapidly dividing cancer cells, the purpose of metronomic chemotherapy is to inhibit angiogenesis by damaging endothelial cells and possibly to modulate the immune system by decreasing levels of regulatory T cells.[49]

Chemotherapy administration may be oral, IV, intramuscular, subcutaneous. Birds have thin and delicate skin, which makes the placement of vascular access ports difficult. A recent report of a vascular access port placement in a chicken suggests, however, that this may be feasible in select cases, making IV chemotherapy administration much more feasible.[50] When administering chemotherapy, personal protective equipment should always be worn, any spills cleaned thoroughly with bleach, and the contaminated materials disposed of appropriately. Closed system devices are now readily available and relatively cheap (eg, Tevadaptor, Equashield, and PhaSeal) and should be used when administering chemotherapy to decrease risk of exposure to hazardous drugs. Sending clients home with oral (liquid or pill/capsule) chemotherapy is not encouraged, because administration can be challenging, and environmental and user contaminations are common. In addition, chemotherapy may be administered directly into a solid tumor (intralesional chemotherapy). The goal of intralesional chemotherapy is to achieve a high concentration of chemotherapy at the tumor site while minimizing systemic uptake and therefore side effects. Although this seems

Table 1
Selected chemotherapy protocols used in birds

Drug	Species	Tumor	Protocol	Response/Duration/Survival	Side Effects	Ref
Carboplatin	Budgerigar (M undulatus)	Renal carcinoma	5 mg/kg IV q 30 d	Clinical improvement after carboplatin #3 but tumor progression and death at 3 mo	None	35
Carboplatin	Mallard duck (Anas platyrhynchos)	Sertoli cell tumor	15 mg/kg diluted in 25 mL 5% dextrose, q 5 wk × 4	Clinical improvement at week 3, recurrence at 12 mo. Died at 13 mo.	None	36
Carboplatin	Yellow-naped Amazon parrot (Amazona auropalliata)	SCC (choana)	17.2 mg/kg IV × 4 3–10 wk apart	Progressive disease, died at 9 mo	None	43
Carboplatin	Cockatiel (N hollandicus)	SCC (cutaneous, multifocal)	27 mg/kg q 4 wk × 4 (received cryotherapy prior)	Progressive disease, death at 3 mo	None	43
Carboplatin	Spectacled Amazon parrot (Amazona albifrons)	SCC (cutaneous, multifocal)	24 mg/kg q 3–4 wk × 9	Survived 1 y	None	43
Chlorambucil	Java sparrow (Lonchura oryzivora)	Thymic lymphoma	2 mg/kg po twice a week until week 19 (d/c due to anorexia), then prednisolone 2.2 mg/kg po bid	Partial remission from 3–20 wk, died at 61 wk	Anorexia (no blood monitoring)	32
Chlorambucil	Double yellow-headed Amazon parrot (Amazona ochrocephala oratrix)	T-cell chronic lymphocytic leukemia	2 mg/kg po twice weekly	No response at 40 d — euthanasia	None	3

(continued on next page)

Table 1
(continued)

Drug	Species	Tumor	Protocol	Response/Duration/Survival	Side Effects	Ref
Chlorambucil + vincristine	Umbrella cockatoo (*Cacatua alba*)	Nonepitheliotropic B-cell cutaneous lymphoma and leukemia	Chlorambucil (2 mg/kg po twice weekly) + Vincristine (0.1 mg/kg IV q 1–3 wk)	Partial remission week 9 (treatment d/c at week 17 due to anemia) —complete response at week 29 and ongoing (>8 y)	Myelosuppression	15
Multiple protocols	Green-winged macaw (*Ara chloropterus*)	Chronic lymphocytic leukemia	Chlorambucil 1 mg/kg po twice weekly (6 wk d/c due to thrombocytopenia) + prednisone 1 mg/kg po q 24 h THEN Cyclophosphamide 5 mg/kg po × 4 d q 21 d (week 8.5)	Unknown to chlorambucil Stable disease on cyclophosphamide	Thrombocytopenia (chlorambucil)	33
Multiple protocols	Black swan (*Cygnus atratus*)	Chronic T-cell lymphocytic leukemia with coelomic organ involvement	Chlorambucil 2 mg po q 48 h (until day 150), then L-Spar 400 IU/kg SQ + CCNU 60 mg/m² po q 3 wk, then prednisone added 0.5 mg/kg po q 24 h, then whole-body radiation	No response to chlorambucil L-Spar/CCNU/prednisone. Partial response to whole-body radiation. Died at day 450.	None	2

Abbreviations: d/c, discontinued; L-Spar, L-asparaginase.

effective in certain cases, it cannot be emphasized enough that strict precautions should be taken if this technique is to be undertaken. It is the authors' opinion that intralesional chemotherapy should not routinely be offered or performed due to risk of extremely hazardous contamination. Direct contact and aerosolization are inevitable for the staff involved in administering the chemotherapy as well as for bird owners. Risks and benefits should be carefully discussed with clients and a consent form signed by both parties prior to performing intralesional chemotherapy.

Response to chemotherapy should be monitored closely and objectively. The canine Response Evaluation Criteria in Solid Tumors criteria[51] is used in canine and feline patients to assess tumor response and could be used in avian patients. A complete response is defined as a complete disappearance of all lesions; a partial response is defined as at least a 30% decrease in the sum of the longest diameter of target lesions; progressive disease is defined as a 20% increase in the sum of the longest diameter of target lesions; and stable disease is neither a partial response nor progressive disease. If a chemotherapy treatment is ineffective, it should be discontinued and further options should be discussed.

Steroids are routinely used in the treatment of hematopoietic cancers. Birds are sensitive to steroids and may develop secondary fungal and/or bacterial infections caused by the immunosuppressive effects of steroids. In an attempt to prevent this, antibiotics and antifungal drugs should be considered concurrently with chemotherapy.

Photodynamic therapy
Photodynamic therapy (PDT) uses an IV or intratumoral photosensitizing agent, activated by a light source. Once activated, oxygen radicals are produced and destroy the neoplastic cells. This technique has most commonly been used for the treatment of cutaneous SCC in cats and equine periocular SCC.[52–55] In birds, use of PDT has been reported for treatment of SCC.[56,57] In a 5-year-old ringed-necked parakeet (*Psittacula krameri*), an ulcerated SCC on the medial aspect of the postpatagial area of the right wing was treated with PDT.[57] This resulted in necrosis of the tumor and reduction in tumor burden but not complete resolution. In a 33-year-old great hornbill (*Buceros bicornis*), PDT was used to treat SCC of the rostral casque. A partial response was noted, but the tumor then progressed and the bird was euthanized.[56] These 2 reports suggest that PDT may be a useful tool to treat sold tumors in birds; however, further studies are necessary to determine optimal technique and indications.

Cryotherapy
Cryotherapy used extremely cold temperatures to achieve destruction of tissues. There are many different techniques described (open-spray, closed-spray, and cryoprobe) using single or multiple freeze-thaw cycles and most commonly using liquid nitrogen. Cryotherapy is commonly used for the treatment of superficial small lesions, most commonly on the head/face area in dogs and cats.[58] In birds, cryotherapy has been used successfully after treatment with intralesional cisplatin in an African penguin (*Spheniscus demersus*) with choanal SCC.[34] Advantages of cryotherapy are the ease of treatment and low morbidity associated with it and the possibility of performing repeat treatments if necessary. The disadvantage is that it is only suitable for superficial lesions of small diameter.

Antihormonal therapy
The administration of long-acting synthetic gonadotropin-releasing hormone (GnRH) supra-agonists (eg, leuprolide acetate and deslorelin acetate) leads to a reduction

of gonadal hormone secretion by overriding the physiologic pulsatile GnRH released from the hypothalamus.[59] Sustained-release GnRH superagonists have been used in avian medicine to treat neoplasia of the reproductive tract in male and female birds. Several case reports exist on the use of leuprolide and deslorelin in birds with malignant ovarian, oviductal, and gonadal neoplasia.[59–62]

Tamoxifen is an antiestrogen drug used in the treatment and prevention of certain estrogen-receptor positive breast cancers in women. It is a selective inhibitor of estrogen receptors and a potent antiestrogen drug. It has been evaluated in dogs with mammary tumors; however, side effects were common, including vulvar edema, purulent vaginal discharge, pyometra, and retinitis.[63] It has been evaluated in budgerigars (*M undulatus*). The most common adverse effect was reversible leukopenia. Antiestrogenic effects were suggested by the observation of a change in color of the cere from white/brown to blue.

COMMON NEOPLASMS
Integumentary and Soft Tissue Tumors

SCCs are a malignant tumor of the epithelial cells lining certain tissues or organs. These can occur anywhere on the body and are commonly seen on the feathered skin,[44,57] beak,[21] uropygial gland,[64] and phalanges and in the upper gastrointestinal tract (in particular affecting the crop).[65–67] Cockatiels, Amazon parrots, and conures are commonly affected.[68] SCCs present as pink, raised, infiltrative, and proliferative masses. They are usually ill defined and can be ulcerated. Diagnosis can be obtained by cytology (SCCs exfoliate well) or histopathology. They behave in a locally invasive fashion and have a low metastatic rate. They are best treated surgically, with the goal of achieving a complete surgical excision.[68] Local radiation therapy using a single treatment with a strontium probe has been used successfully as the sole treatment in 2 budgerigars (*M undulatus*) with uropygial gland carcinoma and in a cockatiel (*Nymphicus hollandicus*) with a uropygial gland adenoma.[69] Complete resolution of the neoplastic lesions occurred and all three birds were disease-free at the time of reporting, 8 months, 9 months, and 2 months post-treatment, respectively.[69] Preliminary data from a multi-institutional retrospective study on outcome of SCC in 85 birds treated with surgery, chemotherapy, or radiation therapy (orthovoltage or strontium) indicate that complete surgical excision was associated with a more positive outcome.[68] Radiation, however, penetrates only a few millimeters with strontium therapy and may not be appropriate for more invasive tumors. As in other species, SCCs are radiation resistant, making the treatment of larger or deeper lesions difficult. Intralesional chemotherapy, using carboplatin or cisplatin chemotherapy, and cryotherapy have yielded some mixed success.

Lipomas

Lipomas are benign neoplasms of adipose tissue and are the most common skin tumor in avian species. Lipomas are usually well circumscribed, but infiltrative lipomas have been reported in psittacines.[70,71] Lipomas occur frequently in obese birds, specifically budgerigars, Quaker parrots, Amazon parrots, and macaws (**Fig. 7**).

Lipomas are most commonly found in the subcutaneous tissues and can arise anywhere on the body, including inside the thoracic or coelomic cavity. A recent study[18] reported that lipomas were the most common neoplasm referred for a surgical procedure in birds. Most lipomas were present subcutaneously in the pericloacal area (see **Fig. 7**B). Cytology can yield a population of well-differentiated adipocytes (**Fig. 8**). They are prone to lysis, however, during sampling and their content dissolves

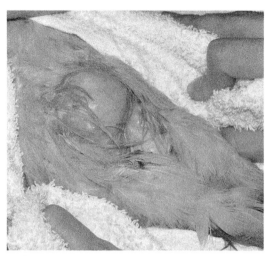

Fig. 7. Subcutaneous lipomas in a blue-and-yellow macaw (*Ara ararauna*). (*Courtesy of* Christoph Mans, Madison, WI.)

during the staining process. The slide, therefore, can look devoid of material despite a seemingly copious sample visible at the time of slide preparation. Treatment depends on tumor size and location. Dietary changes and increase in exercise are appropriate for many obese avian patients. Lipomas can resolve once the obesity has been corrected. In a pilot study, supplementation with L-carnitine (1000 mg/kg of pellets) has been shown to reduce subcutaneous lipoma size and body weight in budgerigars compared with the control group.[72] Further research is necessary to fully understand the possible benefits of this supplement. If the tumor is growing fast or causing discomfort, surgical excision should be performed and the tissue submitted for histopathologic analysis to obtain a definitive diagnosis. A differential diagnosis for lipomas is a liposarcoma.[73,74] These do not result from malignant transformation of a lipoma. They are composed of immature adipocytes and are typically less well circumscribed

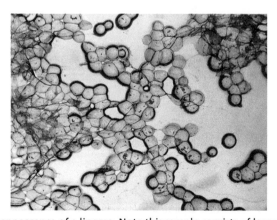

Fig. 8. Cytologic appearance of a lipoma. Note this sample consists of large clusters of intact well-differentiated adipocytes, which is consistent with a lipoma. Subcutaneous fat has the same appearance; therefore, the interpretation depends on clinician confidence that these cells are representative of the mass sampled. (*Courtesy of* Cecilia Robat, Madison, WI.)

and more invasive. They act more aggressively and recurrence rates are high and metastasis common.[74]

Fibrosarcomas

Fibrosarcomas are a type of soft tissue sarcoma (**Fig. 9**). They are a malignant tumor of fibrous tissue. They are locally invasive, and metastasis is uncommonly reported.[75,76] They are most commonly seen in the facial/oral regions and bones and can be seen in the coelomic cavity or cloaca[77] as well. They tend to have a high recurrence rate after conservative surgery due to their invasive nature and the need for wide surgical margins. Postoperative radiation therapy with or without intralesional chemotherapy should be considered and has been described as effective, if radical surgery and complete excision are not achievable.[28,29]

Myxosarcomas

Myxosarcomas are uncommon soft tissue sarcomas, mostly reported in chickens and in a kori bustard.[31] The authors diagnosed a metastatic myxosarcoma in a severe macaw (**Fig. 10**). This neoplasm produces abundant mucinous stroma, which can readily be sampled on fine-needle aspirate (see **Fig. 10**). They are locally invasive with a low metastatic rate. Wide surgical margins are necessary for adequate tumor control.

Xanthomas

Xanthomas are dermal non-neoplastic masses composed of lipid-laden macrophages and cholesterol (ie, cholesterol granuloma). Xanthomas are more common in the skin and subcutaneous tissues of gallinaceous birds and psittacines.[78] Grossly, they are friable and well-vascularized yellow/orange masses, located on the dorsum, wings, and thighs and, therefore, can easily be mistaken as a neoplastic mass. Cytologic examination of a fine-needle aspirate shows multinucleated giant cells and cholesterol clefts. Xanthomas are thought to develop secondary to obesity and hyperlipidemia with concurrent trauma.[79] A diet supplemented in vitamin A or precursors may help treat these masses; however, no treatment is necessary unless the mass in causing functional problems or being traumatized.

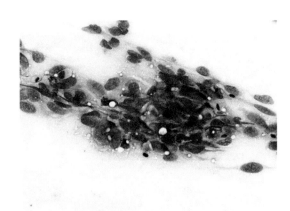

Fig. 9. Cytologic appearance cells aspirated from a mass on the wing of 3-year-old budgerigar (*M undulatus*). Note the large mesenchymal cells, with high nuclear:cytoplasmic ratios, up to 5-fold anisocytosis and anisokaryosis, and prominent multiple nucleoli, consistent with a sarcoma, most likely a soft tissue sarcoma (magnification ×600). (*Courtesy of* Melanie Ammersbach, Guelph, Ontario.)

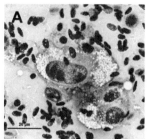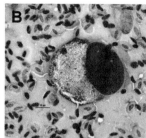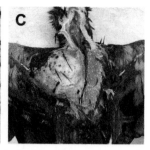

Fig. 10. A 36-year-old severe macaw (*Ara severus*) that presented with a large mass over the right sternal area. (*A, B*) Cytologic aspirate of the mass revealed a pleomorphic mesenchymal population with moderate to high nuclear:cytoplasmic ratios, abundant pale basophilic cytoplasm, and (*A*) numerous clear punctate vacuoles and (*B*) fine magenta granules consistent with a malignant mesenchymal tumor. (*C*) Postmortem diagnosis was a myxosarcoma, with metastasis to the lungs. (*Courtesy of* Ruth Houseright, Madison, WI.)

Musculoskeletal Tumors

Musculoskeletal tumors in birds are infrequently reported in the literature. The most common are osteosarcoma and chondrosarcoma. They most commonly arise from long bones but are also reported in the ribs and skull bones. Clinical signs include lameness, pain, or presence of a mass. Diagnosis is suspected based on radiographic findings of osteolysis with or without proliferation; however, a definitive diagnosis can only be achieved on histopathology. Although osteosarcoma commonly metastasizes to the lungs in dogs, it seems infrequent in birds, and in 10 reported cases, 4 tumors metastasized (only 1 to the lungs).[80] As in other species, chondrosarcomas are locally invasive with a low metastatic rate (see **Fig. 2**).[80] A synovial cell sarcoma arising at the site of a previous fracture, associated with an intramedullary pin,[81] has recently been described. Other nonmalignant neoplasms of bone, such as chondromas and osteomas, have also been reported. Leiomyosarcoma is a tumor of smooth muscle. It is most commonly reported in intracoelomic organs, such as the spleen and gastrointestinal tract. It is locally invasive and infrequently metastasizes.[82] Rhabdomyosarcomas are malignant tumors of skeletal muscle. They are most common in the muscles of the shoulder and wing but can arise from any skeletal muscle.[11,12,83] Surgery is the treatment of choice although behavior of this neoplasm and expected outcome are not described in birds.

Hematopoietic Tumors

Lymphoma is one of the most common neoplasms in companion birds and the most frequent neoplastic condition diagnosed at the authors institution in avian patients. Lymphoma can manifest in birds as a visceral, cutaneous, retrobulbar or periorbital, oral, or leukemic disease (**Figs. 11–13**).[2–4,13,27,33] Cutaneous lymphoma most commonly occurs around the head/periocular/neck area (see **Fig. 12**) and may present as diffuse swelling or as multifocal nodules.[14,15] Lymphoma may either occur in organs or tissues, solely in the blood (leukemia), or in both (leukemic lymphoma) (see **Fig. 12**). Clinical signs reported are progressive weight loss and lethargy, feather loss, self-mutilation, a distended coelomic cavity (secondary to hepatosplenomegaly) (see **Fig. 13**), and diarrhea, among others. Blood work may reveal anemia, lymphocytosis, or elevated liver values. These changes are nonspecific for lymphoma; however, a severe lymphocytosis should raise suspicion for a leukemic process (see **Fig. 12**D). Rarely, paraneoplastic hypercalcemia[4] and monoclonal hyperglobulinemia[84] have been reported.

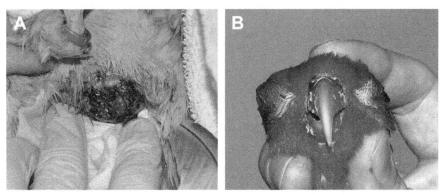

Fig. 11. Clinical presentation of lymphoma in companion birds. (*A*) Amazon parrot (*Amazona spp*) with severe swelling and ulceration of the pericloacal skin and cloacal opening. (*B*) Red lory (*Eos bornea*) with unilateral severe periocular swelling and exophthalmos. In both cases the diagnosis of lymphoma was made by cytology. (*Courtesy of* Christoph Mans, Madison, WI.)

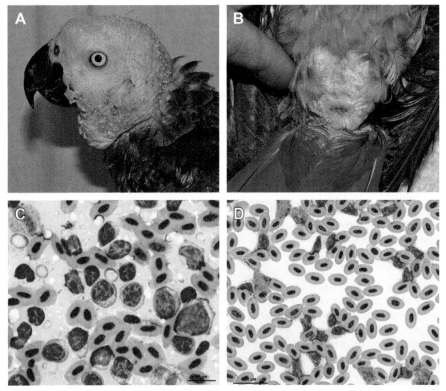

Fig. 12. A 22-year-old Congo African gray parrot (*P erithacus*) diagnosed with leukemic cutaneous lymphoma. (*A*) Alopecia and scabbing affecting skin of the head and (*B*) pericloacal area. (*C*) Cytologic examination of samples collected from the skin of the head reveal an increased number of lymphocytes, a majority of which are medium-sized with a lower number of small and large lymphocytes (magnification ×1000). (*D*) Blood smear showing marked lymphocytosis. The absolute lymphocyte count was 192 × 10³/uL (magnification ×600). (*Courtesy of* Christoph Mans and Ruth Houseright, Madison, WI.)

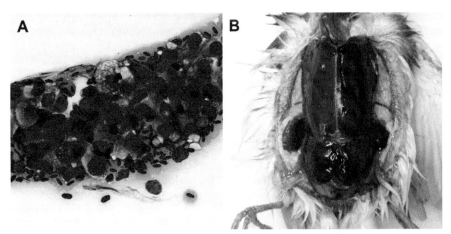

Fig. 13. Multicentric lymphoma in a Gouldian finch (*Erythrura gouldiae*). (*A*) Cytology of a fine-needle aspirate of the enlarged liver, showing hepatocytes and large neoplastic lymphocytes, which is consistent with hepatic lymphoma (magnification ×1000). Treatment with high dose L-asparaginase (1600 U/kg intramuscularly) and prednisolone did not result in clinical improvement. (*B*) Postmortem photograph showing the severely enlarged liver. Multicentric lymphoma was the final diagnosis. Neoplastic lymphocytes were found in the liver, spleen, lungs, intestine, bone marrow, and skeletal muscle, among many other tissues. (*Courtesy of* Cecilia Robat, Madison, WI.)

Diagnosis is obtained via cytologic or histopathologic diagnosis. Further characterization using immunocytochemistry/histochemistry to obtain information on immunophenotype should be considered, although the prognostic significance of this information in birds is currently unknown. The commonly used T-cell lymphoid marker, CD3, seems to cross-react between most species, with a less consistent observation with B-cell markers (BLA36 and CD79a).[85] Full staging should be performed, when possible, including blood work, whole-body imaging, and bone marrow investigation.

Treatment of systemic disease is performed with chemotherapy; local disease control can be achieved with surgery with or without radiation therapy. Various chemotherapy agents have been used in birds with lymphoma, including chlorambucil, vincristine, cytoxan, doxorubicin, L-asparaginase, and prednisone or dexamethasone. Responses are variable and data are mostly lacking on treatment and prognosis.

Respiratory Tumors

Respiratory neoplasia is uncommon in birds (see **Fig. 3**). SCC of the nasal cavity and infraorbital sinus has been reported.[86,87] Air sac and bronchial adenocarcinoma and cystadenocarcinoma have been reported in Psittaciformes. Most patients present with advanced respiratory clinical signs, weakness, and lethargy. Air sac cystadenocarcinoma was reported in 6 cockatoos.[88] All cases presented with severe respiratory clinical signs, which were rapidly fatal. Extensive neoplastic invasion of the lungs, major airways, and/or humerus was present in all cases. Respiratory tumors in birds seem to be highly locally invasive and diffuse metastatic disease to intracavitary organs and bones is common.[8,88–94] A unique and incompletely characterized form of pulmonary tumors seems to develop in cockatiels.[95] It has been reported as pulmonary bimorphic tumor, undifferentiated pulmonary tumor, or pulmonary sarcoma. These tumors have a unique histologic appearance. They are very aggressive and locally invasive into surrounding structures but appear less metastatic. A respiratory hamartoma was reported in a cockatiel.[96] Hamartomas are focal malformations of an organ, resulting from a developmental anomaly. This patient presented with coelomic distention, and the mass was successfully removed surgically.

Gastrointestinal Tumors

Adenocarcinomas

Adenocarcinomas of the proventriculus or ventriculus are described in birds, the most common site being the isthmus.[97–99] Clinical signs are associated with the presence of tissue proliferation inhibiting the normal digestive process. Affected birds often regurgitate/vomit, are hyporexic and may pass undigested food and have melena. Anemia and hypoproteinemia are common. Antemortem diagnosis is only possible is larger species, in which endoscopic biopsies can be performed. In others, these tumors are usually diagnosed at the time of necropsy. Distant metastases are described.[97] Treatment is not described. In dogs, treatment of gastric carcinoma is not rewarding and the prognosis is poor.

Cholangiocarcinomas

Cholangiocarcinomas have most commonly been described in Amazon parrots.[100–103] These are aggressive tumors that are known to metastasize. One report has suggested a link between papillomatosis and bile duct carcinoma; however, these findings should be interpreted with caution, because numbers were low in that study.[102] Clinical signs are usually nonspecific as are biochemical changes. Antemortem diagnosis is uncommon; however, lesions may be seen on ultrasound imaging and should be sampled for cytologic diagnosis. Prognosis is poor. Carboplatin has been used successfully in a yellow-naped Amazon parrot (*Amazona ochrocephala*).[104]

Urogenital Tumors

Ovarian and oviductal neoplasms of companion birds include adenocarcinoma, adenoma, carcinomas, cystadenocarcinomas, granulosa cell tumors, and hemangiosarcoma.[105–107] The most common tumor seems to be ovarian tumors of stromal cell origin (granulosa cell tumor) and oviductal adenocarcinomas. These occur in budgerigars at a frequency of 4% to 14%. Clinical signs include persistent breeding behavior, egg retention, and coelomic distention secondary to ascites (**Fig. 14**) or organomegaly, and sometimes no clinical signs are present at all. Polyostotic hyperostosis has been described in patients with ovarian tumors and is thought to be associated with secreting large amounts of estrogens[108]; however, the association has been refuted in another publication.[109] Diffuse coelomic metastasis is common, because these tumors are commonly diagnosed late in the course of the disease. Diagnosis is obtained via imaging and pathology. No effective treatment is reported for ovarian tumors unless disease is localized and surgical excision possible, which is uncommon.[110] Leuprolide acetate was reported to provide a partial clinical response in 2 cockatiels with ovarian tumors.[61] For oviductal tumors, surgical removal may be attempted but carries high anesthetic and surgical risk, in particular in small patients. Therefore, treatment with GnRH supra-agonists (eg, leuprolide acetate and deslorelin acetate) is frequently performed to improve clinical signs (**Figs. 15 and 16**).[106]

Testicular tumors arise from Sertoli cells (Sertoli cell tumor), spermatogenic epithelium (seminoma), or interstitial cells (interstitial cell tumor). They are most commonly reported in budgerigars. Clinical signs include tachypnea, coelomic distention, and tachypnea secondary to and enlarged testicle. Estrogen-producing Sertoli cell tumors lead to feminization of male birds, predominately budgerigar. Affected animals often have a change of color of the cere from blue to brown, widening of the pubic bones,

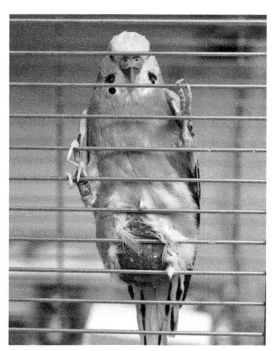

Fig. 14. Female budgerigar (*M undulates*) with severe coelomic distension. (*Courtesy of* Christoph Mans, Madison, WI.)

a broad-based stance, and an enlarged cloacal opening (**Fig. 17**). Radiographs reveal an increase in soft tissue opacity in the coelom and hyperostosis secondary to hyper-estrogenism. Unilateral paresis/paralysis due to the compression of the sciatic nerve root may occur. Seminomas have been reported to form metastases in birds.[6,111] Surgical excision is the treatment of choice but is usually a high-risk procedure, in

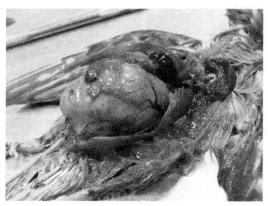

Fig. 15. Postmortem photograph of a female cockatiel (*N hollandicus*) with a large coelomic mass, diagnosed as an oviductal adenocarcinoma. (*Courtesy of* University of Wisconsin, School of Veterinary Medicine, Madison, WI; with permission.)

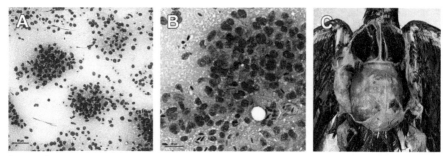

Fig. 16. (*A, B*) Cytologic appearance of an ultrasound-guided fine-needle aspirate of a large coelomic mass in a 13-year-old female eclectus parrot (*Eclectus roratus*). Note the clusters of cells with round to oval nuclei, abundant basophilic cytoplasm with punctate clear vacuolation and indistinct cytoplasmic boarders most consistent with a neuroendocrine or epithelial neoplasm. (*C*) Postmortem diagnosis was ovarian adenocarcinoma with carcinomatosis. (*Courtesy of* Ruth Houseright, Madison, WI.)

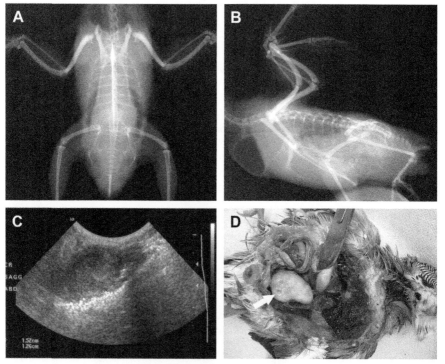

Fig. 17. Sertoli cell tumor in a budgerigar (*M undulatus*). (*A, B*) Ventrodorsal and lateral survey radiograph showing increased soft tissue opacity in the coelom and hyperostosis of all bones and an increased distance between the pubic bones, secondary. (*C*) Coelomic ultrasound identifying a left-sided intracoelomic mass. (*D*) Postmortem examination revealing a large gonadal mass (*arrow*), later confirmed as a Sertoli cell tumor. Note the severely enlarged vent opening, secondary to hyperestrogenism. (*From* Mans C, Pilny A. Use of GnRH-agonists for medical management of reproductive disorders in birds. Vet Clin North Am Exot Anim Pract 2014;17:23–33.)

particular in small birds. In 1 report, surgical removal of a testicular tumor was attempted in 5 budgerigars. Two died perioperatively, 2 survived and were asymptomatic 3 years later, and 1 had incomplete surgical excision followed by carboplatin chemotherapy but failed to respond to chemotherapy.[111] Clinical signs associated with Sertoli cell tumors have been successfully managed in budgerigars using deslorelin implants.[62] Deslorelin acetate implants (4.7 mg) were placed subcutaneously in the knee fold under general anesthesia.[62] A response to treatment was reported in 7 of 9 budgerigars, evident by a change of cere color from brownish to blue. Further improvements included resolution of previously diagnosed lameness (3/3) and an improved general condition (7/8).[62] Initial clinical improvement was noted after several days to 4 weeks. Reoccurrence of clinical signs was noted on average 19 weeks after initial deslorelin administration. Deslorelin implants were repeatedly administered after reoccurrence of clinical signs and the effect of deslorelin lasted on average 20 weeks. Treatment of suspected Sertoli cell tumors in budgerigars with deslorelin implants was found effective by temporarily treatment the clinical signs, secondary to abnormal estrogen production, and no significant side effects were reported.[62]

Renal carcinomas are the most common renal neoplasms reported. Other renal neoplasms reported include renal adenomas, nephroblastomas and cystadenoma, among others.[112] Budgerigars are overrepresented and renal neoplasms account for 17% to 20% of all neoplasms described in this species.[113] A retroviral origin was suggested but a recent publication refutes that theory.[114] Affected birds usually present with unilateral non–weight-bearing leg lameness, due to compression of the lumbar or sacral nerve plexus (**Fig. 18**). Other clinical signs may include coelomic distention, lethargy, regurgitation, and emaciation due to the intracoelomic mass. Renal neoplasms rarely metastasize. Clinical signs and signalment are usually strongly suggestive for a renal neoplasm. Diagnostic imaging can be used to attempt to diagnose the underlying disease, but histopathology is necessary to confirm the diagnosis. When arising from the cranial division of the kidney, the tumor can be mistaken for a gonadal tumor. Renal tumors can be very cystic. Metastatic rate is usually low. No effective therapy is recognized in birds. Carboplatin resulted in a short-lived clinical improvement in 1 patient.[35]

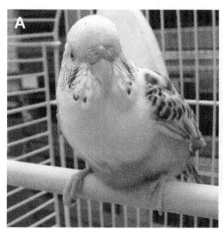
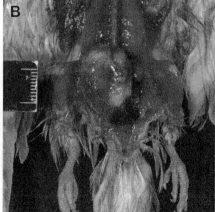

Fig. 18. (A) Budgerigar (M undulatus) with paralysis of the right leg secondary to renal adenocarcinoma. (B) Gross image showing renal adenocarcinoma that is compressing ischiatic plexus. (*Courtesy of* D. Sanchez-Migallon Guzman and D.A. Goldsmith, Davis, CA.)

Ocular Tumors

Neoplasms involving the eyes and adjacent structures are uncommon in birds. Various intraocular neoplasms (eg, medulloepitheliomas,[115,116] lymphoreticular tumors,[27] melanocytic tumors,[117] rhabdomyosarcomas,[6] and osteosarcomas[26]) as well as neoplasms of the adnexal ocular structures (ie, conjunctiva, eyelids, and orbit), such as periorbital liposarcoma,[74] retrobulbar adenocarcinoma,[118] and orbital lymphoma,[119] have been reported. Retrobulbar or orbital lymphoma is among the most common ocular neoplasms (see **Fig. 11B**). In a recent retrospective review of avian ocular neoplasms, approximately half of the cases were metastatic lesions affecting the globe and not primary neoplasms.[120] Of the primary ocular tumors in this review, none of the observed primary ocular tumors was identified as having metastasized to regional or distant locations.[120]

REFERENCES

1. Filippich LJ. Tumor control in birds. J Exot Pet Med 2004;13(1):25–43.
2. Sinclair KM, Hawkins MG, Wright L, et al. Chronic T-cell lymphocytic leukemia in a black swan (Cygnus atratus): diagnosis, treatment, and pathology. J Avian Med Surg 2015;29(4):326–35.
3. Osofsky A, Hawkins MG, Foreman O, et al. T-cell chronic lymphocytic leukemia in a double yellow-headed Amazon parrot (Amazona ochrocephala oratrix). J Avian Med Surg 2011;25(4):286–94.
4. de Wit M, Schoemaker NJ, Kik MJ, et al. Hypercalcemia in two Amazon parrots with malignant lymphoma. Avian Dis 2003;47(1):223–8.
5. Latimer KS, Ritchie BW, Campagnoli RP, et al. Metastatic renal carcinoma in an African grey parrot (Psittacus erithacus erithacus). J Vet Diagn Invest 1996;8(2):261–4.
6. Saied A, Beaufrere H, Tully TN Jr, et al. Bilateral seminoma with hepatic metastasis in a cockatiel (Nymphicus hollandicus). J Avian Med Surg 2011;25(2):126–31.
7. Nakano Y, Une Y. Hemangiosarcoma with widespread metastasis that originated on the metatarsal pad of a Java sparrow (Padda oryzivora). J Vet Med Sci 2012;74(5):621–3.
8. Azmanis P, Stenkat J, Hubel J, et al. A complicated, metastatic, humeral air sac cystadenocarcinoma in a timneh African grey parrot (Psittacus erithacus timneh). J Avian Med Surg 2013;27(1):38–43.
9. Vali Y, Molazem M, Madani SA. Use of 3D ultrasonography in diagnosing ovarian adenocarcinoma in a common mynah (Acridotheres tristis). J Avian Med Surg 2015;29(2):142–5.
10. João Felipe Rito Cardoso MGBL. Pathological and Immunohistochemical diagnosis of an intestinal leiomyosarcoma in a zebra finch. Braz J Vet Path 2014;7(2):89–92.
11. Gulbahar MY, Ozak A, Guvenc T, et al. Retrobulbar rhabdomyosarcoma in a budgerigar (Melopsittacus undulatus). Avian Pathol 2005;34(6):486–8.
12. Maluenda AC, Casagrande RA, Kanamura CT, et al. Rhabdomyosarcoma in a yellow-headed caracara (Milvago chimachima). Avian Dis 2010;54(2):951–4.
13. Souza MJ, Newman SJ, Greenacre CB, et al. Diffuse intestinal T-cell lymphosarcoma in a yellow-naped Amazon parrot (Amazona ochrocephala auropalliata). J Vet Diagn Invest 2008;20(5):656–60.

14. Burgos-Rodriguez AG, Garner M, Ritzman TK, et al. Cutaneous lymphosarcoma in a double yellow-headed Amazon parrot (Amazona ochrocephala oratrix). J Avian Med Surg 2007;21(4):283–9.

15. Rivera S, McClearen JR, Reavill DR. Treatment of nonepitheliotropic cutaneous B-cell lymphoma in an umbrella cockatoo (Cacatua alba). J Avian Med Surg 2009;23(4):294–302.

16. Suedmeyer WK, Witter RL, Bermudez A. Hemangiosarcoma in a Golden Pheasant (Chrysolophus pictus). J Avian Med Surg 2001;15(2):126–30.

17. Tell LA, Woods L, Mathews KG. Basal cell carcinoma in a blue-fronted amazon parrot (Amazona aestiva). Avian Dis 1997;41(3):755–9.

18. Castro PF, Fantoni DT, Miranda BC, et al. Prevalence of neoplastic diseases in pet birds referred for surgical procedures. Vet Med Int 2016;2016:4096801.

19. Larue SM, Gordon IK. 12-Radiation Therapy A2-Page. In: Stephen J, Withrow David M, Vail Rodney L, editors. Withrow and MacEwen's small animal clinical oncology. 5th edition. St Louis (MO): W.B. Saunders; 2013. p. 180–97.

20. Barron HW, Roberts RE, Latimer KS, et al. Tolerance doses of cutaneous and mucosal tissues in ring-necked parakeets (Psittacula krameri) for external beam megavoltage radiation. J Avian Med Surg 2009;23(1):6–9.

21. Manucy TK, Bennett RA, Greenacre CB, et al. Squamous cell carcinoma of the Mandibular Beak in a Buffon's Macaw (Ara ambigua). J Avian Med Surg 1998; 12(3):158–66.

22. Poirier VJ, Kaser-Hotz B, Vail DM, et al. Efficacy and toxicity of an accelerated hypofractionated radiation therapy protocol in cats with oral squamous cell carcinoma. Vet Radiol Ultrasound 2013;54(1):81–8.

23. Guthrie AL, Gonzalez-Angulo C, Wigle WL, et al. Radiation therapy of a malignant melanoma in a thick-billed parrot (Rhynchopsitta pachyrhyncha). J Avian Med Surg 2010;24(4):299–307.

24. Kimberly P, Freeman KAH, Adams WH, et al. Radiation Therapy for a Hemangiosarcoma in a Budgerigar. J Avian Med Surg 1999;13(1):40–4.

25. Filippich LJ, Bucher AM, Charles BG, et al. Intravenous cisplatin administration in sulphur-crested cockatoos (Cacatua galerita): clinical and pathologic observations. J Avian Med Surg 2001;15(1):23–30.

26. Fordham M, Rosenthal K, Durham A, et al. Case report: intraocular osteosarcoma in an umbrella cockatoo (Cacatua alba). Vet Ophthalmol 2010;13(Suppl):103–8.

27. Paul-Murphy J, Lowenstine L, Turrel JM, et al. Malignant lymphoreticular neoplasm in an African gray parrot. J Am Vet Med Assoc 1985;187(11):1216–7.

28. Lamberski N, Theon AP. Concurrent irradiation and intratumoral chemotherapy with cisplatin for treatment of a fibrosarcoma in a blue and gold macaw (Ara ararauna). J Avian Med Surg 2002;16(3):234–8.

29. Ramsay EC, Bos JH, McFadden C. Use of intratumoral cisplatin and orthovoltage radiotherapy in treatment of a fibrosarcoma in a Macaw. J Assoc Avian Med 1993;7(2):87–90.

30. Cutler DC, Shiomitsu K, Liu CC, et al. Comparison of calculated radiation delivery versus actual radiation delivery in military Macaws (Ara militaris). J Avian Med Surg 2016;30(1):1–7.

31. Sander SJ, Hope KL, McNeill CJ, et al. Metronomic chemotherapy for Myxosarcoma treatment in a Kori Bustard (Ardeotis kori). J Avian Med Surg 2015;29(3):210–5.

32. Yu PH, Chi CH. Long-term management of thymic lymphoma in a java sparrow (Lonchura oryzivora). J Avian Med Surg 2015;29(1):51–4.

33. Hammond EE, Guzman DS, Garner MM, et al. Long-term treatment of chronic lymphocytic leukemia in a green-winged macaw (Ara chloroptera). J Avian Med Surg 2010;24(4):330–8.

34. Ferrell ST, Marlar AB, Garner M, et al. Intralesional cisplatin chemotherapy and topical cryotherapy for the control of choanal squamous cell carcinoma in an African penguin (Spheniscus demersus). J Zoo Wildl Med 2006;37(4):539–41.

35. Macwhirter P, Pyke D, Wayne J. Use of carboplatin in the treatment of renal adenocarcinoma in a budgerigar. Exotic Dvm 2002;4(2):11–2.

36. Childs-Sanford SE, Rassnick KM, Alcaraz A. Carboplatin for treatment of a Sertoli cell tumor in a mallard (Anas platyrhynchos). Vet Comp Oncol 2006; 4(1):51–6.

37. Price GS, Frazier DL. Use of body surface area (BSA)-based dosages to calculate chemotherapeutic drug dose in dogs: I. Potential problems with current BSA formulae. J Vet Intern Med 1998;12(4):267–71.

38. Antonissen G, Devreese M, De Baere S, et al. Comparative pharmacokinetics and allometric scaling of carboplatin in different avian species. PLoS One 2015;10(7):e0134177.

39. Filippich LJ, Bucher AM, Charles BG. Platinum pharmacokinetics in sulphur-crested cockatoos (Cacatua galerita) following single-dose cisplatin infusion. Aust Vet J 2000;78(6):406–11.

40. Filippich LJ, Charles BG, Sutton RH, et al. Carboplatin pharmacokinetics following a single-dose infusion in sulphur-crested cockatoos (Cacatua galerita). Aust Vet J 2004;82(6):366–9.

41. Gilbert CM, Filippich LJ, Charles BG. Doxorubicin pharmacokinetics following a single-dose infusion to sulphur-crested cockatoos (Cacatua galerita). Aust Vet J 2004;82(12):769–72.

42. Gilbert CM, Filippich LJ, McGeary RP, et al. Toxicokinetics of the active doxorubicin metabolite, doxorubicinol, in sulphur-crested cockatoos (Cacatua galerita). Res Vet Sci 2007;83(1):123–9.

43. Zehnder A, Hawkins M, Koski M, et al. Therapeutic considerations for squamous cell carcinoma: an avaian case series. Paper presented at: 31st Annual Proc Assoc Avian Vet. San Diego, August 2–5, 2010.

44. Klaphake E, Beazley-Keane SL, Jones M, et al. Multisite integumentary squamous cell carcinoma in an African grey parrot (Psittacus erithacus erithacus). Vet Rec 2006;158(17):593–6.

45. Ficken MD, Barnes HJ. Effect of cyclophosphamide on selected hematologic parameters of the turkey. Avian Dis 1988;32(4):812–7.

46. Fulton RM, Reed WM, Thacker HL, et al. Cyclophosphamide (Cytoxan)-induced hematologic alterations in specific-pathogen-free chickens. Avian Dis 1996; 40(1):1–12.

47. Ratnamohan N. Feather lesions in cyclophosphamide-treated chickens. Avian Dis 1981;25(2):534–7.

48. MD. Adriamycin chemotherapy in a blue-fronted Amazon with osteosarcoma. Paper presented at: Proc Annu Conf Assoc Avian Vet. Boca Raton, 1994.

49. Elmslie RE, Glawe P, Dow SW. Metronomic therapy with cyclophosphamide and piroxicam effectively delays tumor recurrence in dogs with incompletely resected soft tissue sarcomas. J Vet Intern Med 2008;22(6):1373–9.

50. Doneley RJ, Smith BA, Gibson JS. Use of a vascular access port for antibiotic administration in the treatment of pododermatitis in a chicken. J Avian Med Surg 2015;29(2):130–5.

51. Nguyen SM, Thamm DH, Vail DM, et al. Response evaluation criteria for solid tumours in dogs (v1.0): a Veterinary Cooperative Oncology Group (VCOG) consensus document. Vet Comp Oncol 2015;13(3):176–83.

52. Giuliano EA, MacDonald I, McCaw DL, et al. Photodynamic therapy for the treatment of periocular squamous cell carcinoma in horses: a pilot study. Vet Ophthalmol 2008;11(Suppl 1):27–34.

53. Giuliano EA, Johnson PJ, Delgado C, et al. Local photodynamic therapy delays recurrence of equine periocular squamous cell carcinoma compared to cryotherapy. Vet Ophthalmol 2014;17(Suppl 1):37–45.

54. Bexfield NH, Stell AJ, Gear RN, et al. Photodynamic therapy of superficial nasal planum squamous cell carcinomas in cats: 55 cases. J Vet Intern Med 2008; 22(6):1385–9.

55. Ferreira I, Rahal SC, Rocha NS, et al. Hematoporphyrin-based photodynamic therapy for cutaneous squamous cell carcinoma in cats. Vet Dermatol 2009; 20(3):174–8.

56. Suedmeyer WK, McCaw D, Turnquist S. Attempted photodynamic therapy of squamous cell carcinoma in the casque of a great hornbill (Buceros bicornis). J Avian Med Surg 2001;15(1):44–9.

57. Suedmeyer WK, Henry C, McCaw D, et al. Attempted photodynamic therapy against patagial squamous cell carcinoma in an African rose-ringed parakeet (Psittacula krameri). J zoo Wildl Med 2007;38(4):597–600.

58. De Queiroz GF, Matera JM, Zaidan Dagli ML. Clinical study of cryosurgery efficacy in the treatment of skin and subcutaneous tumors in dogs and cats. Vet Surg 2008;37(5):438–43.

59. Mans C, Pilny A. Use of GnRH-agonists for medical management of reproductive disorders in birds. Vet Clin North Am Exot Anim Pract 2014;17(1):23–33.

60. Nemetz L. Deslorelin acetate long-term supression of ovarian carcinoma in a cockatiel (Nymphicus hollandicus). Proc Annu Conf Assoc Avian Vet 2012;37–42.

61. Keller KA, Beaufrère H, Brandão J, et al. Long-term management of ovarian neoplasia in two cockatiels (Nymphicus hollandicus). J Avian Med Surg 2013; 27(1):44–52.

62. Straub J, Zenker I. First experience in hormonal treatment of sertoli cell tumors in budgerigars (M. undulates) with absorbable extended release GnRH chips (Suprelorin®) 1st International Conference on Avian, Herpetological and Exotic Mammal Medicine. Wiesbaden (Germany), April 20–26, 2013. p. 299–301.

63. Tavares WL, Lavalle GE, Figueiredo MS, et al. Evaluation of adverse effects in tamoxifen exposed healthy female dogs. Acta Vet Scand 2010;52:67.

64. Beaufrere H, Brasseur G, Heimann M. What is your diagnosis? Squamous cell carcinoma of the uropygial gland. J Avian Med Surg 2007;21(4):321–4.

65. Murtaugh RJ, Ringler DJ, Petrak ML. Squamous cell carcinoma of the esophagus in an Amazon parrot. J Am Vet Med Assoc 1986;188(8):872–3.

66. Malka S, Keirstead ND, Gancz AY, et al. Ingluvial squamous cell carcinoma in a geriatric cockatiel (Nymphicus hollandicus). J Avian Med Surg 2005;19(3): 234–9.

67. Youl JM, Gartrell BD. Multidrug-resistant bacterial ingluvitis associated with squamous cell carcinoma in a budgerigar (Melopsittacus undulatus). Vet Clin North Am Exot Anim Pract 2006;9(3):557–62.

68. Zehnder A, Swift L, Sundaram A, et al. Multi-instiutional survey of squamous cell carcinoma in birds. Paper presented at: 35th Annu Conf Assoc Avian Vet. New Orleans (LA), August 2–6, 2014.

69. Nemetz L, BM. Strontium-90 therapy for uropygial neoplasia. Paper presented at: Proc Annu Conf Assoc Avian Vet 25th Annual Conference. New Orleans (LA), August 17–19, 2004.

70. Mehler SJ, Briscoe JA, Hendrick MJ, et al. Infiltrative lipoma in a blue-crowned conure (Aratinga acuticaudata). J Avian Med Surg 2007;21(2):146–9.

71. Rosenhagen N, Whittington JK, Hsiao SH. Infiltrative spinal lipoma in a canada goose (Branta canadensis). J Avian Med Surg 2016;30(1):60–5.

72. De Voe RS, Trogdon M, Flammer K. Preliminary assessment of the effect of diet and L-carnitine supplementation on lipoma size and bodyweight in budgerigars (Melopsittacus undulatus). J Avian Med Surg 2004;18(1):12–8.

73. Tully TN, Morris JM, Veazey RS, et al. Liposarcomas in a monk parakeet (Myiopsitta monachus). J Assoc Avian Med 1994;8(3):120–4.

74. Graham JE, Werner JA, Lowenstine LJ, et al. Periorbital Liposarcoma in an African Grey Parrot (Psittacus erithacus). J Avian Med Surg 2003;17(3):147–53.

75. Burgmann PM. Pulmonary fibrosarcoma with hepatic metastases in a cockatiel (Nymphicus Hollandicus). J Assoc Avian Med 1994;8:81–4.

76. Riddell C, Cribb PH. Fibrosarcoma in an African Grey Parrot (Psittacus erithacus). Avian Dis 1983;27(2):549–55.

77. Palmieri C, Cusinato I, Avallone G, et al. Cloacal fibrosarcoma in a canary (Serinus canaria). J Avian Med Surg 2011;25(4):277–80.

78. Souza MJ, Johnstone-McLean NS, Ward D, et al. Conjunctival xanthoma in a blue and gold macaw (Ara ararauna). Vet Ophthalmol 2009;12(1):53–5.

79. Lipar M, HD. Prukner-radovcic. Subcutaneous xanthoma in a cockatiel (Nymphocus hollandicus)- a case report. Veterinarski Arhiv 2011;81(4):535–43.

80. Dittmer KE, French AF, Thompson DJ, et al. Primary bone tumors in birds: a review and description of two new cases. Avian Dis 2012;56(2):422–6.

81. Nakano Y, Une Y. Synovial sarcoma associated with indwelling intramedullary pin in a peach-faced lovebird (Agapornis roseicollis). J Avian Med Surg 2016; 30(1):23–9.

82. Reavill DR, Dorrestein GM. Pathology of aging psittacines. Vet Clin North Am Exot Anim Pract 2010;13(1):135–50.

83. Fernandez-Bellon H, Martorell J, Rabanal R, et al. Rhabdomyosarcoma in a racing pigeon (Columba livia). Avian Pathol 2003;32(6):613–6.

84. Lennox A, Clubb S, Romagnano A, et al. Monoclonal hyperglobulinemia in lymphosarcoma in a cockatiel (Nymphicus hollandicus) and a blue and gold macaw (Ara ararauna). Avian Dis 2014;58(2):326–9.

85. Woodhouse SJ, Rose M, Desjardins DR, et al. Diagnosis of retrobulbar round cell neoplasia in a macaroni penguin (Eudyptes chrysolophus) through use of computed tomography. J Avian Med Surg 2015;29(1):40–5.

86. Diaz-Figueroa O, Tully TN, Williams J, et al. Squamous cell carcinoma of the infraorbital sinus with fungal tracheitis and ingluvitis in an adult solomon eclectus parrot (Eclectus roratus solomonensis). J Avian Med Surg 2006;20(2):113–9.

87. Noonan BP, de Matos R, Butler BP, et al. Nasal adenocarcinoma and secondary chronic sinusitis in a hyacinth macaw (Anodorhynchus hyacinthinus). J Avian Med Surg 2014;28(2):143–50.

88. Raidal SR, Shearer PL, Butler R, et al. Airsac cystadenocarcinomas in cockatoos. Aust Vet J 2006;84(6):213–6.

89. Loukopoulos P, Okuni JB, Micco T, et al. Air sac adenocarcinoma of the sternum in a Quaker parrot (Myiopsitta monachus). J Zoo Wildl Med 2014;45(4): 961–5.

90. Baumgartner WA, Guzman DS, Hollibush S, et al. Bronchogenic adenocarci-noma in a hyacinth macaw (Anodorhynchus hyacinthinus). J Avian Med Surg 2008;22(3):218–25.
91. Rettenmund C, Sladky KK, Rodriguez D, et al. Pulmonary carcinoma in a great horned owl (Bubo virginianus). J Zoo Wildl Med 2010;41(1):77–82.
92. Fredholm DV, Carpenter JW, Shumacher LL, et al. Pulmonary adenocarcinoma with osseous metastasis and secondary paresis in a blue and gold macaw (Ara ararauna). J Zoo Wildl Med 2012;43(4):909–13.
93. Andre Jean-Pierre DM. Primary bronchial carcinoma with osseous metastasis in an african grey parrot (Psittacus erithacus). J Avian Med Surg 1999;13(3): 180–6.
94. Marshall K, Daniel G, Patton C, et al. Humeral air sac mucinous adenocarci-noma in a salmon-crested cockatoo (Cacatua moluccensis). J Avian Med Surg 2004;18(3):167–74.
95. Garner MM, Latimer KS, Mickley KA, et al. Histologic, immunohistochemical, and electron microscopic features of a unique pulmonary tumor in cockatiels (Nymphicus hollandicus): six cases. Vet Pathol 2009;46(6):1100–8.
96. Rosenwax AC, Gabor M, Reece RL. Respiratory hamartoma in a cockatiel (Nymphicus hollandicus). Aust Vet J 2013;91(12):531–3.
97. Campbell TW, Turner O. Carcinoma of the ventriculus with metastasis to the lungs in a sulphur-crested cockatoo (Cacatua galerita). J Avian Med Surg 1999;13(4):265–8.
98. Yonemaru K, Sakai H, Asaoka Y, et al. Proventricular adenocarcinoma in a Humboldt penguin (Spheniscus humboldti) and a great horned owl (Bubo virgin-ianus); identification of origin by mucin histochemistry. Avian Pathol 2004;33(1): 77–81.
99. Leach MW, Paul-Murphy J, Lowenstine LJ. Three cases of gastric neoplasia in psittacines. Avian Dis 1989;33(1):204–10.
100. Coleman CW. Bile duct carcinoma and cloacal prolapse in an orange-winged amazon parrot. J Assoc Avian Med 1991;5(2):87–9.
101. Potter KCT, Galina AM. Cholangiocarcinoma in a yellow-faced amazon parrots (Amazona xanthops). Avian Dis 1983;27(2):556–8.
102. Hillyer EV, Moroff S, Hoefer H, et al. Bile duct carcinoma in two out of ten Amazon Parrots with cloacal papillomas. J Assoc Avian Med 1991;5(2):91–5.
103. Tennakoon AH, Izawa T, Fujita D, et al. Combined hepatocellular-cholangiocarcinoma in a Yellow-headed Amazon (Amazona oratrix). J Vet Med Sci 2013;75(11):1507–10.
104. Zantop DW. Treatment of bile duct carcinoma in birds with carboplatin. Exot DVM 2000;2(3):76–8.
105. Carleton RE, Garner MM. Oviductal adenocarcinoma with osseous and myeloid metaplasia associated with sternal hyperostosis in a cockatiel (Nymphicus hol-landicus). J Avian Med Surg 2002;16(4):309–13.
106. Reavill DRaRS. Tumors of the psittacine ovary and oviduct: 37 cases. Paper pre-sented at: Proc Annu Conf Assoc Avian Vet. Pittsburgh (PA), August, 2003.
107. Mickley K, Buote M, Kiupel M, et al. Ovarian hemangiosarcoma in an orange-winged Amazon parrot (Amazona amazonica). J Avian Med Surg 2009;23(1): 29–35.
108. Stauber E, Papageorges M, Sande R, et al. Polyostotic hyperostosis associated with oviductal tumor in a cockatiel. J Am Vet Med Assoc 1990;196(6):939–40.
109. Baumgartner R, Hatt J-M, Dobeli M, et al. Endocrinologic and pathologic find-ings in birds with polyostotic hyperostosis. J Avian Med Surg 1995;9(4):251–4.

110. Jones R. The surgical management ofan ovarian sex cord stromal cell tumour in a northern goshawk (Accipiter gentilis) Paper presented at: ICARE. Paris (France), April 18–23, 2015.
111. Drury Reavill MSE, Schmidt R. Testicular Tumors of 54 Birds and Therapy in 6 Cases. Paper presented at: Association of Avian Veterinarians. New Orleans, August 16–19, 2004.
112. Schimdt RE, Reavill DR, Phalen DN. Pathology of pet and aviary birds. Ames (IA): Iowa State Press; 2003.
113. Simova-Curd S, Nitzl D, Mayer J, et al. Clinical approach to renal neoplasia in budgerigars (Melopsittacus undulatus). J Small Anim Pract 2006;47(9):504–11.
114. Simova-Curd SA, Huder JB, Boeni J, et al. Investigations on the diagnosis and retroviral aetiology of renal neoplasia in budgerigars (Melopsittacus undulatus). Avian Pathol 2010;39(3):161–7.
115. Bras ID, Gemensky-Metzler AJ, Kusewitt DF, et al. Immunohistochemical characterization of a malignant intraocular teratoid medulloepithelioma in a cockatiel. Vet Ophthalmol 2005;8(1):59–65.
116. Schmidt RE, Becker LL, McElroy JM. Malignant intraocular medulloepithelioma in two cockatiels. J Am Vet Med Assoc 1986;189(9):1105–6.
117. Hvenegaard AP, Safatle AMV, Guimarães MB, et al. Retrospective study of ocular disorders in Amazon parrots. Pesquisa Veterinária Brasileira 2009;29: 979–84.
118. Watson VE, Murdock JH, Cazzini P, et al. Retrobulbar adenocarcinoma in an Amazon parrot (Amazona autumnalis). J Vet Diagn Invest 2013;25(2):273–6.
119. Hartcourt-Brown N. Periorbital liposarcoma in an African grey parrot. Paper presented at: 10th EAAV and 8th ECAMS Conference. Antwerp, March 17–21, 2009.
120. Rodriguez-Ramos Fernandez J, Dubielzig RR. Ocular and eyelid neoplasia in birds: 15 cases (1982–2011). Vet Ophthalmol 2015;18:113–8.

Oncology of Reptiles
Diseases, Diagnosis, and Treatment

 CrossMark

Jane Christman, DVM[a], Michael Devau, DVM, DACVR (Radiation Oncology)[a],
Heather Wilson-Robles, DVM, DACVIM (Oncology)[a], Sharman Hoppes, DVM, DABVP (Avian)[a],
Raquel Rech, DVM, MS, PhD[b], Karen E. Russell, DVM, PhD, DACVP (ClinPath)[a],
J. Jill Heatley, DVM, MS, DABVP (Avian, Reptilian & Amphibian), DACZM[a],*

KEYWORDS

• Lizard • Chelonian • Snake • Cancer • Neoplasia • Chemotherapy • Radiation

KEY POINTS

• There is a lack of prospective research on treatment modalities for reptile species.
• Secondary treatment modalities and treatment of metastatic or systemic neoplasia that have been used in reptiles include chemotherapy (local and systemic), radiation, electro-chemotherapy, laser therapy, cryotherapy, and photodynamic therapy.
• Husbandry considerations including proper nutrition and housing requirements specific to each species are important in the management of reptile patients affected by neoplasia.

INTRODUCTION

Reptiles are a diverse class of animals for which there are unique anatomic consider-ations as well as complex physiologic and pathophysiologic processes. However, they are prone to the diseases and disorders that are common to the animal kingdom, including neoplasia. Based on necropsy review, captive reptiles have an incidence of neoplasia comparable with that of mammals and birds.[1] Some reports have sug-gested an increasing incidence of neoplasia in reptiles.[2–4] However, neoplastic pro-cesses have even been noted with some frequency in ancient reptile ancestors, including several extinct dinosaur species.[5] Recently, advances in medical knowledge and diagnostic capabilities in veterinary medicine have improved antemortem diag-nostics and neoplasia is now a more commonly diagnosed clinical problem affecting

Disclosure: The authors have nothing to disclose.
[a] Department of Small Animal Clinical Sciences, College of Veterinary Medicine and Biomedical Sciences, Texas A&M University, 408 Raymond Stotzer Parkway, College Station, TX 77843-4474, USA; [b] Department of Veterinary Pathobiology, College of Veterinary Medicine and Biomedical Sciences, Texas A&M University, 400 Raymond Stotzer Parkway, College Station, TX 77843-4467, USA
* Corresponding author.
E-mail address: jheatley@cvm.tamu.edu

a wide variety of reptilian species.[2–4,6–10] Reptiles are becoming increasingly popular in the United States as pets,[11] and continue to be maintained in zoologic and research settings. Modern reptile owners are more likely to be interested in pursuing advanced diagnostics and treatments. Therefore, updating current information on diagnostic and treatment modalities for neoplastic processes is essential. However, the diagnosis of a malignant neoplasm in a reptilian patient continues to be challenging for exotic animal clinicians, because primary research in specific tumor types is lacking. For this reason, best practice often remains unknown.

Although reptiles differ considerably in their anatomy and physiology from other taxa, most cancer treatments are adapted from clinical and basic science research and clinical oncology practice in companion mammals. A lack of knowledge in reptile oncology regarding effective treatment protocols makes translational medicine combined with good clinical judgment a necessity to provide the best outcomes for reptiles with cancer. Therefore, veterinary clinicians seeing reptile patients must be generally familiar with diagnosis, treatment, and prognosis of various neoplastic processes in companion animal species. Consultation and collaboration with companion mammal veterinary oncologists is highly recommended for these cases.

This article provides exotic animal veterinary practitioners with a review of current literature, including case reports and primary research on neoplasia in reptiles, and gives an overview of the available diagnostic and treatment tools for use in reptiles with these conditions. It is hoped that this review will facilitate diagnosis of neoplasia in reptiles and challenge veterinary practitioners to document and report treatment of neoplasia in these species, independent of outcome, to advance the knowledge of, and improve standards of care for, these species (**Fig. 2**).

DISEASES

In the last 10 years, numerous case reports and several case series have described neoplasia across various reptile species. Most modern reports describe a specific tumor type occurring in a specific reptile species. Limited data exist describing a range of tumor types in a single species or a single tumor type across multiple species. Case reports of reptile neoplasia from the last 10 years, including tumor type, species group, location, and treatment performed, are listed in **Table 1**. This information, along with

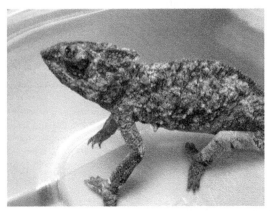

Fig. 1. Multiple cutaneous papillomas in a chameleon (*Chamaeleo* sp). This lizard also has dysecdysis. (*Courtesy of* Michael Garner, DVM, DACVP, Northwest ZooPath.)

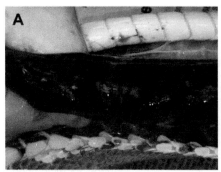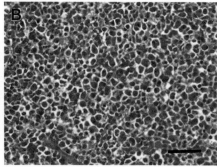

Fig. 2. Round cell tumor in a green tree python (*Morelia viridis*). (*A*) Off white nodular mass in the coelom. (*B*) Histologic appearance of the tumor in in A. Note the sheets of rounds cells with eccentric nuclei and amphophlic cytoplasm resembling plasma cells. A reliable B cell marker has not been found for reptile lymphoid tumors. (Hematoxylin and eosin stain, bar=150 um). (*Courtesy of* Michael Garner, DVM, DACVP, Northwest ZooPath.)

previously published reviews,[2–4] provides veterinary clinical practitioners a foundation of the types of tumors reptiles acquire and their relative prognosis.

Although most tumors in reptiles are spontaneous in origin, as in other species, some tumor types have a known cause as causing tumors in a variety of mammals. Specific to reptiles, several viruses have been identified for their carcinogenic potential in association with tumors. Viruslike eosinophilic intranuclear inclusions were found in the neoplastic lymphocytes of a California king snake (*Lampropeltis getulus californiae*).[67] The association between a herpesvirus and fibropapillomatosis in green sea turtles (*Chelonia mydas*),[68,69] a papovavirus and papillomatosis in the European green lizards (*Lacerta viridis*) and Bolivian side-neck turtles (*Platemys platycephala*),[70] and a poxvirus causing brown papules in 1 tegu (*Tupinambis teguexin*) have been documented (see **Fig. 8**).[71] C-type virus particles within primary tumor tissues of a corn snake (*Elaphe guttata*) with a chondrosarcoma, suggest a viral cause. Other carcinogens suspected to induce neoplastic disease in reptiles include ultraviolet light irradiation and arenavirus (**Fig. 3**).[72–75]

Factors predisposing to tumor development in reptiles continue to be elucidated. A genetic predisposition is suspected in several recent reports of genetically related reptiles, including renal adenocarcinoma occurring in 3 Cape coral snakes[76] and chondrosarcoma in 2 related monitor lizards.[30] Hormone profile alterations may also predispose reptiles to neoplastic disease. Iatrogenic hormonal alternations after incomplete elective castration surgeries are a suspected cause of ovarian cancer in dogs and cats[77] and similar hormone derangements have been a suggested cause of ovarian tumors in reptiles as well. A granulosa cell tumor in a green iguana was accompanied by an altered hormone profile after incomplete ovariosalpingectomy (**Fig. 4**).[43] Multicentric cutaneous papillomas are occasionally seen in lizards, especially chameleons. These lesions typically occur on the dorsum and flanks. The etiology has not been determined despite fairly extensive trasmission electron microscopy and currently available immunohistochemical and molecular techniaques. Viral and solar etiologies have been considered but not proven. Importantly, these papillomas have potential for undergoing dysplastic change or malignant neoplastic transformation to squamous cell carcinoma, and the latter can be invasive and difficult to completely excise (**Fig. 1**; Garner, M. NW Zoo Path, personal communication, 2016).

Based on animals submitted to diagnostic pathology services, the reported incidence of neoplasia in reptiles varies from 12% to 26%.[2–4,6–10] Variation in these

Table 1
Case reports of neoplasia in reptilian species published since 2004 and their treatment and relative outcome, if reported

Year	Site	Species	Tumor Type	Tumor Location	Treatment	Outcome	Reference
Snake							
2011	Bone	Woma python	Osteosarcoma	Bone	None	Euthanasia	13
2012		Corn snake	Chondrosarcoma	Bone	None	Euthanasia	14
2012	Cardiac	Corn snake	Hemangioma	Cardiac	Surgical excision	Euthanasia	29
2010		Reticulated python	Fibrosarcoma	Cardiac	None	Euthanasia	15
2011	Hematopoietic	Red-tailed boa	Lymphoblastic lymphoma	Hematopoietic	None	Died	12
2012	Cutaneous	Diamond python	Papilloma	Cutaneous	None	Spontaneous regression	20
2007		Yellow-bellied racer	Chromatophoromas	Cutaneous	Surgical excision	No recurrence	18
2013		Diamondback rattlesnake	Squamous cell carcinoma	Cutaneous	Surgical excision	No recurrence	22
2013	Hepatobiliary	Madagascar tree boa	Anaplastic sarcoma	Gallbladder, intracoelomic fat	Surgical excision	Died	26
2008		Madagascar tree boa	Biphasic undifferentiated mesenchymal tumor	Hepatic, multicentric	None	Died	21
2014	Gastrointestinal	Diamond python	Adenocarcinoma	Gastric wall	Surgical excision	Died	28
2015		Boa constrictor	Melanoma	Oral	None	Euthanized	24
2015		Jararaca	Fibrosarcoma	Oral	Surgical excision	Unknown	45
2015		Black rat snake	Ameloblastoma	Oral	None	Euthanasia	25
2013		Madagascar ground boa	Squamous cell carcinoma	Oral	Radiation	Euthanasia	19
2010	Endocrine	Everglades rat snake	Cystadenoma	Pituitary	None	Euthanasia	27

	Year	Species	Diagnosis	Location	Treatment	Outcome	Ref.
	2014	Northern water snake	Adenocarcinoma	Splenopancreas	None	Euthanasia	23
	2012	Western hognose	Adenocarcinoma	Splenopancreas	Surgical excision	Euthanasia	17
Lizard							
Bone	2013	Spiny tailed monitor	Chondroblastic osteosarcoma	Bone	None	Euthanasia	30
	2007	Uromastyx	Periosteal chondroma	Juxtacortical bone	None	Euthanasia	62
Cutaneous	2011	Bearded dragon	Squamous cell carcinoma	Cutaneous	Surgical excision	No recurrence	31
	2014	African fat tailed gecko	Mastocytosis	Cutaneous	None	Death	32
	2015	Bearded dragon	Iridiophoroma	Subcutaneous	Surgical excision	Metastasis	33
	2006	Green iguana	Melanophoroma	Cutaneous	Surgical excision	Unknown	34
Hematopoietic	2015	Tokay gecko	Carcinoma	Endolymphatic Sac	None	Euthanasia	35
	2011	Green iguana	Lymphoma (uncharacterized)	Hematopoietic	Radiation (1 treatment), vascular access port, and chemotherapy (doxorubicin, vincristine, cyclophosphamide, and prednisone)	No recurrence	36
	2005	Spiny tailed lizards	B-cell lymphoma	Hematopoietic	None	Euthanasia	50
	2011	Bearded dragon	Leukemia	Hematopoietic	Chemotherapy (cytosine arabinoside)	Death	38
Hepatobiliary	2012	Green iguana	Carcinoma	Hepatic	None	Euthanasia	39
Gastrointestinal	2016	Green iguana	Mast cell tumor	Oral	Surgical excision	Unknown	TAMU 216298
	2013	Black iguana	Fibrosarcoma	Oral	Unknown	Unknown	40

(continued on next page)

Table 1
(continued)

Year	Site	Species	Tumor Type	Tumor Location	Treatment	Outcome	Reference
2016		Mexican spiny tailed iguana	Squamous cell carcinoma	Oral, Head	Surgical excision	Incomplete resection	TAMU 228256
2005		Leopard gecko	Adenocarcinoma	Colon	None	Euthanasia	41
2010	Reproductive	Fiji island banded iguana	Teratoma	Ovarian	Surgical excision	No recurrence	85
2010		Green iguana	Teratoma	Ovarian	Surgical excision	No recurrence	85
2011		Green iguana	Granulosa cell tumor	Ovarian	Surgical excision, Intracoelomic carboplatin	Metastasis	43
2013		Monitor lizard	Granulosa cell tumor	Ovarian	Surgical excision	Metastasis	44
2004		Green iguana	Cystadenocarcinoma	Ovarian	Surgical excision	Euthanasia	37
2016		Savannah monitor	Adenocarcinoma	Ovary, cardiac	Surgical excision	Euthanasia	TAMU 184555
2014	Periorbital	Bearded dragon	Myxosarcoma	Periorbital	Surgical excision and radiation	Recurrence	46
2013		Bearded dragon	Adenocarcinoma	Periorbital	Surgical excision	Recurrence	47
2014	Pulmonary	Beaded lizard	Melanophoroma	Pulmonary	Surgical excision	No recurrence	48
2012	Endocrine	Diplodactylid geckos	Carcinoma	Thyroid	Surgical excision	No recurrence	49
2006	Miscellaneous	Yemenite chameleon	Ganglioneuroblastoma	Unknown	Unknown	Unknown	42
Chelonian							
2015	Bone	Northern red-bellied cooter	Mucinous melanophoroma	Bone	None	Death	51
		Asian leaf turtle	Adenocarcinoma	Bone	None	Euthanasia	94
2015	Cutaneous	Yellow-bellied slider	Squamous cell carcinoma	Cutaneous	Surgical excision, electrochemotherapy	No recurrence	53

Year	Category	Species	Tumor	Location	Treatment	Outcome	Reference
2013		Desert tortoise	Adenocarcinoma	Cutaneous	Surgical excision	Tumor recurrence	54
2012		Common snapping turtle	Fibroma	Cutaneous	Surgical excision	Unknown	55
2007		Galapagos tortoise	Mast Cell Tumor	Cutaneous	Surgical excision	No recurrence	56
2016		Galapagos tortoise	Osteoma	Subcutaneous, Cervical	Surgical Excision	No recurrence	TAMU 219609
2005		Radiated tortoise	Undifferentiated sarcoma	Subcutaneous	Surgical excision	No recurrence	57
		Hermann's tortoise	Melanophoroma	Cutaneous	Unknown	Unknown	58
2013	Hematopoietic	Chinese box turtle	Lymphoid leukemia	Hematopoietic	None	Euthanasia	59
2013	GI	Mata mata turtle	Adenocarcinoma	Esophageal	None	Death	60
		Red-eared slider	Hemangioma	Esophageal	None	Euthanasia	61
2015	Reproductive	Spur-thighed tortoise	Seminoma	Testicular	None	Euthanasia	64
2009		Mediterranean tortoise	Teratoma	Ovarian	None	Death	63
2009	Endocrine	Florida red-bellied turtle	Harderian adenocarcinoma	Harderian Gland	None	Euthanasia	65
2012	Musculoskeletal	Galapagos tortoise	Rhabdomyosarcoma	Subcarapacial skeletal muscle	Surgical excision	Unknown	66

Abbreviation: TAMU, Texas A&M University.

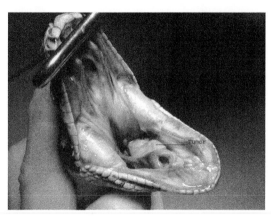

Fig. 3. Ball python (*Python regius*) with spindle cell sarcoma of the oropharyngeal soft tissue adjacent to the tracheal opening. (*Courtesy of* Robert Monaco, DVM, DABVP (Avian).)

estimates may be caused by reporting bias based on differences in location, collection types, institutions, and private practices performing the reviews. Only a few comprehensive reviews are available for neoplasia in reptiles. In chelonians, lizards, and snakes, neoplasms of every nearly every body surface and tumor type have been described. Combining a total of 477 cases from previous published reviews[2–4] and the authors' current review (66 chelonians, 282 snakes, and 129 lizards), the most common systems affected by neoplasia include the hematopoietic (14.9%), hepatobiliary (13.1%), and integumentary system (12.8%).[3–8]

Turtles and tortoises have a relatively low incidence of neoplasia (10.3%),[2–4] and possibly a lower than expected incidence of metastasis.[55–57] Thus less is known regarding neoplasia types in these species. One study found a slightly higher prevalence of neoplasia in turtles and terrapins (3.2%) than in tortoises (1.4%).[2] The skin is the most commonly reported location for neoplasms among chelonian species (21.2%).[53–55,57] Cutaneous squamous cell carcinoma is the most commonly reported neoplasm in chelonians, although mast cell tumors, fibromas, and adenocarcinomas have also been described.[2,53,54,56] Chelonians may also have a higher rate of

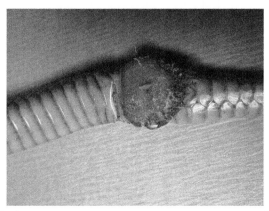

Fig. 4. Garter snake (Natricinae) with ulcerated, cutaneous squamous cell carcinoma of the tail immediately caudal to the cloaca. (*Courtesy of* Robert Monaco, DVM, DABVP (Avian).)

endocrine tumors than other reptiles, as identified in the author's current review (15.1%). Thyroid adenocarcinoma is the most commonly reported single tumor of endocrine origin reported in chelonia.

Snakes are the class of Reptilia most commonly reported as affected by neoplasia.[2–4,6–8] One study found a higher prevalence of neoplasia in colubrids, with decreasing neoplastic prevalences in crotalids, vipers, and boids respectively.[2] The hematopoietic and lymphoid systems are most commonly affected, followed by neoplasia of epithelial origin.[6,7] Snakes have a high incidence of renal adenocarcinoma. Of reviewed renal adenomas and adenocarcinomas in 8 snakes, most tumors had low mitotic index and locally invasive nature.[78] Melanophoroma is the third most common tumor type reported to affect snakes, which commonly presents as a single, often white, cutaneous mass. These tumors of pigment producing cells are locally invasive and have a poor prognosis for the affected snake.[10,24,48] A retrospective study of chromatophoromas in snakes, lizards, and a tortoise showed a higher rate of malignancy for melanophoromas than iridiophoromas. A mucinous subtype of melanophoromas, characterized by a proteoglycan-rich extracellular matrix, described in bearded dragons, a Hermann's tortoise, and a red-bellied cooter, also has a poor prognosis based on local invasion rather than metastasis.[10,33,51,58] Definitive diagnosis and differentiation of chromatophoromas can be attempted with immunohistochemistry. Ovarian adenocarcinomas have been described in several snake species, and typically involve widespread metastasis and a poor prognosis. These tumors may have a hormonal predisposition, although causality has not been established.[79]

Lizards have a median incidence of neoplastic disease compared with snakes, turtles, and tortoises, and the hematopoietic, cutaneous, and hepatic systems are most commonly affected.[2–4,8,9] Bearded dragons (*Pogona vitticeps*) and green iguanas (*Iguana iguana*) are over-represented in recent case reports, likely based on their popularity as pets and increased frequency of visits to veterinarians. In one retrospective pathology study, monitors, skinks, agamids, and geckos had neoplastic prevalences from 7.7% to 9.9%, whereas iguanids and chameleons had lesser prevalences of 3.4% to 3.9%.[2] Lymphoma is the most commonly reported single neoplasia of lizards. Literature review reveals at total of 22 specific cases from 10 *Uromastyx* spp, 4 monitor lizards (*Varanus* spp), 1 desert spiny lizard (*Sceloporus magister*), 2 bearded dragons (*P vitticeps*), 1 Asian water dragon, 2 green iguanas (*I iguana*), a ruin lizard (*Lacerta sicula*), and an east Indian water lizard (*Hydrosaurus amboinensis*). One retrospective pathology study reported the lymphoma prevalence of lizards as 9.3%, included 15 possible additional cases of lymphomatous lizards, and added the chuckwalla (*Sauromalus* spp) **(Fig. 5)**.[2,50,80–82]

Squamous cell carcinoma is also common among reported neoplasms in lizards.[2] Based on literature review as well as a case at Texas A&M University, more than 30 cases of squamous cell carcinoma have occurred in lizard species, including, in order of declining numbers reported, 13 bearded dragons (*P vitticeps*), 6 monitor lizards (*Varanus* spp), 7 sand lizards (*Lacerta agilis*), 2 tegus (*Tupinambis* spp), 2 chameleons, 3 skinks, 2 iguanas, and single cases in the Gila monster (*Heloderma suspectum*), leopard gecko (*Eublepharis macularius*), and tuatara (*Sphenodon punctatus*).[2–4] The authors suspect that many more cases remain unreported. Note that many of these species have pineal eyes and depend on solar or other heat radiation for maintenance of their preferred optimum body temperature. The presenting complaint is usually based on mass visualization or, should the oral cavity be affected, inanition. The foot, ear canal, perivent, perioral, and periocular tissues have been affected and a predilection for tissues in proximity to mucocutaneous junctions to be affected has been

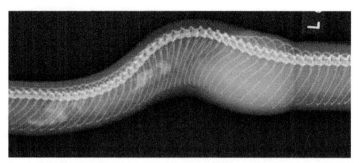

Fig. 5. Radiograph of a circumscribed midcoelomic soft tissue opacity in a 7-year old, female ball python (*P regius*). Subsequent histopathology determined that the mass was an undifferentiated sarcoma. (*With permission* of Texas A&M University Veterinary Medical Teaching Hospital, College Station, TX.)

suggested.[31] In lizards, metastasis of squamous cell carcinomas seems to be rare and has yet to reported, but local invasion should be expected.[2,31,83]

DIAGNOSTICS

Diagnosis of neoplastic disease in reptile patients parallels that recommended for use in humans or domestic animals.[84] As in other species, early diagnosis results in a more effective treatment plan and better long-term prognosis for the patient, especially in reptiles, in which the owner or caretaker may not notice a problem until the patient is extremely debilitated. Additional research is needed to further elucidate the best diagnostic methods for use in reptiles with neoplastic disease. At present, history, physical examination, clinical pathology, imaging, and microscopic evaluation are minimum requirements. Based on oncology principles, staging and grading of tumor types should be included in neoplastic diagnosis but are seldom pursued in reptile medicine. Further, clinicians should be aware that, in reptilian medicine, performing all indicated diagnostics may still only lead to a tentative diagnosis of neoplasia.

A thorough history and physical examination are essential in forming a preliminary diagnosis. Presenting complaints of reptiles are often nonspecific, and neoplasia should be included in the differential diagnosis for lethargic or anorexic reptilian patients. Reptile patients often present with cutaneous masses or nonhealing cutaneous lesions and infectious, traumatic, and degenerative differentials must be considered. Clinical signs most commonly reported in reptiles diagnosed with neoplasia include lethargy, anorexia, dyspnea, cutaneous masses, coelomic distension, constipation, or paresis/paralysis.[2,8,10,22,31,47] Clinical signs vary depending on tumor type and location. Presentation of an aged reptile should increase the clinician's suspicion of neoplasia, especially in combination with other compatible clinical signs. Neoplasia is more common in older reptiles, but has been described in young animals, such as monitor lizards as young as 5 months of age.[30,34] During physical examination of the reptile suspected of having neoplastic disease, clinicians should carefully and completely evaluate the patient for integument abnormalities, or masses, or displaced organs within the coelom. Thorough examination and palpation may reveal masses as an incidental finding. Any observed masses on or within a reptilian patient should be fully evaluated. The differential diagnosis for a mass in a reptile is similar to those of companion mammals and include inflammatory diseases such as abscesses, granulomas (parasitic, fungal, protozoal, or bacterial), nutritional deficiencies such as hypovitaminosis A, and traumatic and degenerative causes (**Fig. 6**).

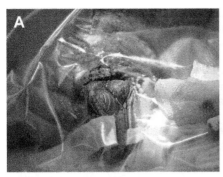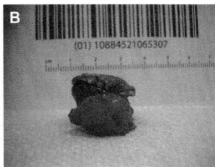

Fig. 6. Subcutaneous mast cell tumor surgically resected from the cutaneous and pharyngeal tissue of a green iguana (*I iguana*). (*A*) During surgery; (*B*) excised gross tumor. (*With permission* of Texas A&M University Veterinary Medical Teaching Hospital, College Station, TX.)

The minimum evaluation of reptilian patients presenting with possible neoplasia includes baseline blood work. Complete blood count and plasma biochemistry results can be used to determine the relative health of the patient, to identify systemic manifestations of disease, and for surgical planning. Paraneoplastic syndromes may manifest via an inflammatory leukogram, and some hematopoietic tumors such as lymphoma and leukemia are associated with severe lymphocytosis.[9,36,38,59,73,80,81] Plasma biochemical abnormalities may be challenging to assess and depend on the tumor type and functionality. Commonly reported abnormalities in reptiles with neoplastic disease include, but are not limited to, hypercalcemia, hypoglycemia or hyperglycemia, hyperphosphatemia, and increased plasma activities of alanine transaminase and creatine kinase.[42,80,81,85-89]

Imaging can facilitate diagnosis and provide information about the tumor type, areas affected, and prognosis. Radiography is the most widely used imaging tool for reptilian patients, based on availability, cost, and adequate veterinary training in classic interpretation. However, the interpretation of radiographs of reptile patients remains a challenge based on the varying radiographic anatomy of these species.[3,52] Attention to proper reptile positioning to provide the best image possible is highly recommended.[52] Because radiographic imaging of reptiles is often performed with only manual restraint or light sedation, this imaging modality can provide quick internal assessment of debilitated patients.[52] Radiographs also provide an excellent way to assess the relationship between internal organs, and to assess obvious changes such as a mass effect within the coelom. However, based on the lack of organ-silhouetting fat, the thick and sometimes scaled skin of these species, and variable species anatomy within this group, the ability to assess individual organ structure or interior anatomy in these species remains poor based on radiographic imaging. Turtles and tortoises present further challenges for radiographic assessment because of their bony carapace.[52] Craniocaudal horizontal beam radiographs are necessary to fully evaluate the coelomic cavity of chelonians. Large metastatic tumors in the pulmonary parenchyma are best evaluated in these horizontal beam views; however, a more detailed full coelomic view is limited in these species.[52]

Ultrasonographic imaging of reptiles is becoming more common in veterinary practice and can provide important information about tumor architecture and organ infiltration. Ultrasonography is superior for the differentiation of fluid and soft tissues and can also be used to guide fine-needle aspirates of coelomic fluid, internal masses, or other abnormal structures for cytologic examination. Results of ultrasonography in reptile medicine depend on the experience and skills of the surveyor. Few imaging studies of reptile species are available to provide expected size or echogenicity of internal organ structures. Evaluation of the contralateral paired organ can be helpful in evaluating abdominal structures for asymmetry in species in which normal reference ranges are not available. For the best ultrasonography assessment of reptiles, high-resolution transducers (7.5–10 MHz) and small probes provide the best detail and quality of images to facilitate diagnosis.[52]

Advanced imaging such as computed tomography and MRI are becoming more widely used in reptile medicine. These modalities can provide three-dimensional volumetric images for evaluation of spatial orientation and relations of neoplasms within the coelom and can provide enhanced organ detail compared with radiographs. Thus detection and assessment of smaller, focal neoplasms and can be used for surgical planning. In the future, as advanced imaging becomes more common, so will the advancement of neoplastic diagnosis and staging of reptiles (**Fig. 7**).[18,19,46,80]

Endoscopy can be used in reptiles to assess internal structures and obtain samples for diagnosis. Endoscopy is often a secondary imaging modality performed after survey radiographs to identify an internal mass or lesion, as well as the best entry points. With the aid of insufflation or saline irrigation for organ visualization, many coelomic structures can be visualized and biopsied, including the lungs, liver, and kidneys. Biopsy of lesions is indicated to determine underlying neoplastic or other cause.[52,90]

Microscopic evaluation of tumor types is an important step in the diagnosis of neoplasia and to differentiate neoplastic processes from infectious or inflammatory causes. Antemortem microscopic evaluation may be performed using cytology of fine-needle aspirates or imprints of resected tumors, or histological examination of resected tumors (biopsy). Cytology may be helpful to assess criteria of malignancy and to rule out inflammatory responses.[84,91] Cytologic evaluation of cellular characteristics (shape and size); cohesiveness; and cytoplasmic and nuclear features may help differentiate potential malignant processes. Cellular shape and arrangement (clusters or aggregates or single cells) may be used to differentiate a carcinoma from a sarcoma. General cellular morphology, such as pleomorphism, anisocytosis,

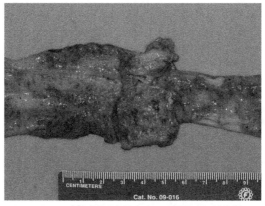

Fig. 7. Colon of a female large eastern pine snake (*Pituophis melanoleucus*) of unknown age submitted for necropsy. Colonic mucosa was thickened by fibrosis and a mucosal mass proliferating and partially obstructing the colonic lumen. Histopathology was consistent with colonic adenocarcinoma. (*Courtesy of* Raquel Rech, DVM, MS, PhD, DACVP.)

anisokaryosis, and variable nuclear:cytoplasmic (N:C) ratios, such as those used on companion mammals, may be equally useful in reptilian patients.[91] However, clinicians must be aware that nondiagnostic cytology results are common in reptile species based on their propensity toward poorly exfoliating tumors and their caseated inflammatory response. Tissue architecture and tumor grade cannot be determined from cytology, which provides only a small window of the area of sample. Should cytology fail to provide a definitive diagnosis, biopsy is almost always indicated in reptile species.

Biopsy is the gold standard for tumor differentiation and allows evaluation of neoplasm architecture and surrounding cells and tissues. Surgically resected tumors should always be submitted for histopathologic analysis to include postsurgical margin assessment. In addition to standard staining, immunohistochemical markers may aid in the determination and differentiation of tumor types.[33,45,59] However, few immunohistochemical or tissue markers of neoplasia that are commonly applied to companion animals are validated or readily available to exotic animal veterinarians.[59] Furthermore, biomarkers used for mammalian species cannot be successfully applied to all reptile species. Immunohistochemistry and the use of other tissue biomarkers has been successfully used for diagnosis of melanophoromas and iridiophoromas with the expression of melan A and S100,[10] gastric neuroendocrine carcinomas in breaded dragons by the expression of somatostatin,[92,93] adenocarcinoma developing from an Asian leaf turtle (*Cyclemys dentata*),[94] hemangioma from a red-eared slider,[61] multiple gall bladder tumors of the bearded dragon with the expression of claudin-7,[95] and cardiac hemangiosarcoma in a Madagascar giant hognose snake (*Leioheterodon madagascariensis*).[96] Consultation with a veterinary pathologist and or oncologist is recommended before obtaining biopsies in order to determine the best tissue preservation methods necessary for histopathology as well as immunohistochemistry specific to the suspected tumor type.

TREATMENT

Cancer treatment guidelines and considerations for reptiles are similar to those of other species. For example, local disease is best treated with local therapy, whereas systemic disease should be treated with systemic therapies. When developing a treatment plan for cancer in reptiles, an individualistic approach for each patient is necessary. Species, age, tumor location, tumor grade, and tumor stage must be accounted for when developing appropriate therapeutic plans. As ectotherms, reptiles affected by neoplasia further require excellent husbandry to include diet, appropriate humidity, and optimum temperature zones.

Surgery is a commonly used and effective means to treat neoplasia and is often curative in cases with easily accessible and resectable tumors. Surgery may be used alone or in combination with other treatments to minimize the chance of recurrence and increase the efficacy of treatment. Surgery must be followed by histopathologic analysis of the resected tissues by a veterinary pathologist for neoplasia determination and margin evaluation. The most common neoplastic complications of surgical intervention are recurrence of the neoplasm at the surgical site, infection, and metastasis.[6,48,53] Surgery and anesthesia have inherent risks in reptiles, and these patients are often debilitated and may have paraneoplastic processes that further complicate anesthesia. Thus anesthetic monitoring and perioperative support must be superior for these patients.

Chemotherapy involves the application of a chemical agent that targets and damages neoplastic and proliferative tissue. Chemotherapeutic dosages may be generated based on body weight or surface area. Chemotherapy may be administered locally or systemically and should be based on the most effective option for that particular patient. Intratumoral chemotherapy (ITCT) is commonly used in exotic species based on ease of administration, and potency at the tumor site.[97–100] However, ITCT is less effective with bulky tumors, and fails to reach systemic concentrations sufficient to treat metastatic disease. Prodrugs, such as cyclophosphamide, should not be used intralesionally. In addition, reptiles may be more sensitive to chemotherapy than mammals or birds based on their lower metabolic rate.[4,38,53,97,98] This increased potential for toxicity in reptiles dictates that chemotherapeutic agents be dosed so as to have the highest efficacy but lowest potential for toxicity. Little prospective research of the appropriate dosages of chemotherapeutic agents has been performed in reptiles. Clinicians must often rely on reported empirical treatments and anecdotal dosages. Consultation with a veterinary oncologist is recommended before embarking on chemotherapy for a reptile.

Chemotherapy may be used with curative or palliative intent. The differences in these protocols generate different dosing strategies in terms of intensity of dosing and frequency of administration of the chemotherapeutic agent.[97,98] Excellent client communication before pursuing chemotherapy in any reptile is imperative to ensure that the goal of chemotherapy is understood. The aim of palliative chemotherapy is to improve short-term quality of life. The current shortage of data available for chemotherapy in reptiles means that neither extension nor improved quality of life can be guaranteed with chemotherapy. However, hope remains, because curative intravenous (IV) chemotherapy has been reported in a single reptilian case.[36] Only through continued trial application of best practice and reporting will knowledge of reptile chemotherapy practice advance. Reptile medicine practitioners are encouraged to report neoplastic disease and chemotherapeutic agent use and outcomes in their patients. Clients, technicians, and veterinarians should be aware of the potential human toxicities of chemotherapeutic agents, use appropriate handling protocols, and adhere to all proper safety recommendations. The intermittent but frequent vascular access necessary to administer systemic chemotherapy may be challenging to obtain in reptile patients. Intravenous catheter placement is hindered by differing local anatomy of various reptile species and by scaled skin, which may obscure vessel visualization. Stabilization and prolonged management of IV catheters may be frustrating in reptiles and frequent replacement may predispose the patient to local scar formation or vasculitis. Surgical placement of vascular access ports provides a reasonable alternative for administration of chemotherapy, with less risk of extravasation of drugs than an IV catheter, in reptile patients.[2,36,38] Vascular access ports are commercially available and provide venous access not only for medication administration but also for sample collection to facilitate monitoring patient response to chemotherapy (**Fig. 8**).

Chemotherapeutic efficacy and appropriate dosing regimens for reptiles remain minimally investigated and poorly understood. As with mammalian patients, chemotherapy carries the risk of immunosuppression. Unlike mammalian species, timelines for the development of leukopenia secondary to administration of chemotherapy agents remain to be elucidated.[97,98] Therefore, frequent monitoring of complete blood counts in reptile patients undergoing chemotherapy is required. Normal bacterial and parasitic flora of reptiles, such as *Salmonella* spp, *Aeromonas* spp, and *Cryptosporidium* spp, may be considered facultative pathogens and have zoonotic potential.[2,101] Thus prophylactic antibiotic therapy may be administered to prevent bacterial infections of the patient secondary to the immunosuppressive effects of chemotherapy; the effects of antibiotic pressure on zoonotic pathogens in reptile patients undergoing chemotherapy must also be considered.

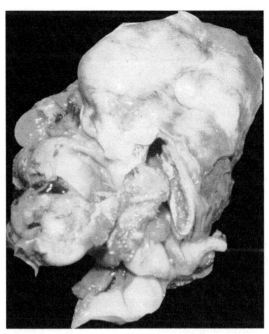

Fig. 8. Gross image of a teratoma removed from the coelomic cavity of a bearded dragon (*P vitticeps*). (*Courtesy of* Dalen Agnew, DVM, PhD, DACVP, Michigan State University.)

Despite all the aforementioned challenges, chemotherapy agents can be systemically administered to reptiles based on the same principles used in dogs and cats. Prednisone remains one of the most frequent chemotherapy agents prescribed in veterinary medicine. Other classes of chemotherapeutic agents include alkylating agents, antimetabolites, antitumoral antibiotics, platinum agents, vinca alkaloids, receptor tyrosine kinase inhibitors, and asparaginase agents.[97] Prednisone remains one of the most frequent chemotherapy agents prescribed in veterinary medicine. Intracoelomic administration of platinum-based chemotherapeutics, including cisplatin and carboplatin, have been used to good effect in reptiles. A granulosa cell tumor in a green iguana was treated with intracoelomic carboplatin at a dose of 10 mg/kg every 3 weeks.[43] Despite some initial reduction in tumor size, the nodule increased in size gradually over time, until quality of life dictated humane euthanasia. Cytosine arabinoside chemotherapy was administered to a bearded dragon diagnosed with monocytic leukemia at a dose of 100 mg/m² IV over a 48-hour period. Despite extensive monitoring and supportive care, the patient died 44 hours after treatment initiation. Necropsy revealed diffuse infiltration of neoplastic cells into several organs and multiple thrombi, suggesting disseminated intravascular coagulation as the cause of death rather than chemotherapeutic toxicity.[38] Cytosine arabinoside has been suggested as causing renal tubular acidosis after administration for the treatment of lymphoma in a rhinoceros viper (*Bitis nasicornis*), suggesting that this drug may not be well tolerated in reptiles.[102] Chemotherapy for and management of lymphoma in a green iguana resulted in successful outcome and neoplasia remission.[36] Cyclophosphamide, vincristine, doxorubicin, and prednisone (CHOP, modified) were administered via a surgically placed vascular access port for 6 months. Clinical remission of neoplastic disease without evidence of recurrence persisted for more than 1000 days after the final treatment (**Fig. 9**).[36]

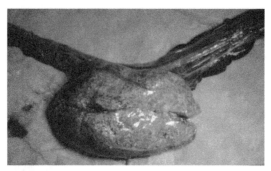

Fig. 9. Gross image of dissected renal tumor from a spitting cobra (*Naja* sp). (*Courtesy of* Dalen Agnew, DVM, PhD, DACVP, Michigan State University.)

Electrochemotherapy involves the administration of a chemotherapeutic agent to the tumor followed by electrical pulses to facilitate drug penetration of the tissues and to prolong drug effects.[53,97,98,103] Agents used include bleomycin and cisplatin based on their ability to locally penetrate neoplastic tissues. The agents are administered locally with uptake provided by a biphasic pulse of 1200 V/cm. The initial procedure is commonly followed with a second or third treatment at intervals of 1 or 2 weeks.[46] Electrochemotherapy has provided acceptable reptile patient outcomes, including fibropapillomas of green sea turtles (*C mydas*).[103] Fibropapillomas failed to recur in 2 sea turtles at 1 year following 2 treatments with intratumoral bleomycin at a dose of 1 U/cm^3 and electrode stimulation at 1000 V over 8 needles 5.0 mm apart.[103] Electrochemotherapy spares normal adjacent tissues based on the hydrophilic nature of the drugs used. Therefore, few side effects occur, and, in the reports described in reptilian patients, no significant side effects were reported. This therapy is likely to provide the best outcomes for patients with tumors that are benign or that have a low risk of metastasis because its effects are limited to localized disease. However, based on the administration of the electrical pulses, electrochemotherapy is considered painful and thus analgesia, heavy sedation, and/or anesthesia must be provided.[103]

Radiation therapy is an effective type of treatment that is used frequently in both veterinary and human medicine. It can be considered a primary or secondary treatment of many types of neoplasia in reptiles and mammalian species. Radiation oncology is a new and evolving field in veterinary medicine. Radiation is administered with different protocols. Ultimately, depending on the client's goals for the patient, palliative or curative radiation can be pursued.[104–107] In reptiles, the use of radiation therapy is uncommon. Few reports document radiation treatment, which is typically reserved for palliation of patients with nonresectable tumors.[20,26] Side effects of radiation are common and include the local effects of vasculitis, cellulitis, and dysecdysis of irradiated tissue as well as systemic effects such as lethargy, inappetence, and death.[104,105] Severe myelosuppression and subsequent infection with *Mycobacterium chelonae* occurred in a boa constrictor secondary to radiation treatment (48 Gy over 21 days) for squamous cell carcinoma combined with intratumoral carboplatin.[19] The higher total dose and hyperfractionated treatment protocol indicated a definitive treatment plan, but secondary infection instead resulted in this patient's demise.[16]

Other local therapies for tumors include laser therapy (hyperthermia), photodynamic therapy, and cryosurgery. Laser therapy involves the application of cautery or a specific wavelength laser to the neoplastic area to discourage growth of neoplastic cells and decrease tumor proliferation. Laser therapy is often reserved for tumors lacking surgical access and for cases in which tumor resection failed to provide complete surgical margins.[97] Photodynamic therapy uses photosensitizers that accumulate within neoplastic cells to destroy the tumor when exposed to a specific wavelength of electromagnetic radiation, and has had most success in the treatment of small, superficial squamous cell carcinomas in mammalian patients.[108] It has even been used with success in the treatment of fibropapillomatosis in 5 green sea turtles using methylene blue as the photosensitizing agent in two 15-minute sessions.[109] Disadvantages of photodynamic therapy include expense, specialized equipment required, and potential posttherapy toxicity. Patients undergoing photodynamic therapy may experience prolonged sensitivity to light, which could render this treatment modality unacceptable for use in some reptile species.[108] Cryotherapy uses freezing agents such as nitrous oxide or liquid nitrogen and is most commonly used for ablation of superficial, easily accessible tumors.[97] Each of these treatment modalities shows promise in treating neoplastic disease in reptiles as long as consideration of the patient, client lifestyle, and tumor type are taken into account.

SUPPORTIVE CONSIDERATIONS FOR REPTILE PATIENTS WITH NEOPLASIA

Reptile patients have many additional hospitalization and supportive care needs compared with companion mammals or birds. As ectotherms, immune response depends on providing the appropriate temperature gradient.[2] As prey species, appropriate places for rest, sleep, and unencumbered natural behaviors must be provided. Hydration and nutrition must be provided in order to obtain the best effects of the drugs and treatments administered. Analgesia and antibiosis must also be carefully considered in these species (**Fig. 10**).

Analgesia must be considered in oncology patients regardless of species. Appropriate pain management appropriately increases longevity and improves the quality of life of oncology patients. Studies of nociception in reptiles have shown similar responses to painful stimuli as those of mammals.[110,111] In reptiles, pain modulation options include local and systemic analgesic medications. Preliminary studies in reptiles, which have been limited to lizard and turtle species, suggest that pain is best managed by full mu receptor opioids, such as morphine, hydromorphone, or tramadol.[109,110] However, because morphine may induce profound respiratory depression in reptiles,

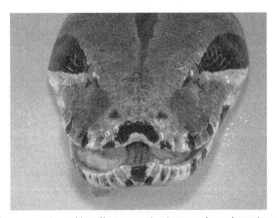

Fig. 10. Bilaterally symmetric and locally aggressive intraoral amelanotic melanoma in a boa constrictor (*Boa constrictor constrictor*). (*Courtesy of* Dalen Agnew, DVM, PhD, DACVP, Michigan State University.)

respiration must be monitored in these patients.[112] Administration of 5-HT3 receptor agonists or dopamine concurrently with morphine may reduce respiratory depression while preserving analgesic effects.[111,112] Because morphine and hydromorphone are controlled substances and must be given parenterally, they are often reserved for use in hospitalized patients, especially perioperatively and postoperatively. For outpatient analgesia, enteral medications such as tramadol and nonsteroidal antiinflammatory drugs are commonly used. Lidocaine and other local anesthetics also deserve consideration for use in reptiles undergoing mass removal, but little research on appropriate doses or toxicity in reptiles is extant.

Nutritional support of oncology patients is of paramount importance regardless of species. Patients with systemic disease are often debilitated, weak, and have decreased appetites and mobility. Providing nutrition may be challenging in reptiles based on anatomy and patient temperament. Assisted or force feedings may be cumbersome, and prolonged force feedings can decrease quality of life for the patient and may also disrupt the human-animal bond based on negative association with the activity.[113] Assisted feedings can be done via simply placing a well-lubricated small prey item into the mouth or cranial esophagus (snakes), syringe feedings into the oral cavity (chelonians, lizards), via tube feeding into the stomach or caudal esophagus (chelonians, lizards, snakes), or by placement of esophagostomy tube. Surgically placed esophagostomy tubes are most commonly used in turtles and tortoises. Placement is fairly simple, follows the same guidelines as placement in companion mammals (although a larger tube is usually used and well accepted), and may be performed in the same anesthesia event as a surgical debulking or treatment procedure.[2] Veterinary diets appropriate for short-term tube feeding in carnivorous, omnivorous, and herbivorous reptiles are now commercially available from multiple companies (eg, Oxbow, Lafeber, Repashy). However, in the short term, use of finely milled human baby foods of appropriate nutritional content may also be acceptable. These highly palatable and high-calorie-content diets can be used to supplement the normal diet or may be used alone for the management of short-term anorexia.[113] Clinicians should carefully observe the reptile patient receiving these diets because their finely milled, highly digestible nature may predispose animals with poorly functional gastrointestinal tracts to undergo excess gas formation, ileus, and bloat.

REFERENCES

1. Effron M, Griner L, Benirschke K. Nature and rate of neoplasia found in captive wild mammals, birds and reptiles at necropsy. J Natl Cancer Inst 1997;59(1): 185–98.
2. Hernandez-Divers SM, Garner MM. Neoplasia of reptiles with an emphasis on lizards. Vet Clin North Am Exot Anim Pract 2004;6:251–73.
3. Mauldin GR, Done LB. Oncology. In: Mader DR, editor. Reptile medicine and surgery. Toronto: Elsevier; 2006. p. 299–322.
4. Sykes JM, Trupkiewicz JG. Reptile neoplasia at the Philadelphia Zoological Garden, 1901-2002. J Zoo Wildl Med 2006;37(1):11–9.
5. Rothschild BM, Tanke DH, Helbling M 2nd, et al. Epidemiologic study of tumors in dinosaurs. Naturwissenschaften 2003;90(11):495–500.
6. Ramsay EC, Munson L, Lowenstine L, et al. A retrospective study of neoplasia in a collection of captive snakes. J Zoo Wildl Med 1996;27(1):28–34.
7. Catão-Dias JL, Nichols DK. Neoplasia in snakes at the National Zoological Park, Washington, DC (1978–1997). J Comp Pathol 1999;120:89–951.

8. Dietz J, Heckers KO, Pees M, et al. Bone tumours in lizards and snakes. A rare clinical finding. Hiemtiere 2015;43(1):31–9.
9. Hernandez-Divers SM, Orcutt CJ, Stahl SJ, et al. Lymphoma in lizards: three case reports. J Herpetol Med Surg 2003;13:14–22.
10. Heckers KO, Aupperle H, Schmidt V, et al. Melanophoromas and iridiophoromas in reptiles. J Comp Pathol 2012;146:258–68.
11. Collins, AC, Fenili RN; The modern U.S. Reptile Industry; Georgetown Economic Services White House Report. 2011.
12. Schilliger L, Selleri P, Frye FL. Lymphoblastic lymphoma and leukemic blood profile in a red-tail boa (*Boa constrictor constrictor*) with concurrent inclusion body disease. J Vet Diagn Invest 2011;23(1):159–62.
13. Cowan ML, Monks DJ, Raidal SR. Osteosarcoma in a woma python (*Aspidites ramsayi*). Aust Vet J 2011;89:520–3.
14. Schmidt RE, Reavill DR. Metastatic chondrosarcoma in a corn snake (*Pantherophis guttatus*). J Herp Med Surg 2012;22(3–4):67–9.
15. Gumber S, Nevarez JG, Cho DY. Endocardial fibrosarcoma in a reticulated python (*Python reticularis*). J Vet Diagn Invest 2010;22(6):1013–6.
16. Langan JN, Adams WH, Patton S, et al. Radiation and intralesional chemotherapy for a fibrosarcoma in a constrictor, *Boa constrictor ortoni*. J Herpetol Med Surg 2001;11(1):4–8.
17. Stern AW, Velguth KE, D'Agostino J. Metastatic ductal adenocarcinoma in a western hognose snake (*Heterodon nasicus*). J Zoo Wildl Med 2010;41(2):320–4.
18. Suedmeyer WK, Bryan JN, Johnson G, et al. Diagnosis and clinical management of multiple chromatophoromas in an eastern yellowbelly racer (*Coluber constrictor flaviventris*). J Zoo Wildl Med 2007;38:127–30.
19. Steeil JC, Schumacher J, Hecht S, et al. Diagnosis and treatment of a pharyngeal squamous cell carcinoma in a Madagascar ground boa (*Boa madagascariensis*). J Zoo Wildl Med 2013;44(1):144–51.
20. Gull JM, Lange CE, Favrot C, et al. Multiple papillomas in a diamond python, *Morelia spilota*. J Zoo Wildl Med 2012;43(4):946–9.
21. Bera MM, Veeramachaneni DN, Pandher K. Characterization of a biphasic neoplasm in a Madagascar tree boa (*Sanzinia madagascariensis*). Vet Pathol 2008;45:259–63.
22. Anderson ET, Kennedy-Stoskoph S, Sandy JR, et al. Squamous cell carcinoma with vascular invasion in a diamondback rattlesnake (*Cortalus adamanteus*). J Zoo Wildl Med 2010;41(1):745–8.
23. Matthews ME, Eshar D, Delk KW, et al. Splenopancreatic ductal adenocarcinoma with multiorgan metastasis in a northern water snake (*Nerodia sipedon*). J Zoo Wildl Med 2014;45(2):437–40.
24. Thompson KA, Campbell M, Levens G, et al. Bilaterally symmetrical oral amelanotic melanoma in a boa constrictor (*Boa constrictor constrictor*). J Zoo Wildl Med 2015;46(3):629–32.
25. Comolli JR, Olsen HM, Seguel M, et al. Ameloblastoma in a wild black rat snake. J Vet Diagn Invest 2015;27(4):536–9.
26. Sharpe S, Lamm CG, Killick R. Intracoelomic anaplastic sarcoma in a Madagascar tree boa (*Sanzinia madagascariensis*). J Vet Diagn Invest 2013;25(1):153–7.
27. Dadone LI, Klaphake E, Garner MM, et al. Pituitary cystadenoma, entrolipidosis, and cutaneous mycosis in an everglades rat snake (*Elaphe obsoleta rossalleni*). J Zoo Wildl Med 2010;41(3):538–41.

28. Baron HHR, Allavena R, Melville LM, et al. Gastric adenocarcinoma in a diamond python (*Morelia spilota spilota*). Aust Vet J 2014;92(10):405–9.

29. Gérard Stumpel JB, del-Pozo J, French A, et al. Cardiac hemangiosarcoma in a corn snake (*Pantherophis guttatus*). J Zoo Wildl Med 2012;43(2):360–6.

30. Needle D, McKnight CA, Kiupel M. Chondroblastic osteosarcoma in two related spiny-tailed monitor lizards (*Varanus acanthursus*). J Exot Pet Med 2013;22:256–69.

31. Hannon DE, Garner MM, Reavill DR. Squamous cell carcinomas in inland bearded dragons (*Pogona vitticeps*). J Herp Med Surg 2011;21(4):101–6.

32. Irizarry Rovira AR, Holzer TR, Credille KM. Systemic mastocytosis in an African fat tailed gecko (*Hemitheconyx caudicinctus*). J Comp Pathol 2014;151:130–4.

33. Brot S, Sydler T, Nufer L, et al. Histologic, immunohistochemical and electron microscopic characterization of a malignant iridiophoroma in a dwarf bearded dragon (*Pogona henrylawsoni*). J Zoo Wildl Med 2015;46(3):583–7.

34. Irizarry-Rovira AR, Wolf A, Ramiros-Vara JA. Cutaneous melanophoroma in a green iguana (*Iguana iguana*). Vet Clin Pathol 2006;35(1):101–5.

35. Sander SJ, Ossiboff RJ, Stokol T, et al. Endolymphatic sac carcinoma in situ in a tokay gecko (*Gekko gecko*). J Herp Med Surg 2015;25(3–4):82–6.

36. Folland DW, Johnston MS, Thamm DH, et al. Diagnosis and management of lymphoma in a green iguana (*Iguana iguana*). J Am Vet Med Assoc 2011;239(7):985–91.

37. Stacy BA, Vidal JD, Osofsky A, et al. Ovarian papillary cystadenocarcinomas in a green iguana (*Iguana iguana*). J Comp Pathol 2004;130:223–8.

38. Jankowski G, Sirninger J, Borne J, et al. Chemotherapeutic treatment for leukemia in a bearded dragon (*Pogona vitticeps*). J Zoo Wildl Med 2011;42(2):322–5.

39. Schilliger L, Selleri P, Gandar F, et al. Adenoid hepatocellular carcinoma accompanied by an uncharacterized eosinophilic intracytoplasmic inclusions in a green iguana (*Iguana iguana*). J Herp Med Surg 2012;22(3–4):70–5.

40. Salinas EM, Aguilar Arriaga BO, Lezama JR, et al. Oral fibrosarcoma in a black iguana (*Ctenosaura pectinata*). J Zoo Wildl Med 2013;44(2):513–6.

41. Patterson-Kane JC, Redrobe SP. Colonic adenocarcinoma in a leopard gecko (*Eublepharis macularius*). Vet Rec 2005;157:294–5.

42. Vasil'ev DB, Solov'ev IuN. Ganglioneuroblastoma in Yemenite chameleon (*Chamaeleo calyptratus*): the first recorded case of a tumor of neuroectodermal histogenesis in reptiles. Arkh Patol 2006;68(4):45–7.

43. Cruz Cardona JA, Conley KJ, Wellehan JF, et al. Incomplete ovariosalpingectomy and subsequent malignant granulosa cell tumor in a female green iguana (*Iguana iguana*). J Am Vet Med Assoc 2011;239(2):237–43.

44. Jacobson ER, Reese DJ, Berry CR, et al. Vet med today: what is your diagnosis. J Am Vet Med Assoc 2013;243(11):1533–5.

45. Santos ED, Silva Filho JR, Machado TP, et al. Oral fibrosarcoma in a jaracara (*Bothrops pubescens*) anatomopathological and immunohistochemical aspects. Pesq Vet Bras 2015;35(7):664–70.

46. Gardhouse S, Eshar D, Lee-Chow B, et al. Diagnosis and treatment of a periocular myxosarcoma in a bearded dragon (*Pogona vitticeps*). Can Vet J 2014;55:663–6.

47. Darrow BG, Johnstone McLean NS, Russman SE, et al. Periorbital adenocarcinoma in a bearded dragon (*Pogona vitticeps*). Vet Ophthalmol 2013;16(1):177–82.

48. Rivera S, Crane MM, McManamon R, et al. Surgical treatment of pulmonary melanophoroma in a beaded lizard (*Heloderma horridum exasperatum*). J Zoo Wildl Med 2015;46(2):397–9.

49. Hadfield C, Clayton LA, Clancy MM, et al. Proliferative thyroid lesions in three diplodactylid geckos: *Nephrurus amyae*, *Nephrurus levis*, and *Oedura marmorata*. J Zoo Wildl Med 2012;43(1):131–40.

50. Gyimesi ZS, Garner MM, Burns RB, et al. High incidence of lymphoid neoplasia in a colony of Egyptian spiny-tailed lizards (*Uromastyx aerogyptius*). J Zoo Wildl Med 2005;36(1):103–10.

51. Bielli M, Forlani A, Nardini G, et al. Mucinous melanophoroma in a northern red-bellied cooter (*Pseudemys rubriventris*). J Exot Pet Med 2015;24:71–5.

52. Schumacher J, Toal RL. Advanced radiography and ultrasonography in reptiles. Sem Av Exotic Pet Med 2001;10(4):162–8.

53. Lanza A, Baldi A, Spugnini EP. Surgery and electrochemotherapy for the treatment of cutaneous squamous cell carcinoma in a yellow-bellied slider (*Trachemys scripta scripta*). J Am Vet Med Assoc 2015;246(4):455–7.

54. Abu-Seida A, Saeid S. Cutaneous adenocarcinoma in a desert tortoise (*Gopherus agassizii*). Int J Vet Sci Med 2013;1:48–50.

55. Gonzales-Viera O, Bauer G, Aguiar LS, et al. Cutaneous fibroma in a common snapping turtle (*Chelydra serpentine*). J Comp Pathol 2012;147:574–6.

56. Santoro M, Stacy BA, Morales JA, et al. Mast cell tumor in a giant Galapagos tortoise (*Geochelone nigra vicina*). J Comp Pathol 2008;138:156–9.

57. Clabaugh K, Haag KM, Hanley CS, et al. Undifferentiated sarcoma resolved by forelimb amputation and prosthesis in a radiated tortoise (*Geochelone radiate*). J Zoo Wildl Med 2005;36(1):117–20.

58. Heckers KO, Schmidt V, Krastel D, et al. Malignant melanophoroma in a Hermann's tortoise (*Testudo hermanni*). Tierarztl Prax Ausg K Kleintiere Heimtiere 2011;39:45–50.

59. Bezjian M, Diep AN, Matos R, et al. Chinese box turtle (*Cuora flavomarginata*) with lymphoid leukemia characterized by immunohistochemical and cytochemical phenotyping. Vet Clin Pathol 2013;42(3):368–76.

60. Lombardini ED, Desoutter AV, Montali RJ, et al. Esophageal adenocarcinoma in a 53-year-old mata mata turtle (*Chelus fimbriatus*). J Zoo Wildl Med 2013;44(3):773–6.

61. Gál J, Jakab C, Szabo Z, et al. Haemangioma in the oesophagus of a red-eared slider (*Trachemys scripta elegans*). Acta Vet Hung 2009;57(4):477–84.

62. Gál J, Jakac C, Balogh B, et al. First occurrence of periosteal chondroma (juxtacortical chondroma) in *Uromastyx maliensis* (Reptilia: Sauria: Agamidae). Acta Vet Hung 2007;55(3):327–31.

63. Martorell J, Soto S, Barrera S, et al. Case report: ovarian teratoma in a Mediterranean tortoise. Compend Contin Educ Vet 2009;31(4):193–6.

64. Pees M, Ludewig E, Plenz B, et al. Imaging diagnosis – seminoma causing liver compression in a spur-thighed tortoise (*Testudo graeca*). Vet Radiol Ultrasound 2015;56(2):E21–4.

65. Gál J, Demeter Z, Palade E, et al. Harderian gland adenocarcinoma in a Florida red-bellied turtle (*Pseudemys nelsoni*) – case report. Acta Vet Hung 2009;57(2):275–81.

66. Eyarefe OD, Antia RE, Abiola OO, et al. Rhabdomyosarcoma in a terrestrial tortoise (*Geochelone nigra*) in Nigeria: a case report. J S Afr Vet Assoc 2012;83(1):300.

67. Jacobson ER, Seely SJ, Novilla MN. Lymphosarcoma associated with virus-like intranuclear inclusions in a California king snake (Colubridae: Lampropeltis). J Natl Cancer Inst 1980;65(3):577–83.
68. Herbst LH. Fibropapillomatosis of marine turtles. Annu Rev Fish Dis 1994;4: 389–425.
69. Jacobson ER, Buergelt C, Williams B, et al. Herpesvirus in cutaneous fibropapillomas of the green turtle Chelonia mydas. Dis Aquat Organ 1991;12:1–6.
70. Marschang RE. Viruses infecting reptiles. Viruses 2011;3(11):2087–126.
71. Waltzek T, Reavill DR, Kelleher SA, et al. Characterization of a novel poxvirus from an argentine tegu (Tupinambis meriana). Assoc Reptilian and Amphibian Veterinarians. Conference Proceedings, 2014.
72. Watson MK, Mitchell MA. Vitamin D and ultraviolet B radiation considerations for exotic pets. J Exot Pet Med 2014;24(4):369–79.
73. Ahmad M, Taqavi IH. Radiation induced leukemia and leukopenia in the lizard Uromastyx hardwickii. Radiobiol Radiother 1978;3:353.
74. Chandra AM, Jacobson ER, Munn RJ. Retroviral particles in neoplasms of Burmese pythons (Python molurus bivittatus). Vet Pathol 2011;38:561–4.
75. Stenglein MD, Sanders C, Kistler AL, et al. Identification, characterization and in vitro culture of highly divergent arenaviruses from boa constrictors and annulated tree boas: candidate etiological agents for snake inclusion body disease. MBio 2012;3(4):e00180–212.
76. Keck M, Zimmerman DM, Ramsay EC, et al. Renal adenocarcinomas in cape coral snakes (Aspidelaps lubricus lubricus). J Herp Med Surg 2011;21(1):5–9.
77. Ball RL, Brichard SJ, Ray LR, et al. Ovarian remnant syndrome in dogs and cats 21 cases (2000-2007). J Am Vet Med Assoc 2010;236(5):548–53.
78. Jacobson ER, Long PH, Miller RE, et al. Renal neoplasia of snakes. J Am Vet Med Assoc 1986;189(9):1134–6.
79. Pereira ME, Viner TC. Oviduct adenocarcinoma in some species of captive snakes. Vet Pathol 2008;45(5):693–7.
80. Schultze AE, Mason GL, Clyde VL. Lymphosarcoma with leukemic blood profile in a Savannah monitor lizard (Varanus exanthematicus). J Zoo Wildl Med 1999; 30:158–64.
81. Romagnano A, Jacobson ER, Boon GD, et al. Lymphosarcoma in a green iguana (Iguana iguana). J Zoo Wildl Med 1996;27(1):83–9.
82. Abou-Madi N, Kern TJ. Squamous cell carcinoma associated with a periorbital mass in a veiled chameleon (Chamaeleo calyptratus). Vet Ophthalmol 2002; 5(3):217–20.
83. Von Deetzen MC, Muller K, Brunnberg L, et al. Non-metastatic squamous cell carcinoma in two Hermann's tortoises. Vet Sci Dev 2012;2(e5):17–9.
84. Frye FL. Diagnosis and surgical treatment of reptilian neoplasms with a compilation of cases 1966-1993. In Vivo 1993;8(5):885–92.
85. Wenger S, Simova-Curd S, Great P, et al. Ovarian teratoma in a Fiji island banded iguana (Brachylopus fasciatus) and a green iguana (Iguana iguana). J Herp Med Surg 2011;20(1):20–4.
86. Stacy NI, Alleman AK, Sayler KA. Diagnostic hematology of reptiles. Clin Lab Med 2011;31:87–108.
87. Suedmeyer K. Noninfectious diseases of reptiles. Sem Av Exot Pet Med 1995; 4(1):56–60.
88. Fereidooni F, Horvath E, Kovacs K. Humoral hypercalcemia of malignancy due to bipartite squamous cell/small cell carcinoma of the esophagus immunoreactive for parathyroid hormone related protein. Dis Esophagus 2003;16:335–8.

89. Eatwell K. Calcium and phosphorus values and their derivatives in captive tortoises (*Testudo* species). J Small Anim Pract 2010;51:472–5.
90. Divers SJ. Reptile diagnostic endoscopy and endosurgery. Vet Clin North Am Exot Anim Pract 2010;13(2):217–42.
91. Alleman RA, Kupprion EK. Cytologic diagnosis of diseases in reptiles. Vet Clin North Am Exot Anim Pract 2007;10(1):155–86.
92. Lyons JA, Newman SJ, Greenacre CB, et al. A gastric neuroendocrine carcinoma expressing somatostatin in a bearded dragon (*Pogona vitticeps*). J Vet Diagn Invest 2010;22(2):316–20.
93. Ritter JM, Garner MM, Chilton JA, et al. Gastric neuroendocrine carcinomas in bearded dragons (*Pogona vitticeps*). Vet Pathol 2009;46(6):1109–16.
94. Gál J, Mándoki M, Sátorhelyi T, et al. In situ complex adenocarcinoma on the femoral part of the hindlimb in an Asian leaf turtle (*Cyclemys dentata*). Acta Vet Hung 2010;58(4):431–40.
95. Jakab C, Rusvai M, Szabó Z, et al. Claudin-7-positive synchronous spontaneous intrahepatic cholangiocarcinoma, adenocarcinoma and adenomas of the gallbladder in a bearded dragon (*Pogona vitticeps*). Acta Vet Hung 2011;59(1): 99–112.
96. Shoemaker M, Barrie M, Holman H, et al. Pathology in practice. J Am Vet Med Assoc 2016;248(2):153–5.
97. Kent MS. The use of chemotherapy in exotic animals. Vet Clin North Am Exot Anim Pract 2004;7:807–20.
98. Graham JE, Kent MS, Theon A. Current therapies in exotic animal oncology. Vet Clin North Am Exot Anim Pract 2004;7:757–81.
99. Gibbons PM. Advances in reptile clinical therapeutics. J Exot Pet Med 2014;23: 21–38.
100. Spugnini EP, Baldi A. Electrochemotherapy in veterinary oncology: from rescue to first line therapy. Methods Mol Biol 2014;1121:247–56.
101. Chinnadurai SK, DeVoe RS. Selected infectious diseases of reptiles. Vet Clin North Am Exot Anim Pract 2009;12(3):583–96.
102. Jacobson E, Calderwood MB, French TW, et al. Lymphosarcoma in an eastern king snake and rhinoceros viper. J Am Vet Med Assoc 1981;179(11):1231–5.
103. Brunner HM, Dutra G, Brunelli C, et al. Electrochemotherapy for the treatment of fibropapillomas in *Chelonia mydas*. J Zoo Wildl Med 2014;45(2):213–8.
104. Siegel S, Cronin KL. Palliative radiotherapy. Vet Clin North Am Small Anim Pract 1997;27(1):149–55.
105. Mauldin GN, Shiomitsu K. Principles and practice of radiation therapy in exotic and avian species. Sem Av Exot Pet Med 2005;14(3):168–74.
106. Leach MW, Nichols DK, Hartsell W, et al. Radiation therapy of a malignant chromatophoroma in a yellow rat snake (*Elaphe obsoleta quadrivittata*). J Zoo Wildl Med 1991;22:241–4.
107. Greenacre CB, Roberts R. Effect of strontium-90 on squamous cell carcinoma in an eastern box turtle (*Terrapene carolina*); discussion of alternative treatment modalities. 3rd International virtual conference in veterinary: diseases of reptiles and amphibians. Athens (GA): Georgia University; 2000.
108. Roberts WG, Klein MK, Loomis M, et al. Photodynamic therapy of spontaneous cancers in felines, canines and snakes with chloro-aluminum sulfonated phthalocyanine. J Natl Cancer Inst 1991;83(1):18–23.
109. Serella FP, Sabino CP, Fernandes LT, et al. Green turtle (*Chelonia mydas*) cutaneous fibropapillomatosis treatment by photodynamic therapy. Mar Turt News 2014;142:6–10.

110. Mosley C. Pain and nociception in reptiles. Vet Clin North Am Exot Anim Pract 2011;14:45–60.
111. Sladky KK, Miletic V, Paul-Murphy J, et al. Analgesic efficacy and respiratory effects of butorphanol and morphine in turtles. J Am Vet Med Assoc 2007;230(9): 1356–62.
112. Manzke T, Guenther U, Ponimaskin EG, et al. 5-HT$_{4(a)}$ receptors avert opioid-induced breathing depression without loss of analgesia. Science 2003;301: 226–9.
113. DeVoe RS. Nutritional support of reptile patients. Vet Clin North Am Exot Anim Pract 2014;17(2):249–61.

Rodent Oncology
Diseases, Diagnostics, and Therapeutics

Samuel E. Hocker, DVM,
David Eshar, DVM, DABVP (Exotic Companion Mammals), DECZM (Small Mammal)*,
Raelene M. Wouda, BVSc, DACVIM (Oncology), MANZCVS (SAIM)

KEYWORDS

- Rodent • Oncology • Guinea pigs • Chinchillas • Hamsters • Mice • Rats • Gerbils

KEY POINTS

- Certain rodent species, such as rats and mice, are more commonly diagnosed with neoplasia compared with other rodents like chinchillas and degus, which seemingly have much lower reported cancer incidence rates.
- Treatment of most rodent neoplasia revolves around surgical excision; however, reports of pharmacologic intervention exist and this is an area of expanding interest.
- All surgically resected tumors should be submitted for histopathologic evaluation to confirm the diagnosis and establish the need for adjuvant therapy.

INTRODUCTION

A general discussion of the most common spontaneous tumors of the pet rodent population, including clinical presentation, diagnostic evaluation, and therapeutic options, is covered in this article. This article is not intended as an all-inclusive review of every tumor histotype that has been reported, but is a review to stimulate exotic animal practitioners to proactively investigate, treat, and report cases of neoplasia. For the purpose of this article, the nomenclature rodent is used to refer to guinea pigs, chinchillas, hamsters, mice, rats, gerbils, degus, and prairie dogs.

GUINEA PIGS (CAVIA PORCELLUS)
Tumors of the Skin and Subcutis

Skin tumors comprise approximately 15% of all neoplasms seen in guinea pigs.[1] The most common skin tumors, accounting for 33% to 89.7% of all skin tumors, are trichofolliculomas (an abortive differentiation of cutaneous pluripotent stem cells toward hair

Disclosure: The authors have nothing to disclose.
Department of Clinical Sciences, Kansas State University, 1800 Denison Avenue, Manhattan, KS 66506, USA
* Corresponding author.
E-mail address: deshar@vet.k-state.edu

follicles).[2,3] These tumors have a tendency to occur on the dorsum, but can arise anywhere on the body. Although these tumors are benign, they can grow large enough to precipitate ulceration and/or rupture.[1,2] Fine-needle aspiration and cytology can reveal significant heterogeneity depending on the area of the tumor sampled, but often keratin, sebum, scant amounts of inflammatory cells, and blood are seen.[4] Complete surgical excision, including removal of the capsule, is considered curative (**Figs. 1** and **2**).[5]

Lipomas are also common in guinea pigs, with an incidence of 25% of all cutaneous tumors reported.[2] Lipomas typically occur on the ventral abdomen, but can occur anywhere on the body. They can be solitary or multifocal.[4] Fine-needle aspiration, incisional biopsy, or complete excisional biopsy can be used to differentiate a benign lipoma from other neoplasia, such as mammary tumors, that may be malignant.[2] Surgical removal of a benign lipoma may be performed for cosmetic purposes or if, as a result of size and position, it is impeding normal ambulation or bodily comfort.

Additional cutaneous tumors that have been reported in guinea pigs include trichoepithelioma (differentiation into all 3 segments of the hair follicle), sebaceous adenoma, fibrosarcoma, lymphoma, and liposarcoma.[2,6–10] Histopathology is required for definitive diagnosis of all cutaneous tumors (**Figs. 3** and **4**).

Tumors of the Mammary Gland

Mammary gland tumors can occur in both boars and sows.[1,5,9] Approximately 30% to 50% of mammary tumors in guinea pigs are malignant, but their metastatic rate is reportedly very low.[1,9] Adenomas and adenocarcinomas are the most common benign and malignant mammary tumors, respectively.[1,5] Several other histologic types of benign and malignant mammary tumors in guinea pigs have been identified.[11] A 2010 retrospective report immunohistochemically evaluated 10 mammary tumors and histologically classified the tumors based on the World Health Organization (WHO) *Histological Classification of Mammary Tumors of the Dog and Cat*.[11,12] Out of the 10 mammary tumors assessed, 7 (70%) were malignant and 86% of these were determined to be simple tubulopapillary carcinomas.[11] All of the tumor samples expressed type alpha estrogen receptors and progesterone receptors.[11]

Mammary tumors must be differentiated from other pathologic lesions that can occur in that area, such as mastitis and lipomas.[2,9] A fine-needle aspiration may be

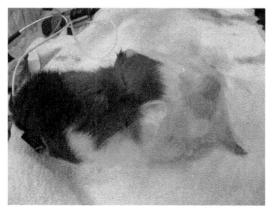

Fig. 1. Trichofolliculoma on the dorsum of a guinea pig. (*Courtesy of* David Eshar, DVM, Dipl. ABVP (Exotic Companion Mammals), Dipl. ECZM (Small Mammal), Manhattan, KS.)

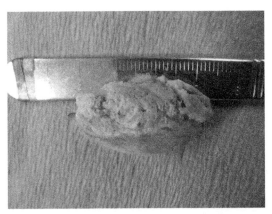

Fig. 2. A trichofolliculoma (in cut section) removed from a guinea pig. (*Courtesy of* David Eshar, DVM, Dipl. ABVP (Exotic Companion Mammals), Dipl. ECZM (Small Mammal), Manhattan, KS.)

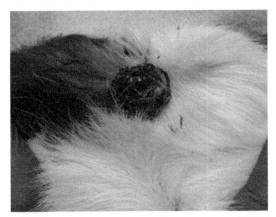

Fig. 3. A soft tissue sarcoma on the dorsum of a guinea pig. (*Courtesy of* David Eshar, DVM, Dipl. ABVP (Exotic Companion Mammals), Dipl. ECZM (Small Mammal), Manhattan, KS.)

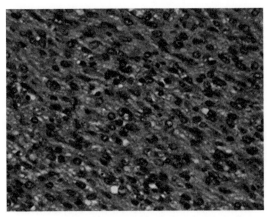

Fig. 4. Histopathology of a soft tissue sarcoma from a guinea pig (hematoxylin-eosin, original magnification ×400). (*Courtesy of* Brad Debey, DVM, PhD, DACVP, Manhattan, KS.)

performed; however, the cytologic appearance may vary greatly depending on the type of mammary tumor.[4] Solid mammary tumors may exfoliate adequate numbers of atypical epithelial cells, whereas tumors with a more cystic component may yield low cellularity with a proteinaceous background.[4] Incisional or excisional biopsy may be performed if the cytology is inconclusive.[9] Mammary tumors should be surgically excised with wide (5–10 mm) margins, along with extirpation of the local lymph node if possible.[5,13] Before surgical resection of the mammary tumor, 3-view thoracic radiographs are warranted to evaluate for pulmonary metastasis.[5] An early-age spay of the unbred sow should be considered as a preventive measure of mammary tumors in guinea pigs.[14]

Tumors of the Reproductive System

Leiomyomas are the most common uterine tumor in guinea pigs.[15–17] In one report, 7 of 83 (8.4%) guinea pigs had uterine leiomyomas at the time of necropsy.[15] The same report suggested an association between uterine leiomyomas and cystic rete ovarii (a common condition in many intact sows); however, this association is yet to be definitively proved (**Fig. 5**).[15] Teratomas are the most common ovarian tumors in sows.[5,16] Teratomas are typically composed of 2 to 3 germinal layers with a high prevalence of neural tissue.[18] They are typically unilateral and rarely metastasize.[5,18]

Uterine and ovarian tumors should be a differential diagnosis in all sows with abdominal distention, a palpable mass, vaginal discharge, and/or abdominal pain.[9,16] Abdominal ultrasonography is beneficial in discerning the origin of the mass.[16,19] Fine-needle aspiration and cytology may also aid in achieving a diagnosis, but certain tumors, such as uterine leiomyomas, exfoliate only low to moderate cellularity.[4] Ovariohysterectomy is recommended for treatment of both uterine and ovarian tumors.[9,16] Histopathologic examination of the removed tissues should be performed to obtain a definitive diagnosis.[16] An early-age ovariohysterectomy of the unbred sow should be considered as a preventive measure for reproductive-system neoplasia in guinea pigs.[14]

Tumors of the Endocrine System

In a recent report, 19 of 236 cases (8.0%) of guinea pig neoplasia were determined to be of thyroid origin.[20] Carcinomas comprise 36.8% to 55.5% of the total thyroid tumor population and in one report a metastatic rate of 5.3% (1 of 19) was documented.[20,21]

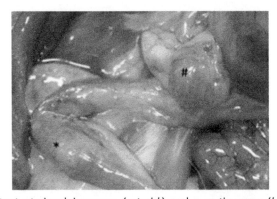

Fig. 5. Concomitant uterine leiomyoma (*asterisk*) and a cystic ovary (*hash symbol*) in a guinea pig. (*Courtesy of* David Eshar, DVM, Dipl. ABVP (Exotic Companion Mammals), Dipl. ECZM (Small Mammal), Manhattan, KS.)

Thyroid tumors in guinea pigs can be nonfunctional or functional (hyperthyroidism).[22] The distribution of adenomas and carcinomas among hyperthyroid guinea pigs is currently not known.[23] Clinical signs associated with thyroid tumors include a ventral neck mass and, if functional, weight loss despite a normal appetite or polyphagia, and hyperactivity.[23–25] Ultrasonography can be used to assess any ventral cervical mass. Thyroid tumors typically appear as heterogeneous cystic masses on ultrasonography.[22,25] Fine-needle aspiration and cytologic evaluation can be used to differentiate neoplasia from other pathologic conditions, such as cervical lymphadenitis, salivary mucocele, or lymphoma.[22] However, cytology does not always definitively distinguish between a benign or malignant thyroid tumor, because cellular atypia and other cytologic markers of malignancy can be minimal in thyroid carcinomas.[22,26] Evaluating serum total thyroxine (T4) levels may support the diagnosis of a functional thyroid tumor.[25,27,28] However, assessing total T4 level can be challenging as a result of normal fluctuations in T4 levels from concurrent systemic illnesses.[27,29,30] Consequently, hyperthyroid guinea pigs may have normal circulating total T4 levels making a diagnosis of hyperthyroidism difficult.[24] Evaluating serum free T4 (fT4) is beneficial because systemic illness is less likely to have an effect on fT4 levels.[24,27,31] Recombinant human thyroid-stimulating hormone may also be used in cases of normal or marginally increased thyroid levels if hyperthyroidism is still suspected.[32] Nuclear scintigraphy using technetium (pertechnetate) has been described as a diagnostic aid for hyperthyroidism.[24] Metastatic thyroid tumors in guinea pigs exist, and thoracic radiographs may show evidence of pulmonary metastasis.[20,21] Treatment of thyroid tumors in guinea pigs is to some degree dictated by the functionality and biological behavior of the tumor.[22] Thyroidectomy of the affected gland has been previously described and can provide an optimal outcome; however, this procedure has been associated with significant postoperative mortality.[20,23,25,33] External beam radiation therapy has been described as a treatment of thyroid neoplasia in humans and dogs, but has yet to be reported in guinea pigs.[27] Radioiodine (I^{131}) therapy has been shown to be effective in the treatment of hyperthyroidism in guinea pigs.[23] This treatment modality is advantageous in that it is noninvasive; can destroy all neoplastic thyroid tissue, including any ectopic tissue; and it has the potential to be curative.[23] Radioiodine has been conventionally performed in those patients that have functional thyroid tumors, but evidence in dogs suggests that it may play a role in treatment of euthyroid patients with thyroid neoplasia.[22,34] The clinical signs associated with a functional thyroid neoplasia can be medically managed with oral or topical antithyroid medications, such as methimazole or carbimazole, which act by blocking thyroid peroxidase, thereby inhibiting synthesis of excessive thyroid hormone.[22,35] Transdermal application of methimazole gel has been used successfully in hyperthyroid guinea pigs, but has been noted to cause depigmentation of the skin.[23,36] Note that antithyroid medications only aid in controlling the clinical signs of hyperthyroidism from a functional thyroid tumor and have no known antineoplastic effects.[37]

Pituitary and adrenal tumors leading to hyperadrenocorticism (HAC) have been uncommonly described in guinea pigs compared with humans and dogs, in which the syndrome is better characterized.[22] Of the guinea pigs that were confirmed to have HAC, all have been middle aged to older and have presented with clinical signs similar to those observed in the canine population with this disorder.[38–41] Clinical signs that have been observed are bilateral symmetric alopecia, thin skin, polyuria, polydipsia, and muscle weakness.[38–40] Diagnosis of HAC can be achieved through endocrine testing. Nevertheless, assessing a baseline plasma cortisol level has no diagnostic value for confirming HAC because of significant fluctuations in cortisol levels attributed to a variety of factors: pulsatile cortisol and adrenocorticotropic hormone (ACTH) release, concurrent diseases, change in environment, or simply the process of collecting a blood sample.[22] Several cases of HAC have been confirmed by an ACTH stimulation test, using saliva as a noninvasive approach to measuring cortisol levels.[39,40,42,43] Abdominal ultrasonography can evaluate the adrenal glands for enlargement or masses, which may support the diagnosis and/or assist in differentiating pituitary-dependent HAC (PDH) from adrenal-dependent HAC.[38,40] One medical treatment option for PDH in guinea pigs is the 3β-hydroxysteroid dehydrogenase inhibitor, trilostane.[37,40] This enzyme is critical for the synthesis of cortisol and other steroids.[37] Supporting literature consists of a single case report in which trilostane was used to treat a guinea pig with clinical signs and diagnostic results consistent with PDH.[40] This patient showed improvement in clinical signs within a couple months of commencing therapy.[40] Surgical excision of a unilateral adrenal tumor has been attempted and the surgical technique has been previously described.[38,44]

Pancreatic beta-cell tumors, or insulinomas, are functional tumors that fail to respond to low glucose levels and subsequently continue to release insulin.[37] Clinical signs associated with insulinomas are related to hypoglycemia and include neurologic signs such as weakness, ataxia, head tilt, lethargy, and seizures (**Fig. 6**).[45,46] Insulinoma should be a differential diagnosis for any middle-aged guinea pig presenting with neurologic signs. A presumptive diagnosis can be made by documenting hypoglycemia and resolution of clinical signs after administration of dextrose.[46] A more definitive method of confirming an insulinoma is to document hypoglycemia with a concurrent normal or increased insulin level.[37,45] However, there are no insulin level reference intervals or validated insulin assays for guinea pigs at this time.[22] Abdominal ultrasonography may visualize a pancreatic nodule, but its absence does not rule out the presence of an insulinoma.[37,45] Treatment in an emergent hypoglycemic crisis should consist of intravenous or intraosseous administration of dextrose, and also orally if catheterization is not possible.[37,45,47] If insulinoma is suspected, dextrose administration should proceed with caution because this intervention can potentiate further pancreatic secretion of insulin and worsen the hypoglycemia.[37] The use of

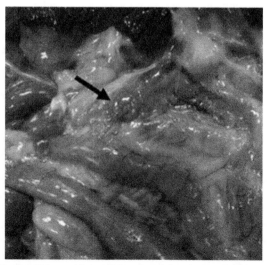

Fig. 6. Pancreatic beta-cell tumor (*arrow*) in a guinea pig. (*Courtesy of* David Eshar, DVM, Dipl. ABVP (Exotic Companion Mammals), Dipl. ECZM (Small Mammal), Manhattan, KS.)

glucagon as a constant rate infusion has shown to be effective in stabilizing a hyperinsulinemic-hypoglycemic dog and ferret.[48,49] In general, long-term medical management of insulinoma is designed to control hypoglycemia through dietary changes, oral glucocorticoids, and sometimes other drugs such as diazoxide. Although this can be effective in dogs and ferrets, guinea pigs are herbivorous animals that require a high-fiber diet throughout day, which is slowly digested by the cecal bacteria, so dietary modification is not feasible.[45] Prednisone use in guinea pigs is controversial based on anecdotal reports of immunosuppression leading to infection, similar to what is hypothesized in rabbits.[50] If prednisone is used, it should be dosed with extreme caution.[45] Diazoxide, a benzothiadiazide diuretic that stimulates hepatic glycogenolysis and gluconeogenesis, inhibits insulin release, and blocks peripheral glucose uptake, has been reported in 1 guinea pig for medical management of an insulinoma.[45,51] Although the treatment of choice in humans and dogs, surgical removal of an insulinoma has yet to be documented in guinea pigs.

Tumors of the Respiratory System

Pulmonary tumors, specifically bronchogenic papillary adenomas, are described as the most common neoplasia identified in guinea pigs overall.[1,16] This assertion has been made from a compilation of multiple reports that are at least several decades old, some of which were evaluating carcinogenic substances in guinea pigs.[52,53] The true incidence of pulmonary tumors should be reevaluated further in a more recent epidemiologic report.

Pulmonary adenomas can be solitary or multicentric and affect multiple lung lobes.[5] These nodules may be mistaken for metastatic neoplasia, abscesses, or granulomas.[5] Ultrasonography-guided aspiration and cytology may help establish a diagnosis.[4]

Tumors of the Hematopoietic System

Lymphoma and/or leukemia has been associated with type C retroviral infections in guinea pigs; however, its role in naturally occurring guinea pig leukemia and lymphoma remains unknown.[5,54] Clinical signs associated with this condition are poor hair coat, lethargy, anorexia, peripheral lymphadenopathy, and possibly hepatomegaly and splenomegaly.[5,9] These patients may have a significant peripheral leukocytosis characterized by an increase in large lymphocytes.[1] Epitheliotropic T-cell lymphoma has also been documented in several guinea pigs.[55–57] These patients all presented with itching, scaling, and alopecia that were unresponsive to treatment.[55–57] Diagnosis may be made from a fine-needle aspiration and cytology of an enlarged lymph node.[4,9] If the diagnosis is elusive on cytology then an incisional or excisional biopsy of an affected lymph node should be performed and submitted for histopathologic examination.[5] In the cases of suspected epitheliotropic lymphoma it is imperative to obtain tissue biopsies to show histologic changes consistent with this form of lymphoma.[55,56] The overall prognosis for patients with lymphoma is poor and the clinical course of this disease is typically only several weeks.[1,5,9] There are no published reports for treatment of lymphoma in guinea pigs; however, doxorubicin and ifosfamide have been experimentally administered to healthy animals of this species.[58,59]

Other Tumors

Other tumor types that have been described in guinea pigs are cardiac leiomyosarcoma,[60] osteosarcoma,[61–66] chondrosarcoma,[67] and gastrointestinal spindle cell sarcoma.[3]

CHINCHILLAS (*CHINCHILLA LANIGERA*)

There is a scarcity of reports in the literature regarding cancer in chinchillas. The limited number of reports may reflect that geriatric conditions like neoplasia went unreported because of chinchillas previously being kept for fur and research purposes.[68] The lack of reports in chinchillas may also indicate a low incidence of cancer compared with other rodent species, and this has been suggested in several retrospective evaluations.[68] Further epidemiologic investigation is needed to confirm this supposition (**Figs. 7** and **8**, **Table 1**).

HAMSTERS

Golden (Syrian) hamster (*Mesocricetus auratus*)
Russian (Djungarian) hamster (*Phodopus sungorus*)
Roborovski hamster (*Phodopus roborovskii*)
Campbell's dwarf hamster (*Phodopus campbelli*)

Tumors of the Skin and Subcutis

The most common anatomic site for tumor development in Djungarian hamsters is the integument, according to one report.[69] The most common tumor histotypes identified

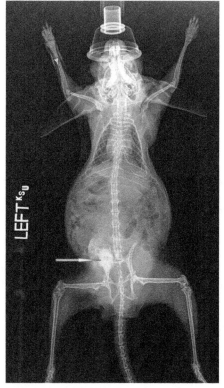

Fig. 7. Pelvic radiograph of a chinchilla with an osteosarcoma (*arrow*). (*Courtesy of* David Eshar, DVM, Dipl. ABVP (Exotic Companion Mammals), Dipl. ECZM (Small Mammal), Manhattan, KS.)

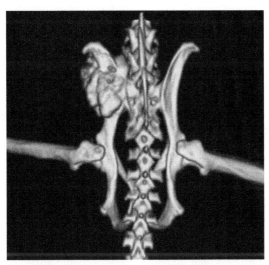

Fig. 8. Computed tomography three-dimensional reconstruction of a pelvic osteosarcoma in a chinchilla. (*Courtesy of* David Eshar, DVM, Dipl. ABVP (Exotic Companion Mammals), Dipl. ECZM (Small Mammal), Manhattan, KS.)

were papillomas (13.3%), squamous cell carcinomas (8%), and atypical fibromas (16%), but a variety of other tumor types have been documented in hamsters with varying frequency.[69]

Mast cell tumors (mastocytomas) have also been identified through cutaneous biopsies in Djungarian hamsters with 8 of 86 (9.3%) in one report.[70] Most of these mast cell tumors were located on the cranial half of the patient, with the head and neck being the most common locations.[70] All but 1 tumor was well differentiated, indicating that mast cell tumors in hamsters may have a more benign clinical course.[70] Fine-needle aspiration and cytology should yield a diagnosis, but an incisional or excisional biopsy may be performed to confirm the diagnosis via histopathology.[70] There are no reports regarding treatment of mast cell tumors in hamsters, but surgical removal may be performed.

Table 1
Reported cases of neoplasia in chinchillas

Site	Histologic Diagnosis	N
Gastrointestinal and hepatobiliary	Salivary gland carcinoma[136]	1
	Gastric adenocarcinoma[137]	1
	Cholangiohepatic carcinoma[138]	1
Hematopoietic	Lymphoma[68]	2
Respiratory	Pulmonary adenocarcinoma[68]	1
Reproductive	Uterine leiomyoma[68]	1
	Uterine leiomyosarcoma[68]	1
Musculoskeletal	Osteosarcoma[139]	1
Miscellaneous	Hemangioma[68]	1
	Pituitary adenoma[68]	1
	Neuroblastoma[16]	1
	Lipoma[16]	1

Syrian hamsters have been noted to develop cutaneous melanomas in their flank organs (pigmented area in male hamsters present on the dorsolateral aspect of the abdomen), head, neck, and back.[71] There is a 10:1 male/female predisposition to melanoma reported from the large compilation of reports regarding hamster neoplasia.[71] Melanomas may show epitheloid or histiocytoid cell morphology and may also display varying degrees of cellular atypia and quantity of melanin present in the cytoplasm.[4] Surgical removal is recommended for treatment of melanoma; however, metastasis has been documented and complete staging with thoracic radiographs and local lymph node aspiration is recommended before surgery.[72]

Atypical fibromas and fibrosarcomas have been reported in Djungarian hamsters, as well as in a Roborovski hamster.[73–76] These tumors arise within the dermis and subcutaneous tissue from ganglion cell–like (GL) cells that are most commonly located on the ventrum, forelimbs, and hindlimbs.[74,75] The quantity of GL cells in the dermis and subcutaneous tissue increases with age and is influenced by circulating androgen levels.[73] Consequently, most atypical fibromas that have been reported occurred in male hamsters older than 7 months of age, corresponding with the onset of sexual maturity.[69,73–75] Fine-needle aspiration and cytology of the mass may show individual oval to spindle-shaped cells with varying degrees of anisocytosis and anisokaryosis.[76] Surgical excision and histopathologic evaluation are recommended. Atypical fibromas have a characteristic immunohistochemical feature of concomitant vimentin and androgen receptor expression.[73,75]

Hamsters that are maintained in an enzootic population infected with hamster polyomavirus (HaPV) or adult hamsters that are infected with HaPV are more susceptible to developing trichoepitheliomas.[54,77,78] There are multiple other reports of tumors occurring in the skin of hamsters, such as a malignant basal cell tumor,[79] hemangiosarcoma,[80] malignant fibrous histiocytoma,[81] and cutaneous plasmacytomas.[82]

Tumors of the Mammary Gland

In a 2008 report, 17 of 78 (21.8%) tumors collected from both Djungarian and Syrian hamsters were mammary gland tumors.[69] Of these, the incidence of malignant and benign tumors was nearly equal.[69] However, in a subsequent report of 12 mammary tumors, 7 of 12 (58.3%) were determined to be simple adenomas when assessed using the *WHO Histological Classification of Mammary Tumors of the Dog and Cat*.[12,83] This report also evaluated immunohistochemical expression of steroid hormone receptors and showed that 5 of 12 (41.7%) expressed estrogen receptor alpha, 10 of 12 (83.3%) expressed androgen receptor, and none expressed progesterone receptors.[83] In contrast, a more recent report suggested that most (28 of 45) hamster mammary tumors were malignant, with the most common histologic type being adenocarcinoma.[84] Mammary tumors may exfoliate an adequate amount of cellularity for a diagnosis, but cytology of the tumor does not always correlate well with histologic findings.[4] Surgical removal of the tumor is warranted from diagnostic and therapeutic perspectives. Staging for evidence of metastatic disease may be necessary with the high percentage of malignant tumors that have been documented, although the true metastatic potential of these tumors in not known.

Tumors of the Reproductive System

Ovarian tumors, such as granulosa cell or thecal cell tumors, have been documented in laboratory hamsters.[16,71] Leiomyosarcoma,[85] leiomyoma,[71] and adenocarcinoma[16] of the uterus have also previously been noted in the hamster. Clinical signs associated with ovarian and uterine tumors include anorexia, lethargy, abdominal distention, and vaginal discharge.[16,85] Abdominal imaging, with radiographs or ultrasonography, can aid in identifying a mass and the organ of origin. Ultrasonography-guided aspiration and cytology of the mass should be the next diagnostic step; however, results may be inconclusive because some tumors, such as leiomyomas, exfoliate low cellularity.[4] Surgical removal and submission of the tumor for histopathology is always recommended.[85] The metastatic rate for malignant ovarian or uterine tumors is not currently known, but in one report of a uterine leiomyosarcoma there was no overt evidence of metastasis at the time of surgery.[85]

Tumors of the Endocrine System

Adrenal tumors are a frequent occurrence in hamsters, and in some reports are the most common tumor identified in laboratory colonies of hamsters.[5,71,77,86] Regardless of the reportedly high incidence ($\sim$30%) of adrenal tumors, there have only been a few clinical HAC cases reported in pet hamsters.[87,88] As with other species, the reported HAC may be pituitary (n = 1) or adrenal dependent (n = 1).[37,87] Clinical signs in these cases included bilaterally symmetric hair loss over the flank, hyperpigmentation, thinning of the skin, abdominal distention, polydipsia, and polyuria.[87,88] The diagnosis of HAC is achieved through a diagnostic approach identical to that described previously for guinea pigs. Note that hamsters secrete both corticosterone and cortisol, but obtaining baseline levels of these hormones is not diagnostic for HAC, because considerable fluctuations in their levels can occur as a result of several variables, such as stress or concurrent illnesses.[89] Given their small body size, obtaining an adequate blood sample volume for endocrine testing in a hamster can be challenging. Consequently, the diagnosis is often simply based on the aforementioned clinical signs.[5] Treatment of HAC has been reported in 3 hamsters with use of metyrapone, ketoconazole, and mitotane, with evidence of success only with metyrapone (n = 1).[87,88] Investigation into the use of trilostane is warranted.

Other endocrine tumors that have been reported are medullary thyroid carcinomas,[90] parathyroid tumors,[71] pheochromocytomas,[71] and pancreatic carcinomas.[71]

Tumors of the Hematopoietic System

Lymphoma is considered one of the most common tumors recognized in hamsters.[77] Three different forms of lymphoma have been described in hamsters.[5,77] One form is induced by hamster polyomavirus and is seen in naive young hamsters, in which it readily produces a multicentric lymphoma that seems to originate in the mesentery and disseminates to the kidney, liver, and possibly thymus.[77,91] This form commonly occurs in research colonies, and only a single report of a young pet hamster with this condition exists.[91] A second form of lymphoma is observed in older hamsters, in which the presentation is multicentric, affecting multiple peripheral lymph nodes and visceral organs.[77] The last form of lymphoma documented is epitheliotropic lymphoma of a T-cell immunophenotype.[92,93] Clinical signs and physical examination findings that have been associated with the multicentric form of lymphoma in hamsters include anorexia, lethargy, ataxia, dyspnea, palpably enlarged peripheral lymph nodes, and palpable abdominal masses.[77,91] Epitheliotropic lymphoma can present with signs similar to those of the multicentric form if the patient is at an advanced stage of disease, but these patients may present with only cutaneous lesions that have not responded to conservative treatment of other skin conditions.[92,93] The primary cutaneous lesions that are noted with this form are patchy or generalized alopecia, pruritus, generalized exfoliative erythroderma, and cutaneous plaques or nodules that may be ulcerated (**Fig. 9**).[92,93] Fine-needle aspiration and cytology of a lymph node may aid in the diagnosis of multicentric lymphoma. The cytologic appearance is similar to that

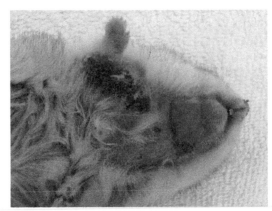

Fig. 9. Multiple cutaneous papules in a hamster with epitheliotropic lymphoma. (*Courtesy* of David Eshar, DVM, Dipl. ABVP (Exotic Companion Mammals), Dipl. ECZM (Small Mammal), Manhattan, KS.)

seen in other mammals.[4] Incisional biopsy and histopathology is necessary to confirm a diagnosis of epitheliotropic lymphoma.[93] There are no published reports regarding the treatment of lymphoma in hamsters. This area warrants further investigation, given that the clinical course of this disease from the time of diagnosis is rapid and overall carries a grave prognosis.[91–93]

Other Tumors

Other tumor histotypes that have been recognized in hamsters include small intestinal adenocarcinomas,[94] hepatocellular carcinomas (HCCs),[16] cholangiomas,[16] and a splenic fibrosarcoma.[95]

MONGOLIAN GERBILS (*MERIONES UNGUICULATUS*)
Tumors of the Skin and Subcutis

Gerbils possess a large ventral abdominal scent gland that is androgen dependent and thus is typically larger in males.[5] This normal gland may be mistaken by owners for a tumor, but in mature gerbils the gland can become neoplastic.[5,77] In such cases, the gland may appear erythematous, inflamed, and ulcerated, and also may have a secondary bacterial infection (**Fig. 10**).[5,96] Fine-needle aspiration and cytology of the mass can be performed.[4] However, it may be best to perform an excisional biopsy with wide surgical margins for therapeutic intervention, and also as a means to obtain a histologic diagnosis and overall prognosis.[5,96] Adenomas, squamous cell carcinomas, and basal cell carcinomas have all been documented to occur at this site.[96–98] Local recurrence and metastasis to inguinal lymph nodes have been documented with malignant tumors occurring in this area.[96,99] Because there seems to be a high incidence of malignant tumors in the ventral scent gland of male gerbils and the scent gland is androgen dependent, castration at the time of tumor removal was advocated.[96,100]

Other skin tumors reported in gerbils include mammary adenocarcinoma,[97] fibrosarcoma,[97] squamous cell carcinoma of the ear,[97] and cutaneous lymphoma.[97,101]

Tumors of the Reproductive System

Testicular teratoma and prostatic adenocarcinoma have both been reported in male gerbils.[97,98] In female gerbils, ovarian tumors have been reported to be the most

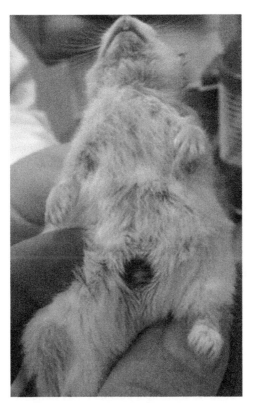

Fig. 10. A neoplastic (undetailed carcinoma) ventral abdominal scent gland in a gerbil. (*Courtesy of* David Eshar, DVM, Dipl. ABVP (Exotic Companion Mammals), Dipl. ECZM (Small Mammal), Manhattan, KS.)

common tumor observed, with varying (9%–44%) incidence rates.[5,77,97,98,102] Gerbils less than 2 years of age seem to develop incipient granulosa cell tumors that are not visible grossly, and this seems to be the most commonly reported ovarian tumor in this species.[103] The metastatic rate described in one report was nearly 18% with the omentum and mesentery being the most common sites affected, and pulmonary metastasis is uncommon.[103] Unbred female gerbils less than 2 years of age have a greater incidence (47.9%) of granulosa cell tumors compared with gerbils that are kept for breeding purposes (23.9%), but the incidence decreases in the unbred population as age increases.[103] It may be reasonable to consider ovariectomy in young nonbreeding gerbils to prevent the development of ovarian tumors.[77] Other tumors that occur within the female reproductive tract are uterine adenocarcinoma, leiomyosarcoma, leiomyoma, ovarian teratoma, and leiomyoma.[97,98,102] Clinical signs that may be noted with female reproductive tumors include vaginal discharge, abdominal distention, lethargy, and anorexia.[5] Abdominal ultrasonography may be used to assess for a suspected reproductive tumor.[99] Ultrasonography-guided fine-needle aspiration with cytology may be attempted under heavy sedation or anesthesia to help obtain a diagnosis. An ovariectomy or ovariohysterectomy is the treatment of choice for ovarian and uterine tumors, respectively.[14,77,104] Evaluation of the entire abdominal cavity should be undertaken during surgery to assess for intra-abdominal metastasis.[103]

Other Tumors

Other tumor types that have been described in gerbils are osteosarcoma,[105] systemic mast cell disease,[106] thyroid adenoma,[107] and a salivary gland sarcoma.[108]

RATS (*RATTUS NORVEGICUS*)

Similar to mice, the incidence of neoplasia in rats varies markedly depending on the age, diet, genetic strain, and environmental settings of the population being studied.[1] Most reports of spontaneous tumors in rats are derived from laboratory populations and in general there is a scarcity of reports from the pet population.

Tumors of the Skin and Subcutis

Rats possess auditory sebaceous glands, called Zymbal glands, that are located ventral to the external ear orifice.[109] Although uncommon and unique to rats, Zymbal gland tumors appear as firm subcutaneous masses just below the ear, and may be ulcerated.[109] These tumors are most often histologically malignant carcinomas, but are reportedly slow to metastasize (**Fig. 11**).[4,109]

Tumors of the Mammary Gland

Mammary fibroadenomas have been reported to be the most common tumor in female rats, with an incidence of 80% to 90%.[1,5,77] Malignant tumors, such as adenocarcinomas, comprise the remaining mammary tumors described.[1,5] Of note, mammary tumors may also occur in male rats.[5] Mammary tumors can grow very large and, because of the extent of mammary tissue in rats, they can appear anywhere from the neck to around the tail base.[1] The masses may become so enlarged that they begin to ulcerate and predispose the rat to a secondary infection.[1,5] Normal ambulation and mobility may become impaired if the mammary tumor is of significant size.[1,5] Cytology from a rat mammary tumor may be difficult to interpret owing to the tumor's typically poor exfoliation, and an inflammatory cell component, from the mass being ulcerated, may also mask the neoplastic element of interest.[4] Surgical removal of the mass is recommended, but recurrence is possible in previously unaffected mammary tissue.[77] The incidence of mammary tumors, in addition to pituitary tumors, has been shown to be markedly decreased in rats that were ovariectomized at 90 days of age compared with those that were not ovariectomized.[110] It has also been suggested

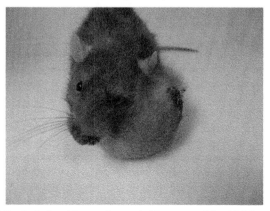

Fig. 11. Ulcerated Zymbal gland tumor in a rat. (*Courtesy of* David Eshar, DVM, Dipl. ABVP (Exotic Companion Mammals), Dipl. ECZM (Small Mammal), Manhattan, KS.)

that performing an ovariectomy (removing the source of estrogens, which are most likely driving development of mammary tumors) in mature rats may decrease the recurrence rate of mammary tumors in other mammary glands.[14,77] This concept is similar to what is practiced in canine and feline oncology. However, no studies exist in rats that show the benefit of neutering at the time of mass removal with regard to recurrence rates, but in theory it should provide benefit as it does in other species. Surgical approach can be through a ventral abdominal incision or via a dorsal ovariectomy.[14,104,111] The use of tamoxifen, an antiestrogen medication, has been discussed for use in rats with mammary tumors, but has been shown to induce liver toxicity and hepatic neoplasia and is not currently recommended.[112] A link between mammary and prolactin-secreting pituitary tumors in rats has been suggested given that the concurrent incidence of both tumors seems to be frequent, but definitive correlation has yet to be established.[5,110]

Tumors of the Endocrine System

Pituitary tumors are a common occurrence in rats.[5] Most of these tumors seem to be prolactin-secreting chromophobic adenomas and the incidence seems to be lower in ovariectomized rats.[110,113] Contributing factors that have been suggested for pituitary tumor development are obesity and high-protein or high-calorie diets.[1,114] Clinical signs of a pituitary tumor are typically consistent with those of central vestibular disease, such as head tilt, ataxia, proprioceptive deficits with normal muscle strength, wide-based stance, knuckling, and an abnormal gait.[115] Other clinical signs that have been noted with a pituitary tumor are visual deficits and behavioral changes.[113]

Advanced imaging with MRI or computed tomography may identify a pituitary lesion.[113,115] Treatment with a dopamine agonist, such as cabergoline (0.6 mg/kg by mouth every 72 hours), has been implemented in 1 case and the patient's clinical signs improved for 8.5 months (**Fig. 12**).[113]

MICE (*MUS MUSCULUS*)

Neoplasia in mice has been extensively researched and the incidence varies widely depending on multiple factors like strain of mice, age, husbandry, parity, diet, and sex.[1,5,16] The pattern of tumor incidence is significantly different between pet mice and inbred strains used in the laboratory, as a result of selective breeding of strains that show variable tumor susceptibility and resistance.[1] Overall, the literature to date typically reflects the incidence of tumors within laboratory mice.

Tumors of the Mammary Gland

Mammary tumors are commonly identified in mice, with an incidence of 30% to 70%.[5,16] Mammary tumors in mice are typically malignant, with a propensity to metastasize.[5] Mice typically present with a subcutaneous mass or masses on their ventrum or flanks, but the tumor can encompass the body from the neck to inguinal region.[5] Fine-needle aspiration and cytology are used to distinguish a mammary tumor from other subcutaneous neoplasia or pathologic lesions.[5] Surgical removal is the best therapeutic option if the tumor is small and amenable to this, but many of these tumors are highly vascular and infiltrative, rendering surgical removal impossible.[1,5] Medical therapies that have been evaluated in experimental settings include tamoxifen and liposomal doxorubicin chemotherapy.[116,117] However, tamoxifen has been shown to induce hepatotoxicity in mice, as is seen in some humans undergoing this treatment.[118] Liposomal doxorubicin (Doxil) administered to retired breeding mice with mammary adenocarcinomas resulted in a mean survival time of 87 days compared

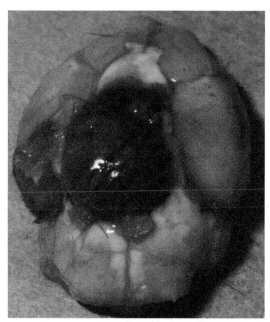

Fig. 12. A large pituitary adenoma in a rat. (*Courtesy of* David Eshar, DVM, Dipl. ABVP (Exotic Companion Mammals), Dipl. ECZM (Small Mammal), Manhattan, KS.)

with 24 days in the untreated group.[117,119,120] There have been no published reports of medical intervention in pet mice.

Other Tumors

One report assessing multiple tumor types in 245 mice identified pulmonary tumors as among the most common tumors in that population.[121] Female mice seemed to have a greater incidence (14%) compared with the male (9%) population.[121] HCCs have been recognized in mice and have been associated with *Helicobacter* spp, which caused chronic active hepatitis and possibly predisposed this group to development of HCC.[122] Lymphoproliferative diseases have also been documented in laboratory mice and have been associated with murine leukemia virus.[1] Other tumors that have been reported are fibrosarcomas,[121] sebaceous adenomas,[121] thyroid adenomas,[121] and intraocular teratoma.[121,123]

BLACK TAILED PRAIRIE DOG (*CYNOMYS LUDOVICIANUS*)
Tumors of the Hepatobiliary System

Hepatobiliary tumors seem to be common in prairie dogs, with one report showing 49% (26 of 53) of tumors evaluated originating from the hepatobiliary system.[124] Most (19 of 26) of these tumors were HCCs.[124] HCC has been documented in other members of the Sciuridae family, like woodchucks and ground squirrels, in which the development of these tumors has been linked to infection with a hepadnavirus (woodchuck hepatitis virus). This finding is similar to what is observed in humans infected with hepatitis B virus.[124–126] The similarity between HCC in prairie dogs and other Sciuridae, as well as humans, suggests that there may be a viral cause responsible for the development of HCCs in prairie dogs, but this has yet to be proved.[125,126] Prairie dogs with HCC may present with lethargy, anorexia, weight loss, acute respiratory distress, and/or a palpable abdominal mass.[124,126] Abdominal radiographs may reveal hepatomegaly and a mass effect, but abdominal ultrasonography better evaluates the origin of the mass and the hepatic echotexture. Furthermore, ultrasonography-guided fine-needle aspiration and cytology may show hepatoid cells with varying degrees of anaplasia.[4] Cytologically these tumors can be difficult to diagnose and a biopsy with histopathology is often needed to confirm the diagnosis and establish the histologic pattern of the HCC.[4] Metastasis can occur and was recognized in 6 of 19 (31.6%) prairie dogs diagnosed with HCC in one report.[124] To date there are no reports of attempted treatment of HCC in a prairie dog. Resection of an isolated liver mass can be considered but might be palliative at best given the suspected viral cause of HCC in sciurids.

Other hepatobiliary tumors that have been reported are hepatocellular adenoma, biliary cystadenoma, and hepatocholangiocarcinoma.[124]

Other Tumors

Pseudo-odontomas are commonly recognized in prairie dogs, but it remains questionable whether these are true neoplasia and thus they are not discussed further in this article.[127]

An assortment of other benign and malignant tumors affecting various body systems have been documented in prairie dogs. These tumors are osteosarcoma,[128] oral squamous cell carcinoma,[124] lymphoma,[129] intestinal leiomyoma,[124] intrathoracic lipoma,[124,130] and several others.[124,131,132]

DEGUS (OCTODON DEGUS)

Degus have a low reported incidence of neoplasia compared with other rodent species.[133,134] In 2 studies assessing pathologic lesions and overall diseases in degus, the incidence of neoplasia ranged from only 2% to 3.7%.[133,134] Although not a true neoplasm, elodontomas are a commonly diagnosed proliferative lesion in degus (**Table 2**).[133,135]

Table 2		
Reported cases of neoplasia in degus		
Site	**Histologic Diagnosis**	**N**
Oral	Melanoma[133]	1
	Fibrosarcoma[133]	1
Skin and subcutis	Myxosarcoma[133]	1
	Malignant histiocytosis[133]	1
	Lipoma[134]	1
Respiratory	Bronchoalveolar carcinoma[140]	1
Urinary	Renal transitional cell carcinoma[141]	1
Hepatobiliary	Hepatocellular carcinoma[134]	2
	Hepatoma[134]	2
Reproductive	Leiomyoma[133]	1
	Leiomyosarcoma[133,142]	2
Hematopoietic	Lymphoma[134]	1
Miscellaneous	Splenic hemangioma[134]	1

REFERENCES

1. Harkness JE, Turner PV, Woude SV, et al. Specific diseases and conditions. In: Harkness JE, Turner PV, Woude SV, et al, editors. Biology and medicine of rabbits and rodents. 5th edition. Ames (IA): Wiley-Blackwell; 2010. p. 249–394.
2. Kanfer S, Reavill DR. Cutaneous neoplasia in ferrets, rabbits, and guinea pigs. Vet Clin North Am Exot Anim Pract 2013;16(3):579–98.
3. Minarikova A, Hauptman K, Jeklova E, et al. Diseases in pet guinea pigs: a retrospective study in 1000 animals. Vet Rec 2015. [Epub ahead of print].
4. Garner MM. Cytologic diagnosis of diseases of rabbits, guinea pigs, and rodents. Vet Clin North Am Exot Anim Pract 2007;10(1):25–49, v-vi.
5. Orr H. Rodents: neoplastic and endocrine disease. In: Keeble E, Meredith A, editors. BSAVA manual of rodents and ferrets. Gloucester (United Kingdom): British Small Animal Veterinary Association; 2011. p. 181–92.
6. Quinton JF, Ollivier F, Dally C. A case of well-differentiated palpebral liposarcoma in a guinea pig (Cavia porcellus). Vet Ophthalmol 2013;16(Suppl 1): 155–9.
7. Steele H. Subcutaneous fibrosarcoma in an aged guinea pig. Can Vet J 2001; 42(4):300–2.
8. Warren S, Gates O. Spontaneous and induced tumors of the guinea pig. Cancer Res 1941;1(1):65–8.
9. Hawkins MG, Bishop CR. Disease problems of guinea pigs. In: Quesenberry KE, Carpenter JW, editors. Ferrets, rabbits, and rodents: clinical medicine and surgery. 3rd edition. St Louis (MO): Elsevier; 2012. p. 302–17.
10. Jelinek F. Spontaneous tumours in guinea pigs. Acta Vet Brno 2003;72:221–8.
11. Suarez-Bonnet A, Martin de Las Mulas J, Millan MY, et al. Morphological and immunohistochemical characterization of spontaneous mammary gland tumors in the guinea pig (Cavia porcellus). Vet Pathol 2010;47(2):298–305.
12. Misdorp W, Else R, Hellme'n E, et al. Histological classification of mammary tumors of the dog and cat, vol. 7. Washington, DC: Armed Forces Institute of Pathology; 1999.
13. Mehler SJ, Bennett RA. Surgical oncology of exotic animals. Vet Clin North Am Exot Anim Pract 2004;7(3):783–805, vii-viii.
14. Capello V. Common surgical procedures in pet rodents. J Exot Pet Med 2011; 20(4):294–307.
15. Field KJ, Griffith JW, Lang CM. Spontaneous reproductive tract leiomyomas in aged guinea-pigs. J Comp Pathol 1989;101(3):287–94.
16. Greenacre CB. Spontaneous tumors of small mammals. Vet Clin North Am Exot Anim Pract 2004;7(3):627–51, vi.
17. Rogers JB, Blumenthal HT. Studies of guinea pig tumors. I. Report of fourteen spontaneous guinea pig tumors, with a review of the literature. Cancer Res 1960;20:191–7.
18. Vink HH. Ovarian teratomas in guinea–pigs: a report of ten cases. J Pathol 1970; 102(3):180–2.
19. Beregi A, Molnar V, Perge E, et al. Radiography and ultrasonography in the diagnosis and treatment of abdominal enlargements in five guinea pigs. J Small Anim Pract 2001;42(9):459–63.
20. Gibbons PM, Garner MM, Kiupel M. Morphological and immunohistochemical characterization of spontaneous thyroid gland neoplasms in guinea pigs (Cavia porcellus). Vet Pathol 2013;50(2):334–42.

21. Hierlmeier B. Tumoröse Veränderungen der Schilddrüse des Meerschweinchens unter besonderer Berücksichtigung der Hyperthyreose. Vienna (Austria): University of Veterinary Medicine Vienna; 2009.
22. Kunzel F, Mayer J. Endocrine tumours in the guinea pig. Vet J 2015;206(3): 268–74.
23. Mayer J, Wagner R, Taeymans O. Advanced diagnostic approaches and current management of thyroid pathologies in guinea pigs. Vet Clin North Am Exot Anim Pract 2010;13(3):509–23.
24. Mayer J, Hunt K, Eshar D, et al. Thyroid scintigraphy in a guinea pig with suspected hyperthyroidism. Exotic DVM 2009;11(1):25–9.
25. Kunzel F, Hierlmeier B, Christian M, et al. Hyperthyroidism in four guinea pigs: clinical manifestations, diagnosis, and treatment. J Small Anim Pract 2013; 54(12):667–71.
26. Meinkoth J, Cowell R, Tyler R. Cell types and criteria of malignancy. In: Cowell R, Tyler R, Meinkoth J, et al, editors. Diagnostic cytology and hematology of the dog and cat. St Louis (MO): Elsevier; 2008. p. 56–150.
27. Brandao J, Vergneau-Grosset C, Mayer J. Hyperthyroidism and hyperparathyroidism in guinea pigs (*Cavia porcellus*). Vet Clin North Am Exot Anim Pract 2013;16(2):407–20.
28. Fredholm DV, Cagle LA, Johnston MS. Evaluation of precision and establishment of reference ranges for plasma thyroxine using a point-of-care analyzer in healthy guinea pigs (*Cavia porcellus*). J Exot Pet Med 2012;21(1):87–93.
29. Peterson ME, Gamble DA. Effect of nonthyroidal illness on serum thyroxine concentrations in cats - 494 cases (1988). J Am Vet Med Assoc 1990;197(9): 1203–8.
30. Peterson ME, Graves TK, Cavanagh I. Serum thyroid-hormone concentrations fluctuate in cats with hyperthyroidism. J Vet Intern Med 1987;1(3):142–6.
31. Thorson L. Thyroid diseases in rodent species. Vet Clin North Am Exot Anim Pract 2014;17(1):51–67.
32. Mayer J, Wagner R, Mitchell MA, et al. Use of recombinant human thyroid-stimulating hormone for evaluation of thyroid function in guinea pigs (*Cavia porcellus*). J Am Vet Med Assoc 2013;242(3):346–9.
33. Kromka MC, Hoar RM. An improved technic for thyroidectomy in guinea pigs. Lab Anim Sci 1975;25(1):82–4.
34. Turrel JM, McEntee MC, Burke BP, et al. Sodium iodide I 131 treatment of dogs with nonresectable thyroid tumors: 39 cases (1990-2003). J Am Vet Med Assoc 2006;229(4):542–8.
35. Daminet S, Kooistra HS, Fracassi F, et al. Best practice for the pharmacological management of hyperthyroid cats with antithyroid drugs. J Small Anim Pract 2014;55(1):4–13.
36. Kasraee B. Depigmentation of brown guinea pig skin by topical application of methimazole. J Invest Dermatol 2002;118(1):205–7.
37. Lunn K, Page R. Tumors of the endocrine system. In: Withrow SJ, Vail DM, Page RL, editors. Small animal clinical oncology. 5th edition. St Louis (MO): Elsevier; 2013. p. 504–31.
38. Gaschen L, Ketz C, Lang J, et al. Ultrasonographic detection of adrenal gland tumor and ureterolithiasis in a guinea pig. Vet Radiol Ultrasound 1998;39(1):43–6.
39. Nowotny I. Hyperadrenokortizismus beim Meerschweinchen. Vienna (Austria): University of Veterinary Medicine Vienna; 2010.

40. Zeugswetter F, Fenske M, Hassan J, et al. Cushing's syndrome in a guinea pig. Vet Rec 2007;160(25):878–80.
41. Behrend EN, Kooistra HS, Nelson R, et al. Diagnosis of spontaneous canine hyperadrenocorticism: 2012 ACVIM consensus statement (small animal). J Vet Intern Med 2013;27(6):1292–304.
42. Fenske M. Saliva cortisol and testosterone in the guinea pig: measures for the endocrine function of adrenals and testes? Steroids 1996;61(11):647–50.
43. Fenske M. The use of salivary cortisol measurements for the non-invasive assessment of adrenal cortical function in guinea pigs. Exp Clin Endocrinol Diabetes 1997;105(3):163–8.
44. Kudsk KA, Miller CL, Sheldon GF. Adrenalectomy in the guinea-pig - operative and perioperative management. Lab Anim Sci 1983;33(2):177–80.
45. Hess LR, Ravich ML, Reavill DR. Diagnosis and treatment of an insulinoma in a guinea pig (Cavia porcellus). J Am Vet Med Assoc 2013;242(4):522–6.
46. Vannevel JY, Wilcock B. Insulinoma in 2 guinea pigs (Cavia porcellus). Can Vet J 2005;46(4):339–41.
47. Powers LV. Techniques for drug delivery in small mammals. J Exot Pet Med 2006;15(3):201–9.
48. Fischer JR, Smith SA, Harkin KR. Glucagon constant-rate infusion: a novel strategy for the management of hyperinsulinemic-hypoglycemic crisis in the dog. J Am Anim Hosp Assoc 2000;36(1):27–32.
49. Bennett KR, Gaunt MC, Parker DL. Constant rate infusion of glucagon as an emergency treatment for hypoglycemia in a domestic ferret (Mustela putorius furo). J Am Vet Med Assoc 2015;246(4):451–4.
50. Graham JE, Kent MS, Theon A. Current therapies in exotic animal oncology. Vet Clin North Am Exot Anim Pract 2004;7(3):757–81, vii.
51. Rosenthal K, Wyre N. Endocrine diseases. In: Quesenberry KE, Carpenter JW, editors. Ferrets, rabbits, and rodents: clinical medicine and surgery. 3rd edition. St Louis (MO): Elsevier; 2012. p. 86–102.
52. Toth B. Susceptibility of guinea pigs to chemical carcinogens: 7,12-dimethylbenz(a)anthracene and urethan. Cancer Res 1970;30(10):2583–9.
53. Manning P. Neoplastic diseases. The biology of the guinea pig. New York: Academic Press; 1976.
54. Kashuba C, Hsu C, Krogstad A, et al. Small mammal virology. Vet Clin North Am Exot Anim Pract 2005;8(1):107–22.
55. Koebrich S, Grest P, Favrot C, et al. Epitheliotropic T-cell lymphoma in a guinea pig. Vet Dermatol 2011;22(2):215–9.
56. Heuer L, Stotter M, Eydner M, et al. Metastasizing epitheliotropic T-cell lymphoma (mycosis fungoides) in two guinea pigs (Cavia porcellus). Berl Munch Tierarztl Wochenschr 2014;127(7–8):333–6 [in German].
57. Martorell J, Such R, Fondevila D, et al. Cutaneous epitheliotropic T-cell lymphoma with systemic spread in a guinea pig (Cavia porcellus). J Exot Pet Med 2011;20(4):313–7.
58. Terasaki T, Iga T, Sugiyama Y, et al. Pharmacokinetic study on the mechanism of tissue distribution of doxorubicin: interorgan and interspecies variation of tissue-to-plasma partition coefficients in rats, rabbits, and guinea pigs. J Pharm Sci 1984;73(10):1359–63.
59. Mancini L, Payne GS, Dzik-Jurasz AS, et al. Ifosfamide pharmacokinetics and hepatobiliary uptake in vivo investigated using single- and double-resonance 31P MRS. Magn Reson Med 2003;50(2):249–55.

60. Vogler BR, Vetsch E, Wernick MB, et al. Primary leiomyosarcoma in the heart of a guinea pig. J Comp Pathol 2012;147(4):452–4.

61. Hong CC, Liu PI. Osteogenic sarcoma in 2 guinea pigs. Lab Anim 1981;15(1): 49–51.

62. Brunetti B, Bo P, Sarli G. Productive osteoblastic osteosarcoma with metastases in a guinea pig. J Am Vet Med Assoc 2013;243(6):801–3.

63. Cook RA, Burk RL, Herron AJ. Extraskeletal osteogenic sarcoma in a guinea pig. J Am Vet Med Assoc 1982;181(11):1423–4.

64. Jolivet MR. Osteosarcoma in a guinea pig. Companion Animal Practice 1988; 2(10):30–1.

65. Leader S. Osteogenic sarcoma of the femur in a guinea pig. Am J Cancer 1937; 29:546–50.

66. Twort C, Twort J. Sarcoma and carcinoma in a guinea-pig. J Pathol Bacteriol 1932;35(6):976.

67. Olcott CT, Papanicolaou GN. Studies on spontaneous tumors in guinea pigs. III. A chondrosarcoma of the iliac bone with metastasis to the mammary region. Cancer Res 1943;3:321–5.

68. Mans C, Donnelly T. Disease problems of chinchillas. In: Quesenberry KE, Carpenter JW, editors. Ferrets, rabbits, and rodents: clinical medicine and surgery. 3rd edition. St Louis (MO): Elsevier; 2012. p. 311–25.

69. Kondo H, Onuma M, Shibuya H, et al. Spontaneous tumors in domestic hamsters. Vet Pathol 2008;45(5):674–80.

70. Nishizumi K, Fujiwara K, Hasegawa A. Cutaneous mastocytomas in Djungarian hamsters. Exp Anim 2000;49(2):127–30.

71. Van Hoosier GL Jr, Trentin JJ. Naturally occurring tumors of the Syrian hamster. Prog Exp Tumor Res 1979;23:1–12.

72. Mangkoewidjojo S, Kim JC. Malignant melanoma metastatic to the lung in a pet hamster. Lab Anim 1977;11(2):125–7.

73. Baba Y, Takahashi K, Nakamura S. Androgen-dependent atypical fibromas spontaneously arising in the skin of Djungarian hamsters (Phodopus sungorus). Comp Med 2003;53(5):527–31.

74. Kashida Y, Ishikawa K, Arai K, et al. Morphological characterization of skin ganglion-like cells in Djungarian hamsters (Phodopus sungorus). Vet Pathol 2003;40(5):548–55.

75. Kondo H, Onuma M, Shibuya H, et al. Atypical fibrosarcomas derived from cutaneous ganglion cell-like cells in 2 domestic Djungarian hamsters (Phodopus sungorus). J Am Assoc Lab Anim Sci 2011;50(4):523–5.

76. Johnson JG 3rd, Blair R, Brandao J, et al. Atypical fibrosarcoma in the skin of a Roborovski hamster (Phodopus roborovskii). Vet Clin Pathol 2014;43(2):281–4.

77. Brown C, Donnelly T. Disease problems of small rodents. In: Quesenberry KE, Carpenter JW, editors. Ferrets, rabbits, and rodents: clinical medicine and surgery. 3rd edition. St Louis (MO): Elsevier; 2012. p. 354–72.

78. Foster AP, Brown PJ, Jandrig B, et al. Polyomavirus infection in hamsters and trichoepitheliomas/cutaneous adnexal tumours. Vet Rec 2002;151(1):13–7.

79. Nakao K, Sato T, Shirai W, et al. Malignant basal cell tumor in a Djungarian hamster. J Vet Med Sci 1999;61(2):191–3.

80. Rosenthal K. Hemangiosarcoma in a hamster. Journal of Small Exotic Animal Medicine 1991;1:15.

81. Endo Y, Sato T, Shirai W, et al. Malignant fibrous histiocytoma in a Djungarian hamster. J Vet Med Sci 2000;62(5):539–41.

82. Kondo H, Takada M, Shibuya H, et al. Cutaneous plasmacytoma in three golden hamsters (*Mesocrietus auratus*). J Vet Med A Physiol Pathol Clin Med 2006; 53(2):74–6.

83. Kondo H, Onuma M, Shibuya H, et al. Morphological and immunohistochemical studies of spontaneous mammary tumours in Siberian hamsters (*Phodopus sungorus*). J Comp Pathol 2009;140(2–3):127–31.

84. Yoshimura H, Kimura-Tsukada N, Ono Y, et al. Characterization of spontaneous mammary tumors in domestic Djungarian hamsters (*Phodopus sungorus*). Vet Pathol 2015;52(6):1227–34.

85. Kondo H, Kimoto H, Shibuya H, et al. Spontaneous uterine leiomyosarcoma in a golden hamster (*Mesocrietus auratus*). J Vet Med A Physiol Pathol Clin Med 2007;54(1):27–9.

86. Tanaka A, Hisanaga A, Ishinishi N. The frequency of spontaneously-occurring neoplasms in the male Syrian golden hamster. Vet Hum Toxicol 1991;33(4): 318–21.

87. Bauck LB, Orr JP, Lawrence KH. Hyperadrenocorticism in three teddy bear hamsters. Can Vet J 1984;25(6):247–50.

88. Martinho F. Suspected case of hyperadrenocorticism in a golden hamster (*Mesocricetus auratus*). Vet Clin North Am Exot Anim Pract 2006;9(3):717–21.

89. Ottenweller JE, Tapp WN, Burke JM, et al. Plasma cortisol and corticosterone concentrations in the golden hamster, (*Mesocricetus auratus*). Life Sci 1985; 37(16):1551–8.

90. DeLellies RA, Wolfe HJ, Mohr U. Medullary thyroid carcinoma in the Syrian golden hamster: an immunohistochemical study. Exp Pathol 1987;31(1):11–6.

91. Simmons JH, Riley LK, Franklin CL, et al. Hamster polyomavirus infection in a pet Syrian hamster (*Mesocricetus auratus*). Vet Pathol 2001;38(4):441–6.

92. Saunders GK, Scott DW. Cutaneous lymphoma resembling mycosis fungoides in the Syrian hamster (Mesocricetus auratus). Lab Anim Sci 1988;38(5):616–7.

93. Harvey R, Whitbread T, Ferrer L, et al. Epidermotropic cutaneous T-cell lymphoma (mycosis fungoides) in Syrian hamsters (*Mesocricetus auratus*). A report of six cases and the demonstration of T-cell specificity. Vet Dermatol 1992;3(1):13–9.

94. Reavill D. Pathology of the exotic companion mammal gastrointestinal system. Vet Clin North Am Exot Anim Pract 2014;17(2):145–64.

95. Yang CC, Liao JW, Yu YC, et al. Case report: splenic fibrosarcoma in a Campbell's Hamster. Taiwan Vet J 2014;40(3):145–9.

96. Jackson TA, Heath LA, Hulin MS, et al. Squamous cell carcinoma of the midventral abdominal pad in three gerbils. J Am Vet Med Assoc 1996;209(4):789–91.

97. Rowe SE, Simmons JL, Ringler DH, et al. Spontaneous neoplasms in aging Gerbillinae. A summary of forty-four neoplasms. Vet Pathol 1974;11(1):38–51.

98. Vincent A, Ash L. Further observations on spontaneous neoplasms in the Mongolian gerbil, *Meriones unguiculatus*. Lab Anim Sci 1978;28(3):297–300.

99. Keeble E. Gerbils. In: Meredith A, Redrobe S, editors. BSAVA manual of exotic pets. 4th edition. Quedgeley, Gloucester, England: British Small Animal Veterinary Association; 2002. p. 34–46.

100. Raflo CP, Diamond SS. Metastatic squamous-cell carcinoma in a gerbil (*Meriones unguiculatus*). Lab Anim 1980;14(3):237–9.

101. Su YC, Wang MH, Wu MF. Cutaneous B cell lymphoma in a Mongolian gerbil (*Meriones unguiculatus*). Contemp Top Lab Anim Sci 2001;40(5):53–6.

102. Meckley PE, Zwicker GM. Naturally-occurring neoplasms in the Mongolian gerbil, *Meriones unguiculatus*. Lab Anim 1979;13(3):203–6.

103. Guzman-Silva MA, Costa-Neves M. Incipient spontaneous granulosa cell tumour in the gerbil, *Meriones unguiculatus*. Lab Anim 2006;40(1):96–101.
104. Miwa Y, Sladky KK. Small mammals: common surgical procedures of rodents, ferrets, hedgehogs, and sugar gliders. Vet Clin North Am Exot Anim Pract 2016;19(1):205–44.
105. Salyards GW, Blas-Machado U, Mishra S, et al. Spontaneous osteoblastic osteosarcoma in a Mongolian gerbil (*Meriones unguiculatus*). Comp Med 2013; 63(1):62–6.
106. Guzman-Silva MA. Systemic mast cell disease in the Mongolian gerbil, *Meriones unguiculatus*: case report. Lab Anim 1997;31(4):373–8.
107. Shumaker RC, Paik SK, Houser WD. Tumors in Gerbillinae: a literature review and report of a case. Lab Anim Sci 1974;24(4):688–90.
108. Toyoda T, Tsukamoto T, Cho YM, et al. Undifferentiated sarcoma of the salivary gland in a Mongolian gerbil (*Meriones unguiculatus*). J Toxicol Pathol 2011; 24(3):173–7.
109. Boorman G, Everitt J. Neoplastic disease. In: Suckow M, Weisbroth S, Franklin C, editors. The laboratory rat. 2nd edition. St Louis (MO): Elsevier; 2006. p. 480–511.
110. Hotchkiss CE. Effect of surgical removal of subcutaneous tumors on survival of rats. J Am Vet Med Assoc 1995;206(10):1575–9.
111. Steele MS, Bennett RA. Clinical technique: dorsal ovariectomy in rodents. J Exot Pet Med 2011;20(3):222–6.
112. Dragan YP, Fahey S, Street K, et al. Studies of tamoxifen as a promoter of hepatocarcinogenesis in female Fischer F344 rats. Breast Cancer Res Treat 1994; 31(1):11–25.
113. Mayer J, Sato A, Kiupel M, et al. Extralabel use of cabergoline in the treatment of a pituitary adenoma in a rat. J Am Vet Med Assoc 2011;239(5):656–60.
114. Turnbull GJ, Lee PN, Roe FJ. Relationship of body-weight gain to longevity and to risk of development of nephropathy and neoplasia in Sprague-Dawley rats. Food Chem Toxicol 1985;23(3):355–61.
115. Vannevel JY. Clinical presentation of pituitary adenomas in rats. Vet Clin North Am Exot Anim Pract 2006;9(3):673–6.
116. Matsuzawa A, Mizuno Y, Yamamoto T. Antitumor effect of the antiestrogen, tamoxifen, on a pregnancy-dependent mouse mammary tumor (TPDMT-4). Cancer Res 1981;41(1):316–24.
117. Vaage J, Mayhew E, Lasic D, et al. Therapy of primary and metastatic mouse mammary carcinomas with doxorubicin encapsulated in long circulating liposomes. Int J Cancer 1992;51(6):942–8.
118. Gao FF, Lv JW, Wang Y, et al. Tamoxifen induces hepatotoxicity and changes to hepatocyte morphology at the early stage of endocrinotherapy in mice. Biomed Rep 2016;4(1):102–6.
119. Kent MS. The use of chemotherapy in exotic animals. Vet Clin North Am Exot Anim Pract 2004;7(3):807–20, viii.
120. Hahn K. Chemotherapy dose calculation and administration in exotic animal species. Seminars in Avian and Exotic Pet Medicine 2005;14(3):193–8.
121. Prejean JD, Peckham JC, Casey AE, et al. Spontaneous tumors in Sprague-Dawley rats and Swiss mice. Cancer Res 1973;33(11):2768–73.
122. Ward JM, Fox JG, Anver MR, et al. Chronic active hepatitis and associated liver tumors in mice caused by a persistent bacterial infection with a novel *Helicobacter* species. J Natl Cancer Inst 1994;86(16):1222–7.

123. Smith RS, Miller JV, Sundberg JP. Intraocular teratoma in a mouse. Comp Med 2002;52(1):68–72.
124. Thas I, Garner MM. A retrospective study of tumours in black-tailed prairie dogs (*Cynomys ludovicianus*) submitted to a zoological pathology service. J Comp Pathol 2012;147(2–3):368–75.
125. Garner MM, Raymond JT, Toshkov I, et al. Hepatocellular carcinoma in black-tailed prairie dogs (*Cynomys ludivicianus*): tumor morphology and immunohistochemistry for hepadnavirus core and surface antigens. Vet Pathol 2004; 41(4):353–61.
126. Une Y, Tatara S, Nomura Y, et al. Hepatitis and hepatocellular carcinoma in two prairie dogs (*Cynomys ludovicianus*). J Vet Med Sci 1996;58(9):933–5.
127. Phalen DN, Antinoff N, Fricke ME. Obstructive respiratory disease in prairie dogs with odontomas. Vet Clin North Am Exot Anim Pract 2000;3(2):513–7, viii.
128. Mouser P, Cole A, Lin TL. Maxillary osteosarcoma in a prairie dog (*Cynomys ludovicianus*). J Vet Diagn Invest 2006;18(3):310–2.
129. Miwa Y, Matsunaga S, Nakayama H, et al. Spontaneous lymphoma in a prairie dog (*Cynomys ludovicianus*). J Am Anim Hosp Assoc 2006;42(2):151–3.
130. Rogers K, Chrisp C. Lipoma in the mediastinum of a Prairie Dog (Cynomys ludovicianus). Contemp Top Lab Anim Sci 1998;37(1):74–6.
131. Sano Y, Matsuda K, Minami S, et al. Cutaneous angioleiomyoma in a black-tailed prairie dog (*Cynomys iudovicianus*). J Comp Pathol 2014;151(1):126–9.
132. Funk R. Medical management of prairie dogs. In: Quesenberry KE, Carpenter JW, editors. Ferrets, rabbits, and rodents: clinical medicine and surgery. 2nd edition. St Louis (MO): Elsevier; 2004. p. 266–73.
133. Jekl V, Hauptman K, Knotek Z. Diseases in pet degus: a retrospective study in 300 animals. J Small Anim Pract 2011;52(2):107–12.
134. Murphy J, Crowell T, Hewes K. Spontaneous lesions in the degu (Rodentia Hystricomorpha: *Octodon degus*. In: Montali R, Migaki G, editors. The comparative pathology of zoo animals. Washington, DC: Smithsonian Institution Press; 1980. p. 437–44.
135. Jekl V, Hauptman K, Skoric M, et al. Elodontoma in a degu (*Octodon degus*). J Exot Pet Med 2008;17(3):216–20.
136. Smith JL, Campbell-Ward M, Else RW, et al. Undifferentiated carcinoma of the salivary gland in a chinchilla (*Chinchilla lanigera*). J Vet Diagn Invest 2010; 22(1):152–5.
137. Lucena RB, Rissi DR, Queiroz DM, et al. Infiltrative gastric adenocarcinoma in a chinchilla (*Chinchilla lanigera*). J Vet Diagn Invest 2012;24(4):797–800.
138. Nobel T, Neumann F. Carcinoma of the liver in a nutria (*Myocastor coypus*) and a chinchilla (*Chinchilla laniger*). Refu Vet 1963;20:161–2.
139. Simova-Curd S, Nitzl D, Pospischil A, et al. Lumbar osteosarcoma in a chinchilla (*Chinchilla laniger*). J Small Anim Pract 2008;49(9):483–5.
140. Anderson WI, Steinberg H, King JM. Bronchioloalveolar carcinoma with renal and hepatic metastases in a degu (*Octodon degus*). J Wildl Dis 1990;26(1): 129–31.
141. Lester PA, Rush HG, Sigler RE. Renal transitional cell carcinoma and choristoma in a degu (*Octodon degus*). Contemp Top Lab Anim Sci 2005;44(3):41–4.
142. Skoric M, Fictum P, Jekl V, et al. Vaginal leiomyosarcoma in a degu (*Octodon degus*): a case report. Veterinarni Medicina 2010;55(8):409–12.

Rabbit Oncology

Diseases, Diagnostics, and Therapeutics

Yvonne van Zeeland, DVM, MVR, PhD, DECZM (Avian, Small mammal), CPBC

KEYWORDS

- Lagomorphs • Neoplasia • Neoplastic disease • Oryctolagus cuniculus
- Lymphoma • Thymoma • Uterine adenocarcinoma • Viral-induced tumors

KEY POINTS

- Rabbits may suffer from similar neoplastic diseases as other companion animals, with a tumor incidence reported of 0.5% to 2.7% across the entire rabbit population.
- Common tumors include uterine adenocarcinoma, lymphoma/leukemia, thymoma, mammary gland tumors, and cutaneous neoplasia; other tumor types may also be diagnosed, but seem to occur less frequently.
- Diagnostic workup follows similar guidelines as in other animals and aims to determine the location, type, and extent of the tumor; the clinical stage; and presence of comorbidities.
- Surgery remains the most commonly used method to treat neoplasia in rabbits, but other therapeutic modalities can be used as primary treatment or in conjunction with surgery.
- Preventive measures include ovariohysterectomy, insect control, and vaccination, which are aimed at reducing the incidence of uterine and mammary neoplasia and transmission of viruses known to cause neoplasia, respectively.

INTRODUCTION

Over the past decades, the popularity of rabbits as pets has risen considerably. Together with the increased quality of (veterinary) care and concomitant increases in the rabbits' life expectancy, this has likely led to an increase in the number of rabbits diagnosed with geriatric diseases and neoplasia. Although the actual incidence of spontaneously occurring neoplasia in the rabbit is difficult to provide, retrospective studies have suggested prevalences of 0.5% and up to 2.7% across the entire rabbit population.[1–3] Similar to other animals, older rabbits are more likely to be diagnosed with tumors, with a profound increase in the incidence of neoplastic disease (from 1.4% to 8.4%) reported after the second year of life.[2] These neoplastic changes predominantly involve the urogenital, hemolymphatic, and integumentary systems, with

Disclosure Statement: The author has nothing to disclose.
Division of Zoological Medicine, Department of Clinical Sciences of Companion Animals, Faculty of Veterinary Medicine, Utrecht University, Yalelaan 108, Utrecht 3584 CM, The Netherlands
E-mail address: Y.R.A.vanZeeland@uu.nl

uterine neoplasia and lymphoid tumors being the 2 most predominant tumor types. Other tumor types have also been reported in rabbits, but their incidence seems to be much lower, with most of the information being derived from anecdotal evidence and case reports. Nevertheless, the knowledge with regard to rabbit oncology has grown considerably over the past years whereby the availability of new, more advanced diagnostic techniques and treatment modalities have greatly improved the abilities to accurately and appropriately diagnose and manage neoplastic disease in the domestic rabbit.

In this article, the different diagnostic steps and therapeutic interventions that can be considered when confronted with a rabbit suspected of a neoplasia are discussed. In addition, an overview will be given of the various spontaneously occurring neoplasia that have been reported in rabbits, whereby the most commonly seen tumors will be discussed in greater detail.

DIAGNOSTIC EVALUATION

As with any disease, the workup of a patient with (suspected) neoplasia starts with a thorough history and full physical examination, followed by additional diagnostic tests. The major goals of this diagnostic evaluation are to assess the following:

- Location of the tumor,
- Size and local invasiveness of the tumor,
- Tumor type, including biologic activity of the tumor,
- Stage of the disease, including regional and distant metastases, and
- Presence of concurrent disease, secondary complications, and paraneoplastic syndromes that may influence the treatment options and outcome.

Signalment, History, and Physical Examination

Various types of neoplasia are known to affect rabbits of a specific age, sex, or breed. Familiarity with these predispositions may aid in the diagnosis. Examples of tumor predilections in rabbits include:

- Age: most tumors are seen in older patients, but lymphomas and papillomas can also be found in rabbits less than 2 years.[3]
- Sex: although mammary tumors may develop in both sexes, females are most prone.
- Breed: uterine tumors are often seen in, for example, Dutch breeds.[3]

Aside from the signalment, the history may also provide information on potential risk factors such as (lack of) neutering and vaccination status. If the patient is presented with an external mass (**Fig. 1**), specific information needs to be obtained regarding the mass' time of onset, duration, growth rate, and (response to) previous treatment. Moreover, the history should include an evaluation of the potential systemic effects of the neoplasia, which will induce changes in, for example, the rabbit's behavior, activity level, appetite, body condition, or breathing. However, in many rabbits the neoplastic process itself will go unnoticed by the owner (eg, in case of an abdominal mass). As a result, the clinical presentation may be more variable, ranging from unspecific signs (eg, inappetance, weight loss, lethargy, depression) to signs resulting from the local or systemic effects of the neoplasia (eg, hematuria, gastric bloat or gut stasis, dyspnea).

Internal and external masses may occasionally be identified as coincidental findings during a routine physical examination (**Fig. 2**). Any mass that is identified

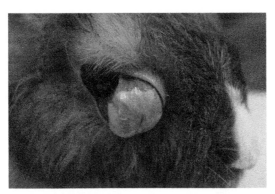

Fig. 1. When a lump or mass is found, such as the one protruding from the third eyelid of this rabbit, the owner will easily associate this with the fact that their rabbit has cancer. Knowledge regarding tumor predispositions will often help to inform the owner adequately and quickly whether and what type of tumor can be involved. In this rabbit, the location and morphologic appearance fit best with a protrusion of the Harderian gland, resulting from a prolapsed third eyelid, although a lymphoma of the Harderian gland cannot be excluded. To differentiate between the 2, cytology or histopathology are required.

should always be evaluated for its location, size, aspect, and association with surrounding tissues because this can provide clues on the involved tumor type and its behavior. Regional lymph nodes will also need to be evaluated for size, consistency, and fixation to adjacent tissues to obtain information on potential metastasis, which is helpful in the staging of the disease. Moreover, a full physical examination is warranted to identify presence of systemic effects (eg, owing to distant metastasis, paraneoplastic syndromes) and comorbidities that may interfere with treatment or negatively influence the prognosis. For example, dyspnea may hint toward the presence of pulmonary metastases and indicate a poor prognosis in does with a uterine adenocarcinoma.

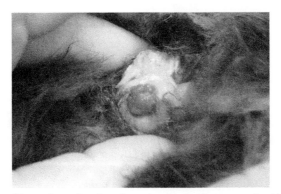

Fig. 2. Neoplasia will not always be directly noticeable by the owner. In this 1-year-old male castrated Flemish giant rabbit, tenesmus was the predominant clinical sign. Only upon closer inspection of the anus, was this anorectal papilloma noticed.

Ancillary Diagnostic Testing

After the history and physical examination, a problem list, and list of differential diagnoses may be constituted to form the basis for planning of further diagnostic steps. Diagnostic modalities that may be used in rabbits are similar to those used in dogs and cats and may include a hematologic and biochemical profile, urinalysis, imaging, and collection of fine-needle aspirates (FNA) or biopsies for cytologic and histopathologic examination.

Hematology and biochemistry

Blood and urinalysis are often performed to establish a baseline of the rabbit's overall health status. Moreover, it can be useful for:

- Diagnosis of leukemia,
- Diagnosis of functional endocrine tumors (eg, hypertestosteronism or prolactinemia in adrenocortical neoplasia or pituitary tumors, respectively),
- Evaluation of paraneoplastic changes such as hypercalcemia[a] (eg, malignant lymphoma) and hyperproteinemia and gammopathy (eg, myeloma), and
- Assessment of organ function (eg, liver, kidneys), especially if these are involved in the primary neoplastic process (eg, generalized lymphoma), or to exclude organ dysfunction before or during a treatment course.

Imaging

Imaging techniques will often provide valuable information with regard to the extent of the tumor and presence of metastases. Similar to other animals, radiography and ultrasonography are most commonly used, because most private practices have easy access to these imaging modalities. In rabbits, radiographs will often aid in the diagnosis of abdominal or mediastinal masses (**Fig. 3**), bony tumors (**Fig. 4**), and pulmonary metastases (**Fig. 5**). In case of abdominal or mediastinal masses, ultrasonography may be used for further evaluating the origin, morphology, and extent of the mass. As in other animals, advanced techniques such as computed tomography

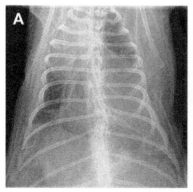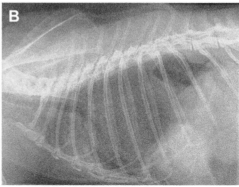

Fig. 3. Ventrodorsal (*A*) and right lateral (*B*) radiographs of a rabbit with progressive dyspnea, displaying a caudal mediastinal mass, and craniolateral displacement of the heart. Histopathology revealed the mass to be a lipoma.

---

[a] In rabbits, hypercalcemia should always be interpreted with caution because high calcium levels are not necessarily pathologic in rabbits owing to their unique calcium-regulating mechanism.

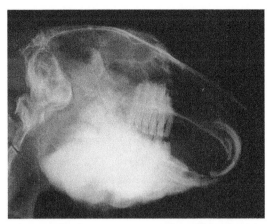

Fig. 4. Radiograph of a mandibular osteosarcoma of a rabbit. Extensive new bone formation may be noted. (*Courtesy of* Evert-Jan de Boer, DVM, Dierenkliniek Wilhelminapark, The Netherlands.)

(CT; **Fig. 6**), MRI, or nuclear scintigraphy (eg, bone scintigraphy) may be required to gain more detailed information on the extent and invasiveness of the tumor to aid in the planning of a surgical intervention or radiation therapy (eg, in case of nasal tumors or thymomas; **Fig. 7**).

Cytology
Cytologic examinations of buffy coat preparations, bone marrow aspirates or FNA from solid masses (**Fig. 8**) or peripheral lymph nodes are often valuable in the diagnosis of primary neoplastic lesions or regional metastases to lymph nodes.[4,5] Owing to the low cytologic yield, this technique is predominantly considered helpful in case of lipomas, and tumors comprising round cells (eg, lymphoma, mast cell tumor) or epithelial cells (eg, squamous cell carcinoma, melanoma, adenocarcinoma).[6,7]

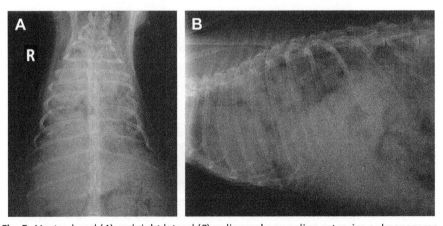

Fig. 5. Ventrodorsal (*A*) and right lateral (*B*) radiographs revealing extensive pulmonary metastases in an intact doe with uterine adenocarcinoma. (*Courtesy of* Evert-Jan de Boer, DVM, Dierenkliniek Wilhelminapark, The Netherlands.)

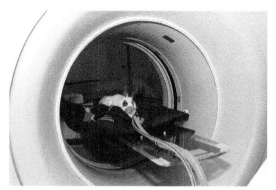

Fig. 6. Advanced imaging techniques, such as computed tomography, are ideal for localizing masses that may remain unnoticed with conventional radiographs (eg, nasal adenocarcinomas).

Histopathology

The collection of biopsies in rabbits follows similar guidelines as those described in dogs and cats.[8–10] However, extra caution is warranted when collecting surface-biting biopsies from the hollow viscera, because these pose an increased risk of perforation, peritonitis and associated mortality owing to their thin-walled and delicate nature.[5] Once tissue samples have been collected, histopathologic evaluation may take place to establish a definite diagnosis and verify whether complete resection has been achieved (in case of excisional biopsies). Classification of the tumor type follows similar guidelines as those used in other animal species, whereby a morphologic diagnosis generally can be obtained based on the primary tumor's site of origin, tissue type, and histologic grade (**Box 1**).[11] Accurate typing of the tumor may furthermore be

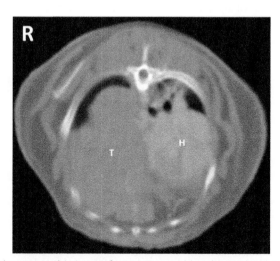

Fig. 7. Computed tomographic image from a 6-year-old male castrated rabbit with clinical signs of progressive dyspnea and bilateral exophthalmos owing to a thymoma. After intravenous administration of iodinated contrast medium, the tumor (T), which occupies approximately one-half of the thorax and causes the heart (H) to deviate to the left, can be identified clearly.

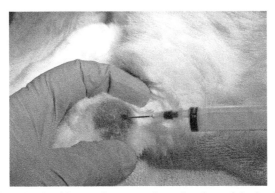

Fig. 8. Fine needle aspiration biopsy of a mass at lateral surface of the hock joint, which was diagnosed as a malignant melanoma. To obtain good quality samples, a needle size of at least 22 Gauge should be used. (*Courtesy of* Evert-Jan de Boer, DVM, Dierenkliniek Wilhelminapark, The Netherlands.)

achieved using tumor markers. These comprise either substances that are produced (in greater amounts) by or in response to the presence of tumor cells in the body or patterns of gene expressions that are characteristic for certain types of cancer (**Table 1**). Tumor markers can be identified in the tissue or bodily excretions (eg, blood, feces, urine) using immunohistochemical stains or laboratory tests Although these are not yet routinely used in exotic animal practice, tumor markers can provide crucial information regarding the nature and behavior of the tumor. As a result, they do not only serve a diagnostic purpose, but also aid in the management, monitoring, and estimation of the prognosis for an oncologic patient.[12]

Tumor staging

Aside from classification of the tumor based on its location, tumor type, and grade, tumors may also be classified by stage using the TNM system (**Box 2**).[13] This type of staging is not applied routinely in rabbit medicine, but may follow similar guidelines to those described in dogs and cats.

THERAPEUTICS

Once the diagnosis and staging have been completed, treatment options may be evaluated and discussed with the owner. The primary goal of any intervention will be to treat the neoplasm without compromising the welfare of the rabbit. Patients at increased risk for morbidity or mortality (eg, rabbits with severe anemia as a result from bleeding tumors) may require stabilization before attempting other treatment options. Moreover, rabbit patients may require close monitoring and supportive care during the treatment course, to prevent them from deteriorating. For patients in which this seems to be unlikely or impossible to achieve, euthanasia should be considered.

Surgical Intervention

Similar to other companion animals, treatment of neoplasia in rabbits often involves surgical intervention. If possible, complete surgical excision, whereby guidelines with regard to margins are comparable with those in other species (ie, 1–3 cm dependent on malignancy of the tissue). However, in smaller rabbits, smaller margins may need to be used because the remaining defect may otherwise be too large to close.

Box 1
Classification of tumors

Classification by site of origin

Anatomic location where the primary tumor originated from

Examples:
- Uterine neoplasia
- Renal tumor
- Liver tumor
- Cutaneous neoplasia
- Mammary gland tumor
- Brain tumor
- Lung tumor

Classification by tissue type

Tumors may be classified into 6 major categories based on the tissue type involved:
- Epithelial tumors: originating from epithelial cells lining the body surface or internal organs (eg, squamous cell carcinoma, adenocarcinoma).
- Mesenchymal tumors: originating in connective and supportive tissues including bone, cartilage, muscle and fat (eg, fibroma; fibrosarcoma, osteosarcoma, lipoma; leiomyoma, rhabdomyosarcoma).
- Hematopoietic tumors originating from the bone marrow:
  - Leukemia: originating from cells that normally mature in the blood stream (eg, myelocytic leukemia, lymphatic leukemia);
  - Lymphoma: originating from cells that normally mature in the lymphatic system, representing solid tumors that may be present in various organs and lymph nodes;
  - Myeloma: originating from plasma cells;
- Germ cell tumors (eg, teratoma); and
- Mixed cell types: composed of 2 or more components (eg, mixed Müllerian duct tumor).

Classification by histologic grade

Differentiation between benign and malignant tumors based on the following criteria:
1. Differentiation (well vs poorly differentiated)
2. Growth rate (slow vs rapid with many mitoses)
3. Growth pattern (expansile vs invasive growth without a capsule)
4. Metastasis (no vs frequent metastasis)
5. Microscopic features (eg, presence of pleiomorphism, hyperchromasia and multiple nucleoli in malignant tumors)

If the tumor is malignant, the degree of malignancy may be determined. Based on the level of tissue differentiation, cellular growth activity and extent of necrosis within the tumor, a grade from 1 to 4 may be assigned.

Grade 1: Low grade; well-differentiated cells that bear close resemblance to the normal cells of the parent tissue.

Grade 2: Intermediate grade; moderately differentiated cells that still bear considerable resemblance to the parent cells and tissue but abnormalities are commonly seen and complex features are often not well-formed.

Grade 3: High grade; poorly differentiated cells that bear little resemblance to the parent tissue. Abnormalities are evident and more complex architectural features are usually rudimentary.

Grade 4: Undifferentiated or anaplastic; cells are immature, primitive, and undifferentiated, and bear no significant resemblance to the corresponding parent cells and tissues.

Similar to dogs and cats, the regional lymph node may also be aspirated, biopsied, or removed as part of the diagnostic workup to enable reliable tumor staging.[14]

If complete resection of the tumor is not feasible, palliative surgery may be considered to relieve the pain and discomfort associated with the tumor. Palliative surgery

Table 1
Examples of tumor biomarkers that have been used in the characterization of neoplasia in rabbits in both experimental and clinical settings

Tumor Marker	Associated Tumor Types
CD3	T-cell lymphoma
CD79α	B-cell lymphoma
Cytokeratin (various types: TPA, TPS, Cyfra21–1)	Many types of carcinoma, some types of sarcoma
Desmin	Smooth muscle sarcoma, skeletal muscle sarcoma, endometrial stromal sarcoma
Immunoglobulin	Lymphoma, leukemia
Keratin (various types)	Carcinoma, some types of sarcoma
Ki-67 (MKI67)	Prostate, brain and mammary carcinomas, nephroblastoma
Melan-A (MART-1)	Melanoma, steroid-producing tumors (adrenocortical carcinoma, gonadal tumors eg, granular cell tumor, testicular interstitial cell tumor)
Osteocalcin	Osteoid containing tumors (eg, osteosarcoma)
Smooth muscle actin	Gastrointestinal stromal tumor, leiomyosarcoma
S100 protein	Melanoma, sarcoma (neurosarcoma, lipoma, chondrosarcoma), astrocytoma, gastrointestinal stromal tumor, salivary gland tumors, some types of adenocarcinoma, histiocytic tumor (dendritic cell, macrophage)
Vimentin	Sarcoma, renal cell carcinoma, endometrial cancer, lung carcinoma, lymphoma, leukemia, melanoma

Box 2
Staging of neoplastic disease based on the TNM system

TNM staging

T: size or direct extent of the primary tumor
   Tx: tumor cannot be evaluated
   T0: no tumor detectable
   T1 to T4: different grades in dimensions of the primary tumor

N: degree of spread to nearby (regional) lymph nodes
   Nx: lymph nodes cannot be evaluated
   N0: absence of tumor cells from the regional lymph nodes
   N1: regional lymph node metastasis present (or spread to closest or small number of regional lymph nodes)
   N2: tumor spread to an extent between N1 and N3
   N3: tumor spread to more distant or numerous regional lymph nodes

M: presence of distant metastasis
   M0: no distant metastasis
   M1: metastasis to distant organs (beyond regional lymph nodes)

Clinical staging

Stage 0: Cancer in situ or limited to surface cells

Stage I: Cancer limited to the tissue of origin

Stage II: Limited local spread of the cancer

Stage III: Extensive local and regional spread of the cancer

Stage IV: Advanced cancer with distant spread and metastasis

may include both debulking surgery and limb amputation, for example, in case of os-teosarcomas. This procedure is generally well-tolerated by rabbits.[15,16] In contrast, explorative laparotomy for gastrointestinal tumors, which often present as acute cases owing to gastrointestinal obstruction and ileus, is often associated with high mortal-ity.[17] Aside from conventional surgical techniques, newer techniques involving laser and electrosurgery may also be used in rabbits, especially if precise cutting and coag-ulating are required (eg, in case of anorectal papillomas; **Fig. 9**).[8] Cryotherapy, which relies on the destruction of cells by repeated freeze–thaw cycles, may be used in treat-ment of small (<1 cm), superficial tumors found on the skin, lips, eyelids, and perianal region, such as trichoblastomas and papillomas.[18]

Chemotherapy

Chemotherapy may be considered as the primary means of therapy in case of nonre-sectable tumors or metastases (eg, lymphoma, leukemia). In addition, chemotherapy may be used as adjunct therapy before or after surgical resection. Various types of chemotherapeutic agents are available for use in rabbits (**Table 2**), which may be administered either systemically or intralesionally. Systemic chemotherapy may be attempted in cases of lymphoma and leukemia, as a good response after this type of treatment has been reported in other species, but thus far no specific protocols have been published regarding their clinical use of efficacy in rabbits. However, exper-imental studies have demonstrated good effects of platinum and pirarubicin in rabbits with induced uterine, bladder, or mammary carcinomas.[19–21] Dosages are usually based on body surface area rather than weight, whereby a recent study determined a reliable method for calculating body surface areas in rabbits based on CT imaging.[22]

In rabbits, reported side effects include inappetance and gastrointestinal stasis, and clinical manifestation of subclinical pasteurellosis or Encephalitozoonosis.[5] If side ef-fects are present, immediate attention and supportive therapy are warranted.[5] Routine monitoring may include a hematologic and biochemical profile to monitor liver and kid-ney function and evaluate bone marrow function. In case of decreased heterophil/lymphocyte counts, chemotherapy should be delayed until white blood cell counts have returned to normal. Subsequent dosages may be reduced by 20% to avoid recurrence of problems.[5] To reduce the risk of systemic effects, intratumoral admin-istration of chemotherapeutic agents may also be considered, especially in solid tu-mors in locations where surgery is less ideal (eg, for cosmetic or functional

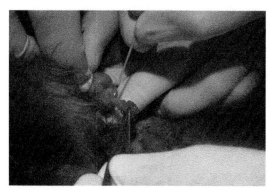

Fig. 9. Removal of an anorectal papilloma using laser surgery. Compared with conventional surgical techniques, laser enables precise cutting and helps to maintain hemostasis by imme-diate coagulation of blood vessels.

reasons). Cisplatin is currently the drug of choice because it is nonnecrotizing and has a good effect on solid tumors (<2 cm) of various types, including squamous cell carcinomas, soft tissue sarcomas, and round cell tumors. In combination with a collagen matrix or water/sesame oil suspension, a high tumor-to-plasma drug concentration ratio will result.[23] Standard protocols include 4 consecutive chemotherapy sessions performed at-1 week intervals during which cisplatin is administered intratumorally at a dose of 1 mg of cisplatin/cm^3 of tissue.[4,23]

Radiation Therapy

In rabbits, radiation therapy (**Fig. 10**) has been used predominantly for the treatment of thymoma, whereby good results have been achieved with both coarse (ie, palliative) and definitive (ie, curative) fractionated radiation therapy using dosages of 24 to 48 Gy.[24,25] Other tumor types that are likely to respond well to radiation therapy include lymphoma, myeloma, seminoma, and nasal adenocarcinoma.[5,26–28] Adverse effects seen after irradiation are similar to those in other species and may include hair loss and discoloration, tissue swelling and associated nerve pain, and skin irritation that—in rare instances—may lead to self-mutilation. Incidentally, more severe side effects, such as radiation-induced myocardial failure and radiation pneumonitis may also be noted, particularly in cases where the thorax is irradiated.[24]

Other Treatment Modalities

Aside from the previously mentioned options, other treatment modalities such as photodynamic therapy,[29] whole body and local hyperthermia,[30,31] and immunotherapy may also be considered in the management of oncologic rabbit patients. Their use in rabbits has, however, been limited to experimental studies.[32–35]

Supportive Care

Neoplastic disease will often induce changes in the metabolism of fat, protein, and carbohydrates, thereby resulting in gradual loss of muscle and fat tissue and, eventually, a state of cachexia. Similarly, anorexia will be a common sequela to neoplastic disease in rabbits, thereby further deteriorating the animal's condition. Provision of high-quality foods and adequate nutritional support will therefore be important in any rabbit presented with a neoplasia. In some rabbits, assisted feeding may be necessary, whereby placement of a nasogastric or esophagostomy tube may be considered for patients that need long-term care. Aside from nutritional support, rabbit patients may also benefit from administration of analgesics (eg, nonsteroidal anti-inflammatory drugs, opioids) to provide pain relief. The use of other drugs (eg, motility-enhancing drugs, gastroprotectants, prednisone, vitamin A) may also be considered as symptomatic treatment, although the potential risks of administering these drugs should be considered. Caution is required particularly when using prednisone or other corticosteroids, because the immunosuppressive effects of these drugs could predispose rabbits to develop secondary pasteurellosis or Encephalitozoonosis.

Follow-up

After treatment, regular checkups are routinely advised because they will facilitate timely diagnosis of recurrent disease or metastases. Guidelines in companion animals suggest rechecks to be scheduled at 1, 2, 3, 5, 7, 9, and 12 months after treatment, with increasing intervals for the years thereafter.[36] During each of these rechecks, a thorough physical examination should be performed, during which the tumor site is carefully examined for evidence of recurrence. Other tests that might be indicated

Table 2
Chemotherapeutic agents used in rabbits

Drug Class	Mechanism of Action	Indications	Side Effects	Dosing Regimen
Alkylating agents (cyclophosphamide, chlorambucil, melphalan, lomustine)	Formation of bonds between alkyl groups in DNA thereby affecting DNA replication (effect is greater in cells with faulty DNA replication). Effect is independent of cell cycle.	Lymphoma	Bone marrow suppression, neutropenia; GI toxicity; hemorrhagic cystitis. Corticosteroids may be given to mitigate side effects. Hepatic and renal toxicity reported when using lomustine.	Cyclophosphamide • 50 mg/m^2 PO q24 h for 2–3 d/wk • 100–200 mg/m^2 IV q1-3 wk (often combined with doxorubicin) Lomustine • 50 mg/m^2 PO q 3–6 wk
Antitumor antibiotics (doxorubicin, mitoxantrone)	Multiple modes of action: affect functionality of DNA and RNA polymerase and topoisomerase I; stimulate formation of free radicals and directly damage DNA/RNA and cell membrane. Action independent of cell cycle.	Lymphoma; leukemia; myeloma; hemangiosarcoma; carcinomas (various types)	Neutropenia; renal failure; GI toxicity; neuropenia; cardiac toxicity (doxorubicin); tissue necrosis at extravasation sites; allergic reactions reported. Corticosteroids and antihistamines may be considered to counteract effects.	Doxorubicin • 1 mg/kg IV q 2–3 wk Mitoxantrone • 5–6 mg/m^2 IV q3 wk
Vinca alkaloids (vincristine, vinblastine)	Inhibition of intracellular microtubule formation (action dependent on phase of the cell cycle).	Lymphoma	Tissue necrosis with extravasation; GI toxicity and neutropenia (at higher dosages); peripheral neuropathy (may result in ileus and constipation).	Vincristine: • 0.5–0.7 mg/m^2 IV q 1–2 wk

Drug	Mechanism	Indications	Adverse effects/Notes	Dose
Platinum products (cisplatin, carboplatin)	Cross-linking between DNA strands (independent of cell cycle).	Carcinoma (various forms); osteosarcoma (alone or in conjunction with doxorubicin)	Severe myelosuppression; neutropenia; GI toxicity; nephrotoxicity. Decrease dose in presence of renal failure. Fluid therapy required before, during and after administration.	Carboplatin: • 150–180 mg/m^2 IV q 3–4 wk
Crisantaspase; L-asparaginase	Degradation of L-asparagine, an amino acid required for protein and DNA synthesis.	Lymphoma; leukemia	Anaphylaxis; pancreatitis and GI toxicity reported in other species.	400 IU/kg IM or SC
Prednisone	Induction of apoptosis in certain lymphoid cell populations. Exact mechanism is not fully understood. Corticosteroids may potentially induce resistance to other chemotherapeutic agents thereby decreasing their effects.	Lymphoma; also effective to treat side effects and as palliative treatment for many other cancer types	Potential immunosuppression which may predispose to pasteurellosis or Encephalitozoonosis. Concurrent use of gastroprotectants (eg, ranitidine or omeprazole) is advised. PU/PD, polyphagia and skin changes may be noted after long-term treatment.	0.5–2.0 mg/kg PO

Body surface area (BSA) can be calculated using the following formula: BSA = 99 × (body weight in grams)$^{2/3}$/10,000.

Abbreviations: GI, gastrointestinal; IM, intramuscularly; IV, intravenous; PO, orally; PU/PD, polyuria/polydipsia; SC, subcutaneous.

Data from Refs.[4,5,19]

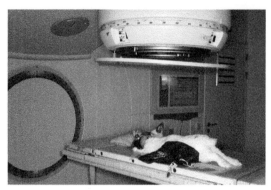

Fig. 10. Radiation therapy in a rabbit with a thymoma. To enable proper positioning, the rabbit was placed on an inflatable cushion whereby landmarks on the rabbit and cushion were used to ascertain that during the consecutive radiation sessions (every 2–3 days for a total of 10 sessions) the rabbit is placed in exactly placed in the same position. A combination of low-dose ketamine (5 mg/kg) and medetomidine (100 μg/kg) produced anesthesia of a depth sufficient to immobilize the rabbit for the duration of the session; supplemental oxygen was provided through a face mask.

include (thoracic and/or abdominal) radiographs, ultrasound, CT-imaging, MRI, bone marrow aspirates, and FNA or biopsy of the original tumor site or regional lymph nodes. Whether and which tests will be performed will depend on the tumor type involved.

DISEASES

Rabbits can suffer from many types of neoplastic disease (**Table 3**). As in other animals, classification is based on their primary site of origin (eg, mammary gland, bone), type of tissue involved (epithelial vs mesenchymal), and growth behavior of the neoplastic cells (benign vs malignant). Although primary neoplasia can originate in any organ system, the degree to which organ and organ systems are affected varies considerably. In both laboratory and pet rabbits, adenocarcinoma of the uterus continues to be the most frequently diagnosed neoplasia, followed by lymphoma/lymphoid leukemia.[3] In laboratory animals, the 2 next most common tumors include embryonal nephroma and bile duct adenoma, whereas in pet rabbits mammary gland tumors and skin tumors are seen more commonly.[3] The differences seen in the frequency with which certain tumor types are seen may, at least in part, be explained by differences in age composition of the groups as well as differences in exposure to pathogens (eg, Shope fibroma virus) or frequency of postmortem examinations performed in apparently healthy animals (resulting in a higher percentage of tumors found by coincidence).

COMMON TUMORS AND THEIR CLINICAL PRESENTATION, DIAGNOSIS AND TREATMENT
Uterine Neoplasia

Uterine adenocarcinoma (**Fig. 11**) is the most commonly diagnosed neoplasia in pet rabbits.[3,37] Although all intact female rabbits are susceptible to develop uterine adenocarcinoma, certain breeds, such as the Tan, French silver, Havana, and Dutch breeds, are considered particularly prone.[37] Incidence significantly increases with age, varying

Table 3
Reported (spontaneous) neoplasia in rabbits

Organ System	Tissue of Origin	Reported Tumor Types	Incidence	Clinical Signs	Diagnosis and Workup	Treatment and Prognosis
Reproductive tract (female)	Ovary; uterus; cervix; vagina; vulva	Uterine adenocarcinoma; leiomyoma/leiomyosarcoma; mixed Müllerian duct tumor; choriocarcinoma; deciduosarcoma; squamous cell carcinoma (vaginal wall); teratoma; hemangioma; granulosa cell tumor; ovarian adenocarcinoma	Entire females; uterine adenocarcinoma is the most common tumor, affecting 50%–80% of does >3 y; certain breeds and family lines may be overrepresented. Other tumors are diagnosed more sporadically.	• Hematuria • Anemia • Firm, irregular uterus on abdominal palpation • Cystic mammary glands • Weight loss, lethargy • Dyspnea (if lung metastases are present)	• Clinical signs (abdominal palpation) • Urinalysis (in patients with hematuria) • Radiography (including thorax to check for lung metastases) • Ultrasonography • Cytology (FNA) • Histopathology • Exploratory laparotomy	Ovariohysterectomy. High rate of metastasis (mainly to lungs and liver but occasionally also to other locations) reported and thus potentially life-threatening without treatment. Up to 3 y may pass from time of diagnosis until metastases-related death occurs.
Reproductive tract (male)	Testes; Prostate	Seminoma; Sertoli cell tumor; interstitial cell tumor (Leydig cell tumor, granular cell tumor); teratoma; adenocarcinoma; Neoplasia of different tumor types can occur simultaneously in both testes and can be nonfunctional or hormone secreting (functional)	Entire males; cryptorchid rabbits are at higher risk; incidence increases with age, but generally considered a rare finding in rabbits.	• Unilateral or bilateral testicular enlargement; contralateral testis may be small • Change in consistency of 1 or both testes • Change in libido and associated behaviors • Reproductive failure • Scrotum skin necrosis (rare) • Gynecomastia (rare) • Gait changes (if testes are severely enlarged) • Weight loss	• Clinical signs • Ultrasonography • Histopathology • Thoracic radiographs to check for lung metastases	Bilateral orchidectomy; palliative care in case surgical intervention is not feasible. Prognosis usually good to excellent after complete excision and lack of metastases.

(continued on next page)

Table 3
(continued)

Organ System	Tissue of Origin	Reported Tumor Types	Incidence	Clinical Signs	Diagnosis and Workup	Treatment and Prognosis
Mammary glands		Adenocarcinoma; papilloma; fibroadenoma	Common in multiparous, intact female rabbits >2 y; often associated with uterine hyperplasia and adenocarcinoma (hyperestrogenism) and prolactin-secreting pituitary adenomas. Reports of familial occurrence in Belgian and English breeds.	• Mammary gland enlargement; single or multiple coalescing firm masses palpable in the mammary glands; usually nonpainful • Brown-red discharge from teat(s); teat(s) may be enlarged with hair loss present around it • General malaise with lethargy, depression, inappetance, weight loss and dyspnea if tumor has metastasized to the lungs	• Cytology (FNA) • Histopathology • Thoracic radiographs to check for lung metastases	Mastectomy and ovariohysterectomy. Prognosis depends on the presence of metastasis (poor if lung metastases are present).

| Hematopoietic and lymphatic systems | Blood; lymph nodes; thymus; spleen; bone marrow; blood vessels | Lymphoma/ lymphosarcoma; lymphoid/myeloid/ erythroid leukemia; thymoma/ thymosarcoma; thymic carcinoma; hemangioma/ hemangiosarcoma/ hemangioepithelioma; epithelioma; histiocytoma; eosinophilic granulocytic sarcoma; plasma cell tumors/ myeloma | Lymphoma/ lymphosarcoma is most common neoplasia in young rabbits <2 y and second most common neoplasia overall; may be of B- or T-cell origin and occur in variety of different tissues (lymph nodes, spleen, liver, bone marrow, eye, skin, GI tract). Thymomas more common in older rabbits. Other tumors are considered very rare in rabbits and generally diagnosed on postmortem examination. | • Highly variable in lymphoma, depends on the site affected (eg, enlarged lymph nodes, reno/spleno/hepatomegaly, general malaise, cutaneous or ocular lesions, diarrhea) • Presenting signs of thymoma may include dyspnea, exercise intolerance and bilateral exophthalmos. • Paraneoplastic syndromes have been reported for both lymphoma (hypercalcemia) and thymoma (exfoliative dermatitis) • Animals with hemangiosarcoma may bleed out from the tumor without premonitory signs | • Clinical signs • Ultrasound, thoracic radiographs or CT imaging • Cytology (FNA) • Histopathology • CBC or blood smear may reveal marked lymphocytosis and neoplastic cells • Protein electrophoresis may reveal monoclonal gammopathy (in case of myeloma) • Necropsy | Similar to other animals, radiation therapy or chemotherapy may be attempted for lymphoid tumors, although no specific chemotherapeutic protocols have been published in rabbits. Surgical treatment of thymomas is possible, but is technically challenging and poses high risks of perioperative mortality. Radiation therapy also poses a risk owing to repeated anesthetic episodes but is considered to have good effect. Chemotherapy is reported as an option in humans. Hemagiosarcomas may require surgical excision followed by (doxorubicin-based) chemotherapy. |

(continued on next page)

Table 3
(continued)

Organ System	Tissue of Origin	Reported Tumor Types	Incidence	Clinical Signs	Diagnosis and Workup	Treatment and Prognosis
Integument	Skin (squamous epithelium, adnexa); ears; eyelids; lips	Basal cell tumor; trichoblastoma; squamous cell carcinoma; sebaceous gland adenoma/ adenocarcinoma; spindle cell sarcoma; collagenous hamartoma; trichoepithelioma; trichoblastoma; malignant melanoma; fibroma/fibrosarcoma; papilloma; apocrine (adeno)carcinoma Viral-induced skin tumors include papilloma, myxoma; shope fibroma	Nonviral skin tumors are reported infrequently and mostly seen in older rabbits; viral-induced tumors may be seen at various ages. Of the nonviral tumors, trichoblastoma appear most frequently diagnosed in rabbits, comprising 20%–25% of all skin neoplasia	• Generally present as solitary, well-circumscribed cutaneous or subcutaneous masses with or without ulceration. Tumors may be pigmented in case of trichoblastoma or melanoma or appear as wartlike growths in case of papillomas. • May be located anywhere on the body surface, although predilection sites may be recognized for some tumors (eg, ear, eyelid, toe or genital area for malignant melanoma; head, neck and limbs for trichoblastoma; head and mucosa for papillomas).	• Clinical presentation • Cytology (FNA) • Histopathology (excisional/incisional biopsy) • Imaging may be required in case of malignant tumors to check for metastases	Treatment of choice is surgical excision of the mass. Adjunct chemotherapy or radiation may be considered depending on the tumor type involved. Prognosis varies depending on the type of neoplasia and location with prognosis for benign tumors such as trichoblastoma generally being excellent, the whereas prognosis for malignant melanoma may be more guarded as tumors tend to be locally invasive and metastasize to the lymph nodes and other tissues, including lung and liver. Adjunct therapy using radiation therapy may thus be necessary. In addition, a melanoma vaccine, developed for dogs, may be used, but its efficacy in rabbits needs to be studied further.

| Gastrointestinal tract | Stomach; small and large intestines; caecum; rectum and anus; liver and bile duct; exocrine pancreas | Bile duct adenoma/adenocarcinoma; hepatic carcinoma; pancreatic hamartoma; pancreatic adenoma/adenocarcinoma; tumors of the stomach and intestines (carcinoma; adenoma/adenocarcinoma, leiomyoma/leiomyosarcoma); papilloma; liver metastases (particularly uterine carcinoma) | Uncommon. Most common tumor includes the bile duct adenoma/adenocarcinoma, which has been speculated to arise as a result from *Eimeria steidae* infection | Bile duct adenomas/adenocarcinomas are often an incidental finding at necropsy. If diagnosed antemortem these may involve solitary growths or multiple masses that are sharply circumscribed from normal liver and may contain honeylike fluid and can be palpated in the abdomen during the physical examination. Animals with gastric or intestinal tumors may present with anorexia, gastric dilatation (bloat), abdominal pain; ileus; diarrhea, ascites, lethargy or chronic wasting. Some animals may present with acute death. Anorectal papillomas present as small, friable fungating masses originating from the anorectal junction. Clinical signs include constipation, discomfort, hematochezia, and occasionally rectal prolapse. | • Clinical presentation (anorectal papillomas)
• Ultrasound, radiography or CT imaging
• Cytology (FNA; often nondiagnostic)
• Histopathology
• Biochemistry may reveal elevated liver enzymes (eg, GGT), increased bile acids, hypoproteinemia and hypoalbuminemia but often only in advanced cases
• Explorative laparotomy
• Necropsy | Surgical excision of solitary growths. Chemotherapy may be attempted for multifocal hepatic tumors or infiltrative lymphomas, but is primarily considered a palliative treatment. Metastasis of hepatic and biliary tumors may occur to the lungs or surrounding tissues (peritoneum, diaphragm, mesentery). Most gastric and intestinal tumors are likely to be diagnosed only in an advanced stage, thereby carrying a grave prognosis. Surgical excision, laser therapy or cryotherapy may be attempted for anorectal papillomas and carry a good prognosis. Spontaneous regression may also occur in asymptomatic cases. |

(continued on next page)

Table 3
(continued)

Organ System	Tissue of Origin	Reported Tumor Types	Incidence	Clinical Signs	Diagnosis and Workup	Treatment and Prognosis
Urinary tract	Kidney; ureters; bladder; urethra	Benign embryonal nephroma; renal carcinoma; leiomyoma	Benign embryonal nephromas are a reportedly common tumor in laboratory rabbits, both in young and older animals (range, 1.5 - >5 y)	• Commonly presented as a coincidental finding at necropsy with no antemortem clinical signs noted; may occur as single or multiple masses in one or both kidneys. • Unilateral renal enlargement. • Acute death or clinical signs resulting from metastases to distant sites.	• Ultrasound, radiography • Necropsy • CBC may reveal secondary polycythemia; kidney values often remain normal (especially in case of unilateral involvement)	Often no therapy indicated for benign embryonal nephromas, although successful nephrectomy has been described in rabbits with secondary polycythemia. Treatment of renal carcinoma may be difficult, with poor response to chemotherapy noted in other species. At the time of diagnosis, metastasis has often occurred to the regional lymph nodes, contralateral kidney, liver, and lungs. Chemotherapy has not been considered effective in these tumors.

				Clinical signs	Diagnosis	Treatment
Respiratory tract	Nasal cavity; sinuses; trachea; lungs	Adenocarcinoma; primary carcinoma; primary epithelioma; pulmonary metastases of any tumor (particularly uterine adenocarcinoma); histiocytic sarcoma	Uncommon	• Unilateral or bilateral nasal discharge; epistaxis; sneezing; snoring. • Progressive dyspnea and tachypnea. • General malaise, including anorexia, lethargy, and depression.	• Radiography or CT imaging (particularly for the upper respiratory tract) • Rhinoscopy and biopsy collection for histopathologic examination • Cytology (FNA)	Surgical excision is often not feasible; certain tumors (eg, adenocarcinoma) may respond well to radiation therapy or chemotherapy; otherwise, palliative treatment may be considered.
Musculoskeletal system (including mesenchymal tissues)	Bone; muscle; joint tissue; tendons and ligaments; connective tissue	Osteosarcoma; osteochondroma; adamantinoma; acanthomatous ameloblastoma; fibroma; fibrosarcoma; spindle cell sarcoma; round cell sarcoma; leiomyoma; leiomyosarcoma; mesothelioma; lipoma/liposarcoma;	Rare, with most tumors involving osteosarcomas of the appendicular skeleton (eg, tibia), ribs, skull or facial bones. Mainly diagnosed in older rabbits (>6 y)	• Swelling of the affected area. • Progressive, unilateral lameness. • In case of facial involvement, anorexia, weight loss, and ocular and nasal discharge may be noted. • Metastasis may occur to the lungs, resulting in dyspnea.	• Biochemistry may reveal elevated alkaline phosphatase activity • Radiographs may reveal proliferative bone density mass and potential lung metastases. • CT imaging may be useful to determine the extent of the tumor (also for surgical planning) • Histopathology	In case of appendicular tumors, amputation of the affected limb is recommended. Hemimandibulectomy has been attempted in cases involving the mandible. Chemotherapy using doxorubicin or platinum compounds may be attempted as adjunct therapy, similar to dogs. Palliative treatment may consist of the use of NSAIDs and other pain medication.

(continued on next page)

Table 3
(continued)

Organ System	Tissue of Origin	Reported Tumor Types	Incidence	Clinical Signs	Diagnosis and Workup	Treatment and Prognosis
Nervous system	Brain; spinal cord; peripheral nerves; eyes	Teratoma; neurinoma; ependymoma; neurofibrosarcoma; peripheral nerve sheath tumor; intraocular sarcoma	Uncommon	Clinical signs will depend on the location of the tumor and may include ataxia, seizures, paresis/paralysis and other neurologic deficits.	• Use of advanced diagnostic techniques such as CT or MRI is generally required • Necropsy	Surgical resection is often not considered feasible unless the tumor is located peripherally, in which case radical surgical resection (eg, amputation of the limb) may be attempted followed by radiation therapy or chemotherapy. Similar to other animals, radiation therapy may be considered as palliative treatment but overall prognosis is considered poor.

| Endocrine system | Pituitary gland; adrenal glands; thyroid gland; endocrine pancreas | Pituitary adenoma/ carcinoma; prolactinoma; adrenocortical adenoma/carcinoma; thyroid carcinoma | Rare; adrenocortical neoplasia have incidentally been reported in older, male (and 1 female) neutered rabbits, | • Recurrence of sexual and aggressive behavior (chasing, biting, mounting).
• Inappropriate urination.
• Enlarged mammary glands (in case of prolactinoma).
• Other tumors often diagnosed as coincidental findings at necropsy, with no obvious clinical signs noted (nonfunctional tumors?). | • CT or MRI may potentially be used in the diagnosis of pituitary adenoma
• Ultrasound
• Hormone analysis
• Necropsy | Adrenalectomy has been successfully used in rabbits with adrenocortical neoplasia. Leuprolide acetate (GnRH agonist) was reported to only have moderate effect on the behavior. Therapy for other tumors has not been described, but most likely follows similar guidelines as those in dogs and cats. |

Abbreviations: CBC, complete blood count; CT, computed tomography; FNA, fine needle aspirate; GGT, gamma-glutamyl transferase; GnRH, gonadotropin-releasing hormone; NSAIDs, nonsteroidal anti-inflammatory drugs.

Data from Refs.[2,3,5,37,64,67]

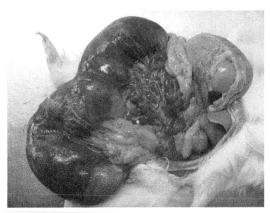

Fig. 11. Severely abnormal uterus of a rabbit. Pathology confirmed this to be a uterine adenocarcinoma. Often the abnormal uterus may be noted on abdominal palpation as a large, firm, irregular mass in the caudal abdomen.

from 4% in 2- to 3-year-old rabbits up to 80% in animals older than 5 years.[38–41] Degree of parity does not affect tumor incidence,[42] whereas the role of hormones (estrogen, progesterone) remains unclear, although involvement of these hormones in the development of tubular or solid uterine carcinomas has been suggested.[43] Aside from uterine adenocarcinomas, adenomas, leiomyomas, leiomyosarcomas, malignant mixed Müllerian duct tumors, deciduosarcomas, hemangiomas, carcinosarcomas, choriocarcinomas, and squamous cell carcinomas (particularly of the vaginosquamo-columnal junction) have also been diagnosed.[3,40,41,44–46]

Clinical signs

In breeder rabbits, reproductive disturbances (eg, decreased fertility, fetal retention, resorption or abortus, still births, reduced litter size) represent one of the first signs of uterine carcinoma.[38] In these animals, clinical detection of the tumor may be delayed by as much as 6 to 10 months.[3] In pet rabbits, hematuria or hemorrhagic vaginal discharge is often the first sign to be noted by the owner (**Fig. 12**).[40,41] In some individuals, mammary gland enlargement may also be observed. However, in many patients, uterine neoplasia will go unnoticed until its presence is discovered during an abdominal palpation or until metastasis to other organs has occurred.[41] At this time, the rabbit may present with a more severe clinical signs such as anorexia, weight loss, depression, dyspnea (in case of pulmonary metastases), or lameness owing to pathologic fractures (in case of bone metastases).

Diagnosis

A tentative diagnosis of uterine carcinoma can usually be made based on the history and clinical examination of the patient, during which the enlarged uterus or uterine masses can be palpated. Radiography or ultrasonography (including FNA for cytology) may be used for confirmation (**Fig. 13**). Thoracic radiographs are indicated to identify pulmonary metastasis. In patients that present with hematuria, urinalysis may be performed to determine whether the patient suffers from true hematuria or porphyria.

Treatment and prognosis

Uterine adenocarcinoma usually comprises a slowly growing tumor, but if left untreated it may locally invade the myometrium and peritoneal cavity or metastasize

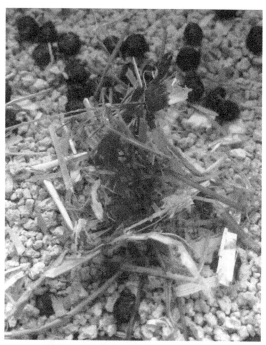

Fig. 12. Hematuria or presence of hemorrhagic vaginal discharge is one of the clinical signs that may be noted in rabbits with uterine pathology.

to the lungs, liver, brain, or bone.[47,48] Treatment of choice therefore consists of ovariohysterectomy (**Fig. 14**), with periodic follow-up recommended to monitor for metastases that were undetectable at the time of surgery. If no metastases have occurred, prognosis is usually good with more than 80% of ovariohysterectomized rabbits reported to still be alive 6 months after surgery.[41] Chemotherapy may be attempted in case of metastases, although this is generally not considered to result in a successful outcome.[5] These cases may therefore better be managed palliatively until euthanasia is warranted (eg, in case of progressive dyspnea owing to advanced metastatic lung disease).

Prevention

Anecdotally, ovariectomy in rabbits less than 6 months or breeding at a young age have been suggested as ways to reduce the risk of uterine adenocarcinoma. However, there are anecdotal reports of diagnosed uterine adenocarcinomas in rabbits despite these measures, suggesting that these do not (completely) eliminate the risk of tumor development (2012, personal communication). Prevention can therefore best be achieved by ovariohysterectomy, which is preferably performed in the first year of life (if the rabbit is not intended to be bred).

Testicular Neoplasia

Tumors of the testicle are infrequently reported in rabbits. Older, intact male rabbits, especially those with undescended testes, are considered to be at greater risk.[3] Reported tumor types in rabbits include seminomas, interstitial (Leydig or granular) cell tumors, Sertoli cell tumors, teratoma, adenocarcinoma, testicular nephroma,

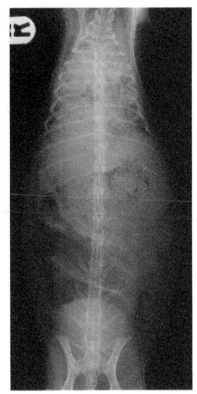

Fig. 13. Ventrodorsal radiograph of a rabbit with a metastasized uterine adenocarcinoma. Both the enlarged uterus and extensive pulmonary metastases may be visualized on this radiograph. (*Courtesy of* Evert-Jan de Boer, DVM, Dierenkliniek Wilhelminapark, The Netherlands.)

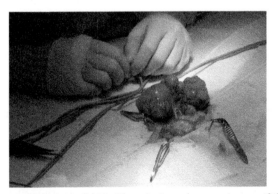

Fig. 14. Ovariohysterectomy in a rabbit with a uterine adenocarcinoma. If the tumor has not metastasized, ovariohysterectomy is the recommended choice of therapy. When performing the surgery, care must be taken to also resect the cervix because tumors have been reported to recur if uterine tissue is left behind.

lymphoma, and mixed cell tumors, also referred to as gonadoblastoma.[3,49–55] Of these, the Leydig cell tumors are the most commonly reported,[53,55] although different tumor types have been reported to occur simultaneously in both testes.[50,51]

Clinical signs

Animals with testicular tumors often present with unilateral or bilateral enlargement of the testes. In general, testicular tumors will present as firm, nodular, nonpainful masses, but occasionally there may be no gross evidence of neoplasia present.[3,49–55] In some animals, fertility may be decreased. If the tumor is functional (eg, estrogen-producing Leydig cell tumors), gynecomastia and behavioral changes (including changes in libido) may be observed.[52] Owing to the negative feedback mechanism, the contralateral testis may be decreased in size in these animals. If the tumor is large, it may interfere with locomotion and/or cause scrotal skin necrosis. Metastases are rare, but have been reported to the regional (sublumbar) lymph nodes and lungs.[56] In these patients, progressive weight loss and other signs of general malaise can also be part of the presenting signs.

Diagnosis

A presumptive diagnosis can usually be made based on the presenting signs and palpation of the testicle. However, to differentiate between a testicular neoplasia and other causes of unilateral or bilateral testicular enlargement (eg, bacterial orchitis, abscesses, testicular torsion, hematoma) further workup will be required. An ultrasound examination may be helpful to evaluate tissue morphology and presence of blood flow. Confirmation of the diagnosis and tumor type will require histopathologic examination.

Treatment and prognosis

Unilateral or bilateral orchidectomy is the recommended choice of treatment for testicular tumors. Prognosis is usually good to excellent unless the tumor has metastasized. If surgery is not an option, palliative care may be considered.

Mammary Gland Neoplasia

Mammary gland tumors have frequently been reported in laboratory rabbits, but are also regularly seen in pet rabbits. Predisposing factors include age (older rabbits with a mean age of 5.5 years; range, 2–14), breed (New Zealand White, English, and Belgian breeds), gender (intact female), and multiparity.[3,57] On various occasions, these tumors have been seen in conjunction with uterine hyperplasia or adenocarcinoma, suggesting a direct link between the two processes.[40,58,59] In addition, their onset may be influenced by hyperestrogenism, prolactinemia, or the presence of prolactin-secreting pituitary adenomas.[3,60,61] Reported tumor types include cystadenoma, fibroadenoma, adenoma, adenocarcinoma, papilloma, carcinoma, and carcinosarcoma, of which malignant tumors (>70%), in particular invasive carcinomas, are the most frequently diagnosed.[3,57,62,63] Development of the tumor seems to be preceded frequently by cystic changes of the mammary gland.[3]

Clinical signs

Mammary tumors often present as mammary gland enlargement and/or presence of 1 or multiple fluctuant or firm masses in the mammary gland(s). Masses can be variable in size, and are often nonpainful on palpation. Other clinical signs that may be noted include alopecia, ulceration, and/or discoloration of the gland(s) and/or teat(s) and milky or amber-colored discharge from the teat(s).[3,64] Rabbits will generally be bright, active, and alert, unless metastasis (to regional lymph nodes, lungs, liver, kidney, pancreas, adrenal glands, ovary, and bone marrow) has occurred, at which time the rabbit will become cachexic, depressed, and lethargic.[64]

Diagnosis

Definite diagnosis can be made after FNA or biopsy. This is particularly important, because differential diagnoses include a number of conditions with similar presentation such as pseudopregnancy, prolactin-driven cystic hyperplasia, bacterial mastitis, cyclosporine-induced hyperplasia, and testicular interstitial cell tumor-induced gynecomastia.[52,65,66] Thoracic radiographs or ultrasound imaging may furthermore be useful to check for potential metastases.

Treatment and prognosis

Mastectomy is the treatment of choice, provided a preoperative screening does not reveal the presence of metastases. If a single small lump is present a nodulectomy may be performed, whereas chain mastectomy may be necessary if multiple mammary glands are affected. In intact females, additional ovariohysterectomy may be considered. Even though this is not necessarily proven to decrease the likelihood of mammary tumor development in future, this may help to prevent the more common uterine neoplasias. However, in females that have been spayed at an older age, additional tumors may still develop as a result of previous hormonal sensitization of the mammary tissue.[3] If complete resection is not feasible, radiation therapy may be considered to stop or slow regrowth.[67] In analogy to dogs and cats, chemotherapy with doxorubicin, antiestrogen medication (eg, tamoxifen), or a cyclooxygenase-2 inhibitor (piroxicam, meloxicam) may be attempted for nonresectable or metastasized mammary gland tumors.[67]

Lymphoid Neoplasia: Lymphoma, Lymphosarcoma, and Leukemia

Lymphoid tumors, including lymphoma, lymphosarcoma, and lymphoid leukemia, are the second most common tumor diagnosed in rabbits. Although these tumors may occur in rabbits of all ages (range, 7 weeks to 9.5 years), they are most commonly seen in rabbits less than 2 years of age.[3,68] Lymphomas have been reported in various breeds, including New Zealand white rabbits, Japanese white rabbits, English breeds, and Dutch dwarf breeds.[64] Lymphoid tumors may either be of B-cell or T-cell origin and can be found in practically any organ or tissue, including the lymph nodes, spleen, liver, kidneys, skin, eye, and lymphoid tissues of the gastrointestinal tract and lungs.[3,69] Systemic forms with multiple organ involvement (in particular the liver, spleen, kidneys, and thoracic and mesenteric lymph nodes) are considered the most common.[3] In addition, leukemias in association with lymphoma in multiple organs have been reported.[70–72]

Clinical signs

Clinical manifestations of lymphoma can be extremely variable, depending on the location of the tumor. Clinical signs observed in rabbits with lymphoma include aspecific signs of generalized illness such as anorexia, anemia, lethargy, weight loss, diarrhea, and depression. In addition, peripheral lymphadenopathy and/or an enlarged liver, spleen, or kidneys may be present. In case of skin involvement, lesions may be localized to bilateral blepharitis or cutaneous nodules or plaques with or without ulceration, crusts, erythema, and/or alopecia.[68,73] Ocular lymphoma and retrobulbar lymphoma of the Harderian gland may present as intraocular (white) masses (**Fig. 15**), or unilateral exophthalmos, whereas bilateral exophthalmos and progressive dyspnea may be noted in case of mediastinal lymphomas.[3,64,72,74–76]

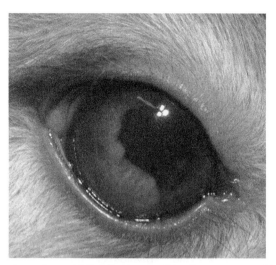

Fig. 15. Ocular lymphoma in a rabbit. After enucleation, the eye was sent in for histopathology revealing the lymphoma to be of T cell origin. (*Courtesy of* Evert-Jan de Boer, DVM, Dierenkliniek Wilhelminapark, The Netherlands.)

Diagnosis

Diagnosis can be achieved by FNA or biopsies of affected lymph nodes or organs. In case of leukemia, increases in total white cell count, lymphocytosis, and/or the presence of lymphoblasts in a blood smear may be observed.[5] In many cases, diagnosis will be made postmortem, revealing hepatosplenomegaly with diffuse small (0.5 mm) pale foci (**Fig. 16**); enlarged, pale kidneys with an irregular lumpy surface; and lymphadenopathy, pale bone marrow, and skin and/or pulmonary nodules.[37,77,78] Confirmation of the diagnosis can be achieved after histopathologic examination, which will reveal the affected lymph nodes and organs to be infiltrated with neoplastic lymphoid cells.

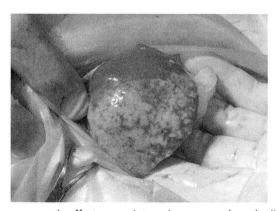

Fig. 16. Lymphoma commonly affects many internal organs, such as the liver in this rabbit. (*Courtesy of* Evert-Jan de Boer, DVM, Dierenkliniek Wilhelminapark, The Netherlands.)

Treatment

In most species, lymphoma is considered to be systemic at the time of diagnosis. Although no chemotherapeutic protocols have been published for rabbits, chemotherapy (using similar chemotherapeutic agents as in other animals) should be considered as the treatment of choice.[5,64] In case of localized forms, surgical excision may be attempted. Similarly, radiation therapy may be considered useful in case of mediastinal masses or after excision of localize masses. Treatment protocols using alpha-interferon and isotretinoin have been reported in rabbits with T-cell lymphomas, but showed no effect.[68]

Thymic Neoplasia

Thymomas are tumors originating from the epithelial cells of the thymus. In contrast with other animal species, the thymus of the rabbit is large and persists into adulthood. In mature animals (median, 6 years; range, 1–10), cells may become neoplastic, giving rise to both benign (thymoma) and malignant (thymic lymphoma [malignant thymoma], thymic carcinoma) tumors, with benign forms being most common.[79] An incidence approaching 8% has been reported.[59] Thymomas tend to be slow growing but may locally invade tissues and metastasize locally to the pleura and other (thoracic and abdominal) organs, although the likelihood of this occurring seems low.[80]

Clinical signs

Clinical signs in rabbits with thymomas may range from an incidental finding of a cranial mediastinal mass on radiographic examination to signs of progressive dyspnea and exercise intolerance owing to the presence of a space-occupying mass in the thorax. Moreover, bilateral exophthalmos; prolapse of the third eyelids; head, neck, and forelimb edema; and pleural effusion associated with cranial vena cava syndrome may be seen (**Fig. 17**).[79,81] Other paraneoplastic syndromes that have been associated with thymomas include systemic immunopathy and/or hemolytic anemia[82,83] and exfoliative dermatitis[84,85] (**Fig. 18**). Hypercalcemia has also been reported in 2 rabbits,[86,87] with 1 rabbit showing resolution of the hypercalcemia after surgical removal of the neoplasia.[87] Nonetheless, caution is warranted when attributing the presence of a hypercalcemia to the neoplastic disease because hypercalcemia may also be present as a result of the rabbit's unique calcium metabolism and dietary influences.[88]

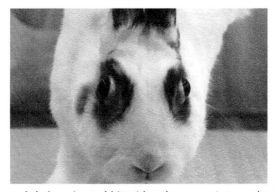

Fig. 17. Bilateral exophthalmos in a rabbit with a thymoma. As a result of the compression on the large veins by the tumor, venous return to the heart is diminished, leading to cranial vena cava syndrome. Typically, the bilateral exophthalmos can be exacerbation by changing the body position.

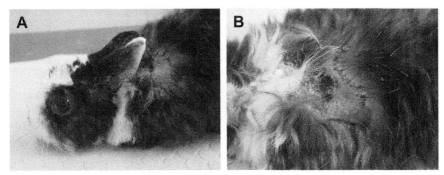

Fig. 18. (*A, B*) A 6-year-old female rabbit was presented with alopecia, scaling, and severe pruritus. Prior treatment against mites and dermatophytosis was unsuccessful. Skin biopsies were consistent with sebaceous adenitis. This skin condition is considered as a potential paraneoplastic syndrome of a thymoma.

Diagnosis

History and clinical signs are usually suggestive of a mass in the cranial mediastinum, especially if the clinical examination reveals one of the following abnormalities: position-dependent worsening or improving of bilateral exophthalmos, decreased compliance of the thoracic wall, absence of breath sounds in the cranial thorax, and caudal displacement of the heart and ictus cordis. The presence of a soft tissue mass in the cranial mediastinum (and potential accompanying pleural effusion) may be confirmed using thoracic radiographs, ultrasound examination, or CT imaging (the latter technique also being helpful in planning of subsequent surgery or radiation therapy; see **Fig. 7**). As lymphoma, abscesses, thymic hyperplasia, and thymic carcinoma are important differential diagnoses, (ultrasound-guided) FNA (**Fig. 19**) or tissue biopsies are required for a definite diagnosis. FNAs will not always be diagnostic, but if the sample contains sufficient material, thymomas can easily be identified by the presence of a mixture of epithelial cells and small, well-differentiated lymphocytes.[25,79]

Treatment

Surgery and radiation therapy are currently the preferred options to treat thymomas. Surgical excision after explorative thoracotomy (**Fig. 20**) is often considered to provide

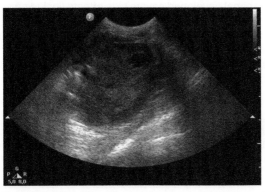

Fig. 19. Ultrasound imaging of a rabbit diagnosed with a mass in the cranial mediastinum. A fine-needle aspirate was collected of the mass for cytology, after which a definite diagnosis of thymoma was obtained.

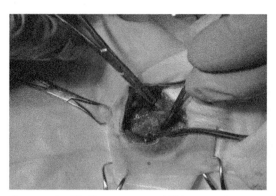

Fig. 20. In rabbits diagnosed with thymomas, a midline sternotomy may be performed to gain access to the thoracic cavity and enable optimal visualization of the tumor. (*Courtesy of* Evert-Jan de Boer, DVM, Dierenkliniek Wilhelminapark, The Netherlands.)

the best chances of removing the entire tumor and long-term control of the disease. However, recurrence has been reported.[79,87] In addition, surgery poses a high risk for perioperative and postoperative morbidity and mortality with reported survival rates varying between 25% and 50%.[79,80] If the decision is made to surgically excise the mass, a median sternotomy is the preferential route to be used, because this provides optimal access and visualization of the thoracic cavity for removal of the mediastinal mass. Owing to the high risks associated with surgery, and the tumor's sensitivity to irradiation, radiation therapy has received growing attention over the past years. Various authors have demonstrated good results of radiation therapy (**Fig. 21**) with resolution of clinical signs seen after 4 to 42 days and a median survival time of 1 to 2 years (range, <14 days to 3 years).[24] Complications that may be seen after the procedure included anesthetic-related death and radiation-induced alopecia, pneumonitis, pulmonary fibrosis, myocardial failure and thrombosis of the thoracic vessels.[24,80] To ameliorate these side effects, the use of nonsteroidal anti-inflammatory drugs or prednisone[b] may be considered.[80] In humans, chemotherapy protocols (eg, using octreotide, ifosfamide, or combinations of eg, cisplatin, doxorubicin, cyclophosphamide, and vincristine) have also been used with good success, with response rates of greater than 79% reported with certain protocols.[89] In rabbits, the use of doxorubicin was attempted in 1 rabbit diagnosed with thymoma, but after its administration the animal developed severe side effects (including anemia, weakness, and collapse), thereby resulting in a discontinuation of the treatment.[80] Aside from doxorubicin, chemotherapy using octreotide has also been attempted in 2 rabbits. Although initial results of this treatment were more promising, treatment in these animals also needed to be discontinued owing to the occurrence of side effects associated with the medication.[5]

Skin Neoplasia

Skin neoplasia can present in various forms (for an overview and description, see Kanfer and Reavill [2013]).[67] Two retrospective studies indicated between 20% to 35% of all submitted skin tumors to comprise trichoblastoma (previously referred to as basal

---

[b] Caution is warranted when using corticosteroids in rabbits owing their potential to induce immunosuppression, thereby rendering the rabbit susceptible to secondary infections. The risks and benefits should therefore be weighed carefully before making a decision whether or not to use these drugs.

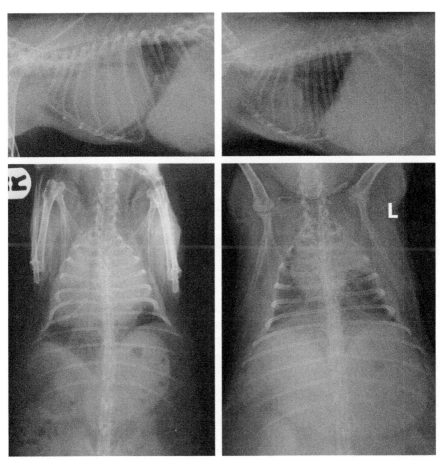

Fig. 21. Ventrodorsal and right lateral radiographs of a rabbit diagnosed with thymoma before (*left*) and after 10 sessions of radiation therapy (administered over a period of 3 weeks), showing a marked decrease in tumor size after treatment (*right*). The total dose of radiation used was 40 Gy. (*Courtesy of* Evert-Jan de Boer, DVM, Dierenkliniek Wilhelminapark, The Netherlands.)

cell tumors; **Fig. 22**).[58,90] Other tumors that were reported as common include collagen nevi (hamartomas), squamous papillomas, squamous cell carcinomas, melanomas, lipomas, and spindle cell sarcomas.[67,90]

Clinical signs
Skin neoplasia generally present themselves as solitary, well-circumscribed cutaneous or subcutaneous masses that are grossly visible to owners and often the reason for presentation to the veterinarian. Their appearance may vary, depending on the type of tumor involved. For example, tumors may be pigmented in case of trichoblastoma or melanoma or appear as wartlike growths in case of papillomas. Ulceration may also be seen. Skin neoplasia may be found anywhere on the body. However, predilection sites have been recognized for specific types of tumors (eg, ear, eyelid, toe, or genital area for malignant melanoma; head, neck, and limbs for trichoblastoma; and head and mucosa for papillomas).[67]

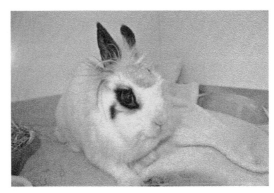

Fig. 22. Trichoblastomas, previously referred to as basal cell tumors, are the most common spontaneous skin tumors found in rabbits. Trichoblastomas can be found anywhere on the body, but the head, neck, and forelegs are favored locations. Generally, they comprise solitary, well-circumscribed tumors. However, they may become very large and ulcerated, as can be seen in this rabbit. (*Courtesy of* Evert-Jan de Boer, DVM, Dierenkliniek Wilhelminapark, The Netherlands.)

Diagnosis

Diagnosis of the type of skin neoplasia involved can usually be made using cytology of FNA or impression smears, or after histopathologic evaluation of excisional or incisional skin biopsies. In case of malignant tumors (eg, malignant melanoma, squamous cell carcinoma), FNA of regional lymph nodes and imaging (radiographs, ultrasound examination, CT imaging) may be considered to check for regional and distant metastases.

Treatment

The treatment of choice for most skin neoplasia is surgical excision. This may be curative in many cases, especially if the tumor is benign and/or wide margins are adhered. However, this may be challenging in small animals, thereby posing a risk for incomplete tumor removal and regrowth. Additional therapy may therefore be considered, depending on the type of tumor and presence of tumor-free margins. In case of tumor regrowth or incomplete excision, adjunct radiation therapy or (intralesional) chemotherapy may be considered. For small tumors (<1 to 2 cm), intralesional chemotherapy, cryotherapy, or photodynamic therapy may be considered as a standalone treatment modality. Prognosis will be highly dependent on the location and type of neoplasia involved.

Bone Neoplasia

Although bone neoplasia has been suggested to be rare in rabbits, in these last few years an increasing number of reports have been published on the presence of osteosarcomas in rabbits. Generally, this type of neoplasia will be found in middle-aged to older rabbits, but osteosarcomas have been diagnosed in rabbits as young as 1 year.[91] No sex or breed predilection has been reported. Osteosarcomas have been reported to affect both the axial (skull, spine, ribs; **Fig. 23**)[91–98] and appendicular (scapula, humerus, tibia, tarsus; **Fig. 24**) skeleton.[16,37,99,100] In addition, extraskeletal osteosarcomas have also been incidentally reported.[101,102] In comparison with dogs, whereby the appendicular skeleton is most commonly involved, osteosarcomas in rabbits seem to involve the facial bones (mandible, frontal bones) in the majority of cases.[100] Various subtypes of osteosarcomas have been reported, of which the

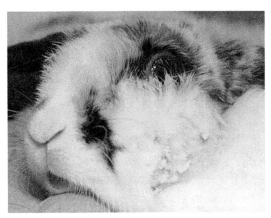

Fig. 23. A 5-year-old female lop-eared rabbit with a significant, painful swelling of the lower jaw, resulting in difficulty with eating. The tumor was diagnosed to be an osteosarcoma. (*Courtesy of* Evert-Jan de Boer, DVM, Dierenkliniek Wilhelminapark, The Netherlands.)

osteoblastic osteosarcoma is reported as the main type to be found in rabbits.[100] Other subtypes reported in rabbits include fibroblastic, giant cell, and poorly differentiated (osteolytic) osteosarcoma.[98,99,102] Similar to dogs, osteosarcomas metastasize rapidly, with multiple (micro)metastases present in the lungs and other tissues (eg, subcutis, pleura, peritoneum, pericardium, heart, liver, kidney, intestines) in more than 50% of animals at the time of diagnosis.[91,93,97,100]

Clinical signs
The clinical signs seen in rabbits with osteosarcoma will often depend on the area that is affected. Appendicular osteosarcomas often present as chronic, progressive lameness, often with a detectable swelling of one of the limbs.[16,37,99,100] Osteosarcomas in other locations also commonly present as a mass or swelling, which may be accompanied by other nonspecific signs, such as decreased appetite, dysphagia, and weight loss.[16,91,93,95,98] Pathologic fractures (**Fig. 25**), bleeding, fever, urine scald, and (severe) pain can also be noted.[16,99,100]

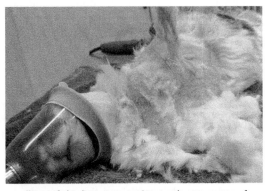

Fig. 24. Significant swelling of the humerus owing to the presence of an osteosarcoma. This rabbit also presented with severe lameness resulting from a pathologic fracture (see **Fig. 25**). (*Courtesy of* Evert-Jan de Boer, DVM, Dierenkliniek Wilhelminapark, The Netherlands.)

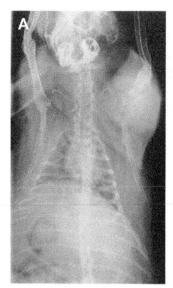
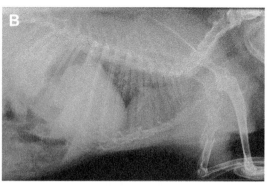

Fig. 25. (A, B) Ventrodorsal and left lateral radiographs of the rabbit from **Fig. 24**, showing the presence of both the neoplastic process and a pathologic fracture of the left humerus. (*Courtesy of* Evert-Jan de Boer, DVM, Dierenkliniek Wilhelminapark, The Netherlands.)

Diagnosis

Radiographs and other advanced imaging techniques (CT, MRI) will usually be helpful in establishing a tentative diagnosis. Radiographic findings may range from lytic to proliferative, sclerotic or mixed lesions.[16,91,95,97–100] In 2 rabbits with appendicular tumors, lesions were found to have crossed the joint space.[99,100] Aside from identifying bone abnormalities at the affected site, imaging is helpful to identify (pulmonary) metastases. Cytologic examination of FNAs has been found useful to obtain a definite diagnosis.[16,100] In case FNA is inconclusive, a histopathologic examination of the biopsied bone (including the use of specific immunohistochemical stains using antiosteocalcin monoclonal antibodies)[99,100] can be used for confirmation. Osteosarcomas have furthermore been associated with increased plasma alkaline phosphatase concentrations, resulting from bone production and remodeling.[16,93,97,99,100] Aside from diagnostic purposes, alkaline phosphatase may also serve as a prognostic indicator,[99] although currently no studies exist with regard to this aspect in rabbits.

Treatment and prognosis

Whenever possible, surgical removal of the tumor is considered most effective. In case of appendicular tumors, amputation of the affected limb is recommended,[16] to which rabbits generally respond favourably.[15,103] In case of tumors involving the mandible, partial mandibulectomy has been found successful.[104] If complete removal is not feasible, debulking surgery followed by radiation therapy or chemotherapy may be attempted. However, in many cases, (micro)metastases may already be present, thereby greatly diminishing the prognosis. Unfortunately, systematic studies into survival times of rabbits with osteosarcoma after surgical intervention (with or without adjunct therapy) are currently lacking. In rabbits with confirmed metastases, palliative treatment using analgesic drugs (nonsteroidal anti-inflammatory drugs, opioids, gabapentin) or irradiation may be considered.

Renal Neoplasia

Renal neoplasia is occasionally found in rabbits. Although malignant tumors (eg, lymphoma, renal carcinoma)[3,105] may occur, benign embryonal nephromas are more commonly reported, especially in laboratory animals where it is the second most common tumor after uterine adenocarcinomas.[3,37,106] Embryonal nephromas have been found in both young and old rabbits, most commonly as an incidental finding during postmortem examinations.[3] Both single and multiple, unilateral or bilateral tumors have been found, with both kidneys being equally affected.[3] Embryonal nephromas are generally slow growing, with metastasis rarely occurring.[107]

Clinical signs

In many rabbits, the presence of renal tumors will go unnoticed, because they do not affect renal function. As a result, these tumors will mainly be diagnosed during postmortem examinations, representing as large whitish, well-circumscribed nodules of 1 to 2 cm in diameter, projecting above the cortical surface of the kidney.[3,108] Incidentally, secondary polycythemia may be present, resulting in hyperemic mucous membranes, lethargy, tachypnea, and exercise intolerance.[109–112] In addition, single or multiple masses in the kidney, or renomegaly, may be noted on abdominal palpation.[64,112]

Diagnosis

In most rabbits with renal tumors, diagnosis will be made postmortem. If an abdominal mass is palpated during a (routine) physical examination, ultrasonography and/or radiography may be helpful to diagnose where the mass originates from. A complete blood count may reveal a marked increase in erythrocytes, most likely resulting from increased erythropoietin production by the tumor.[109–112] Unfortunately, no validated tests exist to confirm these suspicions. Renal function will rarely be affected.

Treatment and prognosis

Treatment is usually not required in case of benign embryonal nephromas. However, in case of secondary polycythemia, resolution of the clinical signs may occur after nephrectomy.[109,112] Before surgery, intravenous urography may be considered to evaluate function of the contralateral kidney.[110,112] Nephrectomy may also be considered in rabbits with renal carcinomas after checking for the presence of metastases, which may be found in either the regional lymph nodes, contralateral kidney, liver, and/or lungs.[64] In these animals, as well as those with bilateral renal involvement, prognosis is generally considered poor, with chemotherapy not considered effective to treat these tumors in other species.[113]

Adrenal Neoplasia

Adrenal neoplasia has infrequently been reported in (older) rabbits, with male rabbits being overrepresented.[114–117] Both functional and nonfunctional adenomas and adenocarcinomas have been diagnosed.[114–118] Similar to ferrets, the disease has been associated with gonadectomy, whereby the loss of negative feedback from the gonads to the hypothalamic–pituitary axis leads to chronically increased plasma luteinizing hormone concentrations that exert a stimulatory effect on the synthesis and secretion of sex steroids by the adrenal gland.[119,120]

Clinical signs

Similar to functional adrenal tumors in ferrets, adrenal neoplasia in rabbits has been linked to increased sexual behavior and aggression. Clinical signs in these animals may include chasing, biting, mounting, and humping on various objects or people's legs.[114–117] In addition, urine spraying and fecal marking have been observed as well as aspecific signs of disease (ie, reduced appetite, weight loss).[114–117] Female rabbits may furthermore present with clitoral enlargement.[117] Nonfunctional adrenal tumors may go unnoticed until they may accidentally be discovered during a physical examination or on abdominal imaging.

Diagnosis

Diagnostic workup of rabbits with suspected adrenal neoplasia include hormone analysis, which may reveal elevated concentrations of sex hormones (ie, progesterone, 17-hydroxyprogesterone, testosterone).[114–117] Moreover, abdominal ultrasound may reveal an unilaterally or bilaterally enlarged adrenal gland.[114–117]

Treatment and prognosis

The treatment of choice for unilateral adrenal neoplasia is adrenalectomy, resulting in alleviation of the clinical signs.[116,117] Similar to ferrets, removal of the right adrenal gland may be challenging owing to the close association with the caudal vena cava,[117,121] whereas removal of the left adrenal gland may be complicated by the close association with the left renal vein.[116] In case of incomplete removal, recurrence of the clinical signs may be noted.[114] Medical management using gonadotrophin-releasing hormone agonists (leuprolide acetate, deslorelin) as well as other drugs used in the treatment of adrenal disease in other companion animals (ie, trilostane, finasteride, flutamide) have been attempted with variable

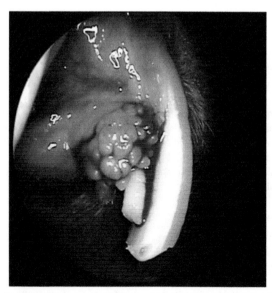

Fig. 26. Endoscopic view of an oral papilloma located just caudal to the upper incisors. Growth of these tumors may be induced by rabbit oral papillomavirus. (*Courtesy of* Evert-Jan de Boer, DVM, Dierenkliniek Wilhelminapark, The Netherlands.)

success.[116,117] More research will therefore be needed to evaluate the efficacy and safety of these drug therapies in rabbits. In case of adenocarcinomas, local metastases to the liver, duodenum, and periadrenal fat and connective tissue have been reported.[114,118]

Viral-Induced Tumors

In rabbits, viral-induced tumors have been reported. Viruses that are known to cause tumors in rabbits include Shope fibroma virus, Shope papilloma virus, or rabbit cutaneous papillomavirus, rabbit oral papilloma virus (**Fig. 26**), and myxomavirus (**Fig. 27**).[5,122–126] More information on the causative agents, routes of transmission, and clinical signs can be found in **Table 4**. In addition to the aforementioned viruses, a malignant rabbit fibromavirus has also been isolated. This virus is closely related to the Shope fibroma virus and the Moses strain of rabbit myxoma virus and presumably causes immunosuppression and malignant tumors.[127,128]

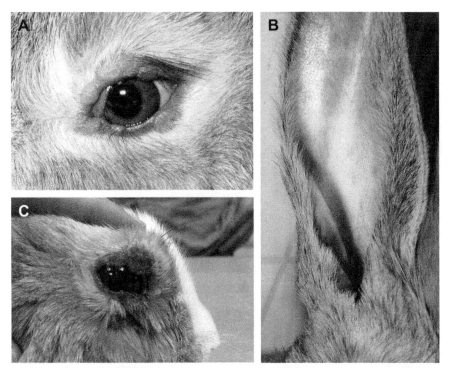

Fig. 27. Rabbit with myxomatosis, a virus from the family Poxviridae, causing a severe and fatal disease in pet rabbits (*Oryctolagus cuniculus*) in Europe. Rabbits with myxomatosis typically develop tumorlike lesions, so-called myxomas, on the eyelids (*A*), ears (*B*), and face, which may subsequently spread to the rest of the body. The virus furthermore induces a severe immunosuppression, rendering the rabbit susceptible to secondary infections (eg, Pasteurellosis) and associated mortality. Vaccination is generally effective to prevent the disease, but may, in rare instances, also result in the formation of self-limiting nodules (*C*). Unlike rabbits with clinical myxomatosis, these rabbits will remain bright, alert, and active, without signs indicative of systemic disease.

Table 4
Viral infections associated with tumor growth in rabbits

Virus	Family	Susceptible Species	Route of Transmission	Clinical Signs	Treatment	Prevention
Shope papilloma virus (also known as cottontail rabbit papillomavirus	Papovaviridae	Pet rabbits (*Oryctolagus cuniculus*); Cottontail rabbits (*Sylvilagus spp.*)	Biting insects; direct contact through skin trauma.	Wartlike, keratinous tumors on or around the head; large tumors may cause problems with food intake	Surgical resection (nodules may become malignant and develop into squamous cell carcinomas); lesions may also spontaneously regress after a few months.	Insect control
Rabbit oral papilloma virus	Papovaviridae	*O cuniculus*	Direct contact with infected rabbits; rabbits may become infected when suckling. Infection may remain latent until trauma of the oral mucosa allows papilloma development.	Oral papillomas; occasionally conjunctival or anal papillomas may also be seen. Generally affects rabbits 2–18 mo of age. May be asymptomatic as well.	Often no treatment indicated; lesions will often regress within 60 d.	Not applicable
Shope fibroma virus	Poxviridae	Wild rabbits (*Sylvilagus spp., Lepus spp.*)	Biting insects	Endemic disease in wild rabbits in North America; may sporadically cause disease in pet rabbits, resulting in fibromatous growths on feet, legs, face and back. Large growths (>7 cm) may interfere with eating and cause mobility problems. In immunocompromised or newborn rabbits, generalized fibromatosis may occur.	Tumors are benign and will usually resolve within 12–24 mo in wild rabbits and more rapidly in *Oryctolagus spp.* Supportive care may be required; surgical intervention may be considered if the size or position of the tumor inhibits normal functioning of the rabbit.	Vaccination (shope fibroma vaccine); insect control

Myxomavirus	Poxviridae	*Oryctolagus cuniculus; Sylvilagus brasiliensis, S bachmani)*	Biting insects or direct contact	Life-threatening systemic disease in *O cuniculus*: edema around the eyelids, nose and face, nodules on body face and legs 10–14 d after infection; high mortality rate associated with viremia and secondary infections. Virus causes mild cutaneous disease in *Sylvilagus spp.* (natural host). Rabbits that have been vaccinated may develop 'atypical myxomatosis' resulting in scabbing around the eyes and nose and multiple nodules over the body, which may regress over time.	Nodules may resolve in 3–4 wk in immunocompetent host. Supportive care, pain relief, and antibiosis may be indicated in affected rabbits. Euthanasia considered in severe cases. Generally no treatment needed for atypical myxomatosis; surgery may be considered if nodules are causing pain or distress to the animal.	Vaccination (bivalent myxomatosis/ rabbit hemorrhagic disease vaccine); Insect control
Malignant rabbit fibroma virus	Poxviridae	*O cuniculus*	Biting insects or direct contact	Rapidly progressing disseminated disease. Development of a large primary tumor with secondary tumors in the extremities including the nose, ears and feet. Tumors resemble myxosarcomas.	Often fatal disease owing to occurrence of metastases and immunosuppression leading to secondary infections (eg, pasteurellosis). Death often occurs within 12–24 d.	Insect control

Data from Refs.[5,122–128]

REFERENCES

1. Bell E, Henrici AT. Renal tumors in the rabbit. J Cancer Res 1916;1:157–67.
2. Weisbroth SH. Neoplastic diseases. In: Manning PJ, Ringler DL, Newcomer CE, editors. The biology of the laboratory rabbit. San Diego (CA): Academic Press; 1994. p. 259–92.
3. Tinkey PT, Uthamanthil RK, Weisbroth SH. Rabbit neoplasia. In: Suckow MA, Stevens KA, Wilson RP, editors. The laboratory rabbit, Guinea pig, hamster, and other rodents. San Diego (CA): Academic Press; 2012. p. 447–501.
4. Graham JE, Kent MS, Théon A. Current therapies in exotic animal oncology. Vet Clin North Am Exot Anim Pract 2004;7(3):757–81.
5. Varga M. Neoplasia. In: Meredith A, Lord B, editors. BSAVA manual of rabbit medicine. Quedgeley, Gloucester (United Kingdom): BSAVA; 2014. p. 264–73.
6. Campbell TW. The cytology of hyperplasia/benign neoplasia. In: Campbell TW, editor. Exotic animal hematology and cytology. 4th edition. Hoboken (NJ): John Wiley & Sons, Inc; 2015. p. 267–75.
7. Campbell TW. The cytology of malignant neoplasia. In: Campbell TW, editor. Exotic animal hematology and cytology. 4th edition. Hoboken (NJ): John Wiley & Sons, Inc; 2015. p. 277–307.
8. Mehler SJ, Bennett RA. Surgical oncology of exotic animals. Vet Clin North Am Exot Anim Pract 2004;7(3):783–805.
9. Withrow S. Biopsy principles. In: Withrow S, MacEwen E, editors. Small animal clinical oncology. Philadelphia: WB Saunders; 2001. p. 63–9.
10. Stone EA. Biopsy: principles, technical considerations, and pitfalls. Vet Clin North Am Exot Anim Pract 1995;25:33–45.
11. Meuten DJ. Tumors in domestic animals. Oxfordshire (United Kingdom): CAB Direct; 2002.
12. Febbo PG, Ladanyi M, Aldape KD, et al. NCCN Task Force report: Evaluating the clinical utility of tumor markers in oncology. J Natl Compr Canc Netw 2011;9(Suppl 5):S1–32.
13. Denoix PF. Enquete permanent dans les centres anticancereaux. Bull Inst Natl Hyg 1946;1(1):70–5.
14. Gilson SD. Clinical management of the regional lymph node. Vet Clin North Am Small Anim Pract 1995;25:149–67.
15. Northrup NC, Barron GHW, Aldridge CF, et al. Outcome for client-owned domestic rabbits undergoing limb amputation: 34 cases (2000–2009). J Am Vet Med Assoc 2014;244(8):950–5.
16. Higgins S, Guzman DSM, Sadar MJ, et al. Coxofemoral amputation in a domestic rabbit (Oryctolagus cuniculus) with tibiofibular osteoblastic osteosarcoma. J Exot Pet Med 2015;24(4):455–63.
17. Harcourt-Brown FM. Gastric dilation and intestinal obstruction in 76 rabbits. Vet Rec 2007;161(12):409–14.
18. Withrow S. Cryosurgery. In: Withrow S, MacEwen E, editors. Small animal clinical oncology. Philadelphia: WB Saunders; 2001. p. 77–83.
19. Hoshi S, Mao H, Takahashi T, et al. Internal iliac arterial infusion chemotherapy for rabbit invasive bladder cancer. Int J Urol 1997;4:493–9.
20. Itamochi H, Kigawa J, Minagawa Y, et al. Antitumor effects of internal iliac arterial infusion of platinum compounds in a rabbit cervical cancer model. Obstet Gynecol 1997;89:286–90.

21. Chen J, Yao Q, Li D, et al. Chemotherapy targeting regional lymphatic tissues to treat rabbits bearing VX2 tumor in the mammary glands. Cancer Biol Ther 2008; 7:721–5.
22. Zehnder A, Hawkins M, Trestail L, et al. A novel method for determining body surface area in domestic rabbits. Proceedings of the annual Association of Exotic Mammal Veterinarians (AEMV) conference. Seattle (WA), August 6–11, 2011. p. 105–6.
23. Theon A. Intralesional and topical chemotherapy and immunotherapy. Vet Clin North Am Equine Pract 1998;14:659–71.
24. Andres KM, Kent M, Siedlecki CT, et al. The use of megavoltage radiation therapy in the treatment of thymomas in rabbits: 19 cases. Vet Comp Oncol 2012; 10(2):82–94.
25. Sanchez-Migallon DG, Mayer J, Gould J, et al. Radiation therapy for the treatment of thymoma in rabbits (Oryctolagus cuniculus). J Exot Pet Med 2006; 15(2):138–44.
26. Mauldin GN, Shiomitsu K. Principles and practice of radiation therapy in exotic and avian species. Semin Avian Exot Pet Med 2005;14(3):168–74.
27. Antinoff N. Mediastinal masses in rabbits: Another therapeutic option. Proceedings of the annual Association of Exotic Mammal Veterinarians (AEMV) conference. Milwaukee (WI), August 12–15, 2009. p. 65.
28. Nakata M, Yasutsugu MIWA, Tsuboi M, et al. Surgical and localized radiation therapy for an intranasal adenocarcinoma in a rabbit. J Vet Med Sci 2014; 76(12):1659–62.
29. Merkel L, Biel M. Photodynamic therapy. In: Withrow S, MacEwen E, editors. Small animal clinical oncology. Philadelphia: WB Saunders; 2001. p. 86–91.
30. Page RL, Thrall DE, Dewhirst MW, et al. Whole body hyperthermia. Rationale and potential use for cancer treatment. J Vet Intern Med 1987;1(3):110–20.
31. Gillette E. Hyperthermia. In: Withrow S, MacEwen E, editors. Small animal clinical oncology. Philadelphia: WB Saunders; 2001. p. 83–6.
32. Gomer CJ, Jester JV, Razum NJ, et al. Photodynamic therapy of intraocular tumors examination of hematoporphyrin derivative distribution and long-term damage in rabbit ocular tissue. Cancer Res 1985;45(8):3718–25.
33. Meyer M, Speight P, Bown SG. A study of the effects of photodynamic therapy on the normal tissues of the rabbit jaw. Br J Cancer 1991;64(6):1093–7.
34. Moroz P, Jones SK, Winter J, et al. Targeting liver tumors with hyperthermia: ferromagnetic embolization in a rabbit liver tumor model. J Surg Oncol 2001; 78(1):22–9.
35. Wissniowski TT, Hänsler J, Neureiter D, et al. Activation of tumor-specific T lymphocytes by radio-frequency ablation of the VX2 hepatoma in rabbits. Cancer Res 2003;63(19):6496–500.
36. Gilson SD, Stone EA. Management of the surgical oncology patient. Compend Contin Educ Pract Vet 1990;12(8):1047–54.
37. Weisbroth SH. Neoplastic disease. In: Weisbroth SH, Flatt RE, Kraus AL, editors. The biology of the laboratory rabbit. San Diego (CA): Academic Press; 1974. p. 331–75.
38. Greene HS. Adenocarcinoma of the uterine fundus in the rabbit. Ann N Y Acad Sci 1959;75:535–42.
39. Ingalls TH, Adams W, Lurie MB, et al. Natural history of adenocarcinoma of the uterus in the Phipps rabbit colony. J Natl Cancer Inst 1964;33:799–806.
40. Walter B, Poth T, Böhmer E, et al. Uterine disorders in 59 rabbits. Vet Rec 2010; 166(8):230–3.

41. Künzel F, Grinninger P, Shibly S, et al. Uterine disorders in 50 pet rabbits. J Am Anim Hosp Assoc 2015;51(1):8–14.
42. Adams WM Jr. The natural history of adenocarcinoma of the uterus in the Phipps rabbit colony. Philadelphia: University of Pennsylvania; 1962 [N Med Sci Thesis].
43. Asakawa MG, Goldschmidt MH, Une Y, et al. The immunohistochemical evaluation of estrogen receptor-alpha and progesterone receptors of normal, hyperplastic, and neoplastic endometrium in 88 pet rabbits. Vet Pathol 2008;45: 217–25.
44. Cooper TK, Adelsohn D, Gilbertson SR. Spontaneous deciduosarcoma in a domestic rabbit (Oryctolagus cuniculus). Vet Pathol 2006;43(3):377–80.
45. Goto M, Nomura Y, Une Y, et al. Malignant mixed Müllerian tumor in a rabbit (Oryctolagus cuniculus): case report with immunohistochemistry. Vet Pathol 2006; 43(4):560–4.
46. Kaufmann-Bart M, Fischer I. Choriocarcinoma with metastasis in a rabbit (Oryctolagus cuniculi). Vet Pathol 2008;45(1):77–9.
47. Raftery A. Letter: Uterine adenocarcinoma in pet rabbits. Vet Rec 1998;142:704.
48. Klaphake E, Paul-Murphy J. Disorders of the reproductive and urinary systems. In: Quesenberry KE, Carpenter JW, editors. Ferrets, rabbits and rodents: clinical medicine and surgery. 3rd edition. St Louis (MO): Elsevier; 2012. p. 217–31.
49. Hoffman JA. Hodendrebs bei einem Kanichen. Berl Munch Tierarztl Wochenschr 1954;67:350–3.
50. Roccabianca P, Ghisleni G, Scanziani E. Simultaneous seminoma and interstitial cell tumor in a rabbit with a previous cutaneous basal cell tumor. J Comp Pathol 1999;121(1):95–9.
51. Veeramachaneni DNR, Vande Woude S. Interstitial cell tumour and germ cell tumour with carcinoma in situ in rabbit testes. Int J Androl 1999;22(2):97–101.
52. Maratea KA, Ramos-Vara JA, Corriveau LA, et al. Testicular interstitial cell tumor and gynecomastia in a rabbit. Vet Pathol 2007;44(4):513–7.
53. Irizarry-Rovira AR, Lennox AM, Ramos-Vara JA. Granular cell tumor in the testis of a rabbit: cytologic, histologic, immunohistochemical, and electron microscopic characterization. Vet Pathol 2008;45(1):73–7.
54. Alexandre N, Branco S, Soares TF, et al. Bilateral testicular seminoma in a rabbit (Oryctolagus cuniculus). J Exot Pet Med 2010;19(4):304–8.
55. Suzuki M, Ozaki M, Ano N, et al. Testicular gonadoblastoma in two pet domestic rabbits (Oryctolagus cuniculus domesticus). J Vet Diagn Invest 2011;23(5): 1028–32.
56. Banco B, Stefanello D, Giudice C, et al. Metastasizing testicular seminoma in a pet rabbit. J Vet Diagn Invest 2012;24(3):608–11.
57. Baum B, Hewicker-Trautwein M. Classification and epidemiology of mammary tumours in pet rabbits (Oryctolagus cuniculus). J Comp Pathol 2015;152(4): 291–8.
58. Burrows H. Spontaneous uterine and mammary tumors in the rabbit. J Pathol Bacteriol 1940;51:385–90.
59. Greene H, Strauss J. Multiple primary tumors in the rabbit. Cancer 1949;2: 673–91.
60. Lipman NS, Zhao ZB, Andrutis KA, et al. Prolactin-secreting pituitary adenomas with mammary dysplasia in New Zealand white rabbits. Lab Anim Sci 1994;44: 114–20.
61. Sikoski P, Trybus J, Cline JM, et al. Cystic mammary adenocarcinoma associated with a prolactin-secreting pituitary adenoma in a New Zealand white rabbit (Oryctolagus cuniculus). Comp Med 2008;58:297–300.

62. Shahbazfar AA, Mohammadpour H, Isfahani HRE. Mammary gland carcinosarcoma in a New Zealand white rabbit (Oryctolagus cuniculus). Acta Sci Vet 2012; 40(1):1025–8.
63. Schöniger S, Horn LC, Schoon HA. Tumors and tumor-like lesions in the mammary gland of 24 pet rabbits: a histomorphological and immunohistochemical characterization. Vet Pathol 2014;51(3):569–80.
64. Heatley JJ, Smith AN. Spontaneous neoplasms of lagomorphs. Vet Clin North Am Exot Anim Pract 2004;7(3):561–77.
65. Petraitiene R, Petraitis V, Bacher J, et al. Cyclosporine A-induced mammary hyperplasia and hyperprolactinemia in New Zealand white rabbits. Comp Med 2001;51:430–5.
66. Blevins S, Gardner K, Wagner A, et al. Mammary gland enlargement and discharge in an adult New Zealand white rabbit. Lab Anim (NY) 2009;38: 258–61.
67. Kanfer S, Reavill D. Cutaneous neoplasia in ferrets, rabbits, and guinea Pigs. Vet Clin North Am Exot Anim Pract 2013;16:579–98.
68. White S, Campbell T, Logan A, et al. Lymphoma with cutaneous involvement in three domestic rabbits (Oryctolagus cuniculus). Vet Dermatol 2000;11:61–7.
69. Van Kampen KR. Lymphosarcoma in the rabbit: a case report and general review. Cornell Vet 1968;58(1):121–8.
70. Cloyd GG, Johnson GR. Lymphosarcoma with lymphoblastic leukemia in a New Zealand white rabbit. Lab Anim Sci 1978;28:66–9.
71. Finnie JW, Bostock DE, Walden NB. Lymphoblastic leukaemia in a rabbit: a case report. Lab Anim 1980;14:49–51.
72. Toth LA, Olson GA, Wilson E, et al. Lymphocytic leukemia and lymphosarcoma in a rabbit. J Am Vet Med Assoc 1990;197:627–9.
73. Hinton M, Regan M. Cutaneous lymphosarcoma. Vet Rec 1978;103:140–1.
74. Pilny AA, Reavill D. Chylothorax and thymic lymphoma in a pet rabbit (Oryctolagus cuniculus). J Exot Pet Med 2008;17(4):295–9.
75. Volopich S, Gruber A, Hassan J, et al. Malignant B-cell lymphoma of the Harder's gland in a rabbit. Vet Ophthalmol 2005;8(4):259–63.
76. Wagner F, Fehr M. Common ophthalmic problems in pet rabbits. J Exot Pet Med 2007;16(3):158–67.
77. Shibuya K, Tajima M, Kanai K, et al. Spontaneous lymphoma in a Japanese white rabbit. J Vet Med Sci 1999;61(12):1327–9.
78. Gomez L, Gasquez A, Roncero V, et al. Lymphoma in a rabbit: histopathological and immunohistochemical findings. J Small Anim Pract 2002;43:224–6.
79. Künzel F, Hittmair KM, Hassan J, et al. Thymomas in rabbits: clinical evaluation, diagnosis, and treatment. J Am Anim Hosp Assoc 2012;48(2):97–104.
80. Morrisey JK, McEntee M. Therapeutic options for thymoma in the rabbit. Semin Avian Exot Pet Med 2005;14(3):175–81.
81. Wagner F, Beinecke A, Fehr M, et al. Recurrent bilateral exophthalmos associated with metastatic thymic carcinoma in a pet rabbit. J Small Anim Pract 2005;46(8):393–7.
82. Fox RR, Meier H, Crary DD, et al. Hemolytic anemia associated with thymoma in the rabbit. Genetic studies and pathological findings. Oncology 1971;25: 372–82.
83. Meier H, Fox RR. Hereditary lymphosarcoma in WH rabbits and hereditary hemolytic anemia associated with thymoma in strain X rabbits. Bibl Haematol 1973;39:72–92.

84. Florizoone K. Thymoma-associated exfoliative dermatitis in a rabbit. Vet Dermatol 2005;16(4):281–4.
85. Rosthaher Prélaud A, Jassies-van der Lee A, Mueller RS, et al. Presumptive paraneoplastic exfoliative dermatitis in four domestic rabbits. Vet Rec 2013; 172(6):155.
86. Vernau KM, Grahn BH, Clarke-Scott HA, et al. Thymoma in a geriatric rabbit with hypercalcemia and periodic exophthalmos. J Am Vet Med Assoc 1995;206: 820–2.
87. Clippinger TL, Bennett A, Alleman R, et al. Removal of a thymoma via median sternotomy in a rabbit with recurrent appendicular neurofibrosarcoma. J Am Vet Med Assoc 1998;213:1140–3.
88. Rosenthal K, Hoefer H, Quesenberry K, et al. Question cause of hypercalcemia in a rabbit. J Am Vet Med Assoc 1995;206(11):1675.
89. Kesler KA, Wright CD, Loehrer PJ. Thymoma: Current medical and surgical management. Semin Neurol 2004;24:63–73.
90. von Bomhard W, Goldschmidt MH, Shofer FS, et al. Cutaneous neoplasms in pet rabbits: a retrospective study. Vet Pathol 2007;44(5):579–88.
91. Mazzullo G, Russo M, Niutta PP, et al. Osteosarcoma with multiple metastases and subcutaneous involvement in a rabbit (Oryctolagus cuniculus). Vet Pathol 2004;33(2):102–4.
92. Salm R, Field J. Osteosarcoma in a rabbit. J Pathol Bacteriol 1965;89(1):400–2.
93. Weisbroth SH, Hurvitz A. Spontaneous osteogenic sarcoma in Oryctolagus cuniculus with elevated serum alkaline phosphatase. Lab Anim Care 1969;19(2): 263–5.
94. Jacobson SA. Comparative pathology of the tumors of bone. Springfield (IL): Charles C Thomas; 1971.
95. Amand WB, Riser WH, Biery DN. Spontaneous osteosarcoma with widespread metastasis in a belted Dutch rabbit. J Am Anim Hosp Assoc 1973;9(6):577–81.
96. Walberg JA. Osteogenic sarcoma with metastasis in a rabbit (Oryctolagus cuniculus). Lab Anim Sci 1981;31(4):407–8.
97. Hoover JP, Paulsen DB, Quallis CW, et al. Osteogenic sarcoma with subcutaneous involvement in a rabbit. J Am Vet Med Assoc 1986;189(9):1156–8.
98. Weiss AT, Muller K. Spinal osteolytic osteosarcoma in a pet rabbit. Vet Rec 2011; 168(10):266.
99. Kondo H, Ishikawa M, Maeda H, et al. Spontaneous osteosarcoma in a rabbit (Oryctolagus cuniculus). Vet Pathol 2007;44(5):691–4.
100. Ishikawa M, Kondo H, Onuma M, et al. Osteoblastic osteosarcoma in a rabbit. Comp Med 2013;62(2):124–6.
101. Renfrew H, Rest JR, Holden AR. Extraskeletal fibroblastic osteosarcoma in a rabbit (Oryctolagus cuniculus). J Small Anim Pract 2001;42(9):456–8.
102. Wijesundera KK, Izawa T, Fujita D, et al. Spontaneous extraskeletal osteosarcoma in a rabbit (Oryctolagus cuniculus): histopathological and immunohistochemical findings. J Toxicol Pathol 2013;26(3):309–12.
103. Fisher PG, Carpenter JW. Neurologic and musculoskeletal diseases. In: Quesenberry KE, Carpenter JW, editors. Ferrets, rabbits and rodents: clinical medicine and surgery. St Louis (MO): Elsevier; 2012. p. 245–56.
104. Risi E, Sauvaget S, Boutoille F, et al. Five successful cases of partial mandibulectomy and their medical follow-up in rabbits suffering from mandibular abscesses or tumors. Proceedings of the annual Association of Exotic Mammal Veterinarians (AEMV) conference, Oakland (CA), October 19–23, 2012. p.72.

105. Kaufman A, Quist K. Spontaneous renal carcinoma in a New Zealand White Rabbit. Lab Anim Care 1970;20(3):530–2.
106. Dobberstein J, Tamaschke C. Die spontantumoren beim kaninchen. New York: Springer-Verlag; 1958.
107. Atasever A, Beyaz L, Deniz K. A case of triphasic nephroblastoma with lung metastases in an angora rabbit. Rev Med Vet 2007;158(6):303–8.
108. Green HSN. The occurrence and transplantation of embryonal nephromas in the rabbit. Canc Res 1943;3(7):434–9.
109. Wardrop KJ, Nakamura J, Giddens WE. Nephroblastoma with secondary polycythemia in a New Zealand white rabbit. Lab Anim Sci 1982;32(3):280–2.
110. Lipman NS, Murphy JC, Newcomer CE. Polycythemia in a New Zealand White rabbit with an embryonal nephroma. J Am Vet Med Assoc 1985;187(11):1255–6.
111. Kubota M, Takaku Y, Saito M, et al. Nephroblastoma with polycythemia in two rabbits. Jpn J Vet Anesth Surg 2006;37:7–10.
112. Hassan J, Katic N, Klang A, et al. Treatment of nephroblastoma with polycythaemia by nephrectomy in a rabbit. Vet Rec 2012;170(18):465–6.
113. Knapp D. Tumors of the urinary system. In: Withrow S, MacEwen E, editors. Small animal clinical oncology. Philadelphia: WB Saunders; 2001. p. 490–9.
114. Lennox AM, Chitty J. Adrenal neoplasia and hyperplasia as a cause of hypertestosteronism in two rabbits. J Exot Pet Med 2006;15(1):56–8.
115. Varga M. Hypersexuality in a castrated rabbit (*Oryctolagus cuniculus*). Comp Anim 2011;16(1):48–51.
116. Baine K, Newkirk K, Fecteau KA, et al. Elevated testosterone and progestin concentrations in a spayed female rabbit with an adrenal cortical adenoma. Case Rep Vet Med 2014;2014:e1–4.
117. Lennox AM. Surgical treatment of adrenocortical disease. In: Harcourt-Brown F, Chitty J, editors. BSAVA manual of rabbit surgery, dentistry, and imaging. Gloucester (United Kingdom): British Small Animal Veterinary Association; 2014. p. 269–72.
118. Hueper WC, Ichniowski CT. Carcinoma of the adrenal cortex in a rabbit. Canc Res 1944;4(3):176–8.
119. Schoemaker NJ, Teerds KJ, Mol JA, et al. The role of luteinizing hormone in the pathogenesis of hyperadrenocorticism in neutered ferrets. Mol Cell Endocrinol 2002;197(1–2):117–25.
120. Bielinska M, Kiiveri S, Parviainen H, et al. Gonadectomy-induced adrenocortical neoplasia in the domestic ferret (*Mustela putorius furo*) and laboratory mouse. Vet Pathol 2006;43(2):97–117.
121. White SW. Adrenalectomy in the rabbit. Aust J Exp Biol Med Sci 1966;44(4):447–9.
122. Shope RE, Hurst EW. Infectious papillomatosis of rabbits with a note on the histopathology. J Exp Med 1933;58(5):607–24.
123. Shope RE. Infectious Fibroma of Rabbits III. The serial transmission of virus myxomatosum in cottontail rabbits, and cross-immunity tests with the fibroma virus. J Exp Med 1936;63(1):33–41.
124. Pulley LT, Shively JN. Naturally occurring infectious fibroma in the domestic rabbit. Vet Pathol 1973;10(6):509–19.
125. Kerr PJ, Best SM. Myxoma virus in rabbits. Rev Sci Tech 1998;17(1):256–68.
126. Munday JS, Aberdein D, Squires RA, et al. Persistent conjunctival papilloma due to oral papillomavirus infection in a rabbit in New Zealand. J Am Assoc Lab Anim Sci 2007;46(5):69–71.

127. Strayer DS, Skaletsky E, Cabirac GF, et al. Malignant rabbit fibroma virus causes secondary immunosuppression in rabbits. J Immunol 1983;130(1):399–404.
128. Strayer DS, Sell S, Leibowitz JL. Malignant rabbit fibroma syndrome. A possible model for acquired immunodeficiency syndrome (AIDS). Am J Pathol 1985; 120(1):170–1.

Ferret Oncology
Diseases, Diagnostics, and Therapeutics

Nico J. Schoemaker, DVM, PhD, DECZM (small mammal & avian), DABVP-Avian Practice

KEYWORDS

- Neoplasia • Neoplasm • *Mustela putorius furo* • Hyperadrenocorticism • Insulinoma
- Lymphoma

KEY POINTS

- Tumors are commonly seen in ferrets after the age of 3 years, and the endocrine, hemolymphatic, and integumentary systems are most commonly affected.
- The 3 most common tumors in ferrets are adrenal tumors, insulinoma, and lymphoma, making up more than 40% of all tumors seen in ferrets.
- It is extremely common for ferrets to have multiple types of tumors simultaneously; ferrets with up to 4 types of concurrent tumors have been seen.
- Although with surgery a neoplasm can be removed, both adrenal tumors and insulinoma can be managed medically with an even better, or similar, mean survival period compared with surgically managed cases.
- Providing ferrets with a depot gonadotrophin-releasing hormone-containing implant and feeding them a diet with a high protein and fat content and a low carbohydrate content have been suggested as measures to prevent the occurrence of adrenal tumors and insulinoma, respectively; however, proof that these measures work has not been published to date.

INTRODUCTION

In recent decades it has become clear that the previous conception that neoplasia in ferrets are rare is false.[1] A large range of case reports have been published on a wide variety of tumors, and more information has become available on the most common neoplasia of ferrets. In addition, ferrets have recently been introduced as lung cancer research models in which lung cancer could be induced after exposure to either tobacco smoke or a specific tobacco carcinogen.[2]

Most tumors in ferrets are seen after the age of 3 years.[3–5] The endocrine, hemolymphatic, and integumentary systems are most commonly affected, with adrenocortical

Disclosure: The author has nothing to disclose.
Faculty of Veterinary Medicine, Division of Zoological Medicine, Department of Clinical Sciences of Companion Animals, Utrecht University, Yalelaan 108, Utrecht 3584 CM, The Netherlands
E-mail address: N.J.Schoemaker@uu.nl

Vet Clin Exot Anim 20 (2017) 183–208
http://dx.doi.org/10.1016/j.cvex.2016.07.004

tumors and insulinoma making up more than 40% of all tumors seen.[4,5] The third most commonly seen neoplasm in ferrets is the lymphoma.[3-5] In up to 20% of ferrets with a tumor, multiple tumors of different origin (up to 4) can be found simultaneously.[3,4,6]

Aside from the 3 common types of neoplasia in ferrets, any other type of tumor may be diagnosed. **Table 1** provides an overview of the different types of spontaneously occurring neoplasia reported in ferrets. For an overview of the general diagnostic and therapeutic options in oncological patients (see van Zeeland's article, "Rabbit Oncology: Diseases, Diagnostics and Therapeutics," in this issue). Examples of the most sophisticated diagnostic techniques available to diagnose oncological disease in ferrets include computed tomography (CT), MRI, and scintigraphy. Although these techniques are not as easily available and are more expensive compared with radiology and ultrasonography, these advanced imaging techniques may enable visualization of masses that otherwise would remain undetected (**Fig. 1**),[16,34] and allow the volume of tissues to be calculated, thereby enabling monitoring of their growth. In addition, CT may help visualize the extent of the tumor and its potential invasiveness in other tissues (**Fig. 2**). Scintigraphy may also help detect neoplasia, whereby the distribution of radiopharmaceutical agents in specific tissues, such as the thyroid gland, can be visualized by using a gamma camera.[43] Specific ferret-related diagnostic and therapeutic options are discussed here in relation to the endocrine, hemolymphatic, and integumentary tumors in this species.

ENDOCRINE TUMORS
Adrenocortical Tumors

Hyperadrenocorticism, also referred to as adrenocortical disease or adrenal gland disease, is the most common endocrine tumor seen in ferrets. Although hyperadrenocorticism is considered similar to hypercortisolism (Cushing disease) in dogs, cats, and humans, in ferrets plasma androstenedione, 17α-hydroxyprogesterone, and estradiol concentrations are increased. In line with the latter three increased hormone concentrations, no atrophy is seen in the nonneoplastic, contralateral adrenal gland.[44] Histologic changes of the adrenal glands range from (nodular) hyperplasia to adenocarcinoma and everything in between. However, an indication of the prognosis based on the histologic diagnosis cannot be given.

Cause

Although early neutering (at the age of 6 weeks) has long been postulated as the cause for the high prevalence of adrenal tumors in ferrets, it is not likely that the time of neutering is the most important factor in the development of these tumors. It is likely that the increased concentrations of gonadotropins, which occur after neutering because of the loss of negative feedback, persistently stimulate the adrenal cortex, which eventually results in adrenocortical growth. Support for this hypothesis can be found in the fact that luteinizing hormone receptors have been detected in the adrenal glands of ferrets with hyperadrenocorticism. These receptors are considered to be functional, because plasma concentrations of adrenal androgens increase after intravenous injection of a gonadotrophin-releasing hormone (GnRH) agonist.[45] In addition, the depot GnRH agonist, deslorelin, is currently used successfully in managing the clinical signs of ferrets with hyperadrenocorticism.

When ferrets are kept indoors, it is likely that the length of (day)light they receive is longer than that received by ferrets that are housed outdoors. Because gonadotropins are secreted during the time when ferrets are kept in light for longer than 12 hours per day, indoor ferrets are longer under the influence of these hormones and may thus

Table 1
Reported (spontaneous) neoplasms in ferrets

Organ System	Tissue of Origin	Reported Tumor Types	Incidence	Clinical Signs	Diagnosis and Work-up	Treatment and Prognosis
Reproductive tract (female)[3-5,7,8]	Ovary; uterus	• Ovarian spindle cell tumors, leiomyoma, leiomyosarcoma, sex cord stromal tumor (including thecoma, granulosa cell tumor [arrhenoblastomal]), adenocarcinoma • Ovarian remnant: thecoma, granulosa cell tumor • Uterine (fibro)leiomyoma, leiomyosarcoma, teratoma, deciduoma, adenocarcinoma	In general, not well reported in the veterinary literature because of neutering	• Most neoplasms of the reproductive tract are clinically silent • Reproductive failure • Ovarian (remnant) tumors may result in symmetric alopecia and a swollen vulva	• Abdominal palpation • Hormone analysis • Radiography • Ultrasonography • Cytology (FNA) • Histopathology • Exploratory laparotomy	Metastatic disease has not been reported and surgical resection of the tumor is usually curative

(continued on next page)

Table 1
(continued)

Organ System	Tissue of Origin	Reported Tumor Types	Incidence	Clinical Signs	Diagnosis and Work-up	Treatment and Prognosis
Reproductive tract (male)[3,4,9–13]	Testicles; prostate; preputial gland	• Testicular seminoma; Sertoli cell tumor; interstitial cell tumor; leiomyosarcoma; mixed germ cell–sex cord–stromal tumor; peripheral nerve sheath tumor. Neoplasms of (up to 4) different tumor types can occur simultaneously • Prostate (adeno) carcinomas • Preputial gland adenocarcinoma	• Testicular tumors not well reported because of frequency of neutering; incidence is considered higher in cryptorchid animals. A ferret that was chemically neutered with a deslorelin-containing implant developed a testicular tumor • Prostate tumors are extremely rare • Preputial gland tumors are frequently seen in (neutered) ferrets	—	• Clinical signs • Ultrasonography • Histopathology	Bilateral orchidectomy. Testicular tumors seldom metastasize Preputial gland tumors are locally invasive and require aggressive surgery in which margins of at least 1 cm are recommended. Radiation therapy has been used in conjunction with surgical resection with varying degrees of success

Mammary glands[3–5,7]	—	Simple and complex mammary adenomas Adenocarcinomas	Rare in ferrets	Mammary gland enlargement	• FNA (cytology) or biopsy (histopathology) • Thoracic radiographs to check for lung metastases	Mastectomy and ovariohysterectomy. Prognosis depends on the presence of metastasis
Hematopoietic and lymphatic systems[3–5,7,14–16]	May be localized in every organ system, but most prominent in lymph nodes, blood, thymus, spleen, liver, bone marrow, GI tract, and skin	Lymphoma; leukemia (lymphoblastic, lymphocytic, myeloid, megakaryocytic myelomonocytic, erythremic); myeloma; myelolipoma; thymoma	Lymphoma is the third most common neoplasia in ferrets and is seen in ferrets <1 y old to adult; may be of B-cell or T-cell origin; T cell is most common	• Highly variable in lymphoma, dependent on the site affected (eg, enlarged lymph nodes, renomegaly/splenomegaly/hepatomegaly, general malaise, cutaneous or ocular lesions, diarrhea) • Coughing and regurgitation may be seen in case of a mediastinal mass	• Clinical signs • Ultrasonography, thoracic radiographs, or CT imaging • FNA (cytology) or biopsy (histology) • CBC or blood smear may reveal marked lymphocytosis and neoplastic cells (lymphoblasts) • Lymphopenia is seen in older ferrets with lymphoma • Hypercalcemia • Necropsy • Gammopathy in case of myeloma	With only 1 anatomic lesion surgical removal may be curative. Median survival without treatment and/or chemotherapy is 6 month

(continued on next page)

Table 1
(continued)

Organ System	Tissue of Origin	Reported Tumor Types	Incidence	Clinical Signs	Diagnosis and Work-up	Treatment and Prognosis
Integument[3–5,7,13,17–23]	Skin; ears; eyelids	Basal cell tumor (sebaceous epithelioma, sebaceous adenoma); mast cell tumor; apocrine sweat gland tumor (see preputial gland adenocarcinoma); ceruminous gland adenocarcinoma; trichoblastoma; hemangioma; hemangiosarcoma; hamartoma; lipoma; liposarcoma; (mucoid) fibroma; (vaccination-site) fibrosarcoma; myxosarcoma; squamous cell carcinoma; adrenocortical-like cutaneous tumor; histiocytoma; melanocytoma; epitheliotropic lymphoma	Most common tumors after the endocrine and hemolymphatic tumors. Basal cell tumors account for approximately 60% of skin tumors. Viruses (eg, papilloma virus) and vaccination may play a role in the cause of some neoplasia (squamous cell carcinoma, fibroma)	• Solitary, well-circumscribed, cutaneous or subcutaneous masses with or without the presence of crusts. Multiple sebaceous epithelioma and piloleiomyomas can be present simultaneously • Tumors may be located anywhere on the body surface, although predilection sites may be recognized for some tumors (eg, prepuce, ear for apocrine gland tumors; along the head, neck, or dorsal midline for piloleiomyosarcoma)	• Clinical presentation • FNA (cytology) or excisional/incisional biopsy (histology)	• Treatment of choice is general surgical excision of the mass. Adjunct chemotherapy or radiation may be considered depending on the tumor type involved. Prognosis varies depending on the type of neoplasia and location • For basal cell, mast cell tumors, hemangioma, hemangiosarcoma, surgical excision is considered curative • Apocrine sweat gland tumors vary in malignancy. Prepuce and perivulvular tumors have a high malignancy. Wide margins are needed during surgical resection. Radiation therapy may have a supplemental effect

System	Sites	Tumor types	Notes	Clinical presentation	Diagnosis	Prognosis
GI tract[3-5,7,24-29]	Oral cavity; stomach; small and large intestines; liver and bile duct; exocrine pancreas	Lymphoma, squamous cell carcinoma; gastric adenocarcinomas; GI stromal tumor; colonic adenomatous polyp. The liver is a common site for metastasis. Hepatocellular adenoma and carcinoma; peliod hepatocellular carcinoma. Biliary cystadenoma; cholangiocellular carcinoma. Pancreatic exocrine adenocarcinoma; salivary gland carcinoma; peritoneal mesotheliomas; malignant mesenchymoma	Lymphoma is the most common tumor of the GI tract. Squamous cell carcinoma is the most common tumor in oral cavity. Biliary cystadenoma is the most common tumor of the biliary tract. A novel *Helicobacter* species has been associated with biliary malignancies	• Squamous cell carcinoma in the oral cavity results in pain and difficulty eating • Animals with GI tumors may present with lethargy, anorexia, and distended abdomen (eg, hepatomegaly)	• Clinical presentation (squamous cell carcinoma in the oral cavity). Abdominal palpation • Ultrasonography, radiography (barium GI series) or CT imaging • FNA or biopsy • Explorative laparotomy • Necropsy	Squamous cell carcinoma: invasive surgical excision. Extensive bone involvement may limit effect of surgery. Most gastric and intestinal tumors are likely to be diagnosed only in an advanced stage, thereby carrying a grave prognosis
Urinary tract[3-5,7,30]	Kidney; bladder	Transitional cell carcinoma; renal carcinoma, adenoma. Nephroblastoma	Tumors of the urinary tract are rare in ferrets	• Hematuria, dysuria, and incontinence • Unilateral renal enlargement	• Ultrasonography, (contrast) radiography • Necropsy	Unilateral nephrectomy may be curative in case of renal neoplasia. Bladder carcinoma has a poor prognosis

(continued on next page)

Table 1
(continued)

Organ System	Tissue of Origin	Reported Tumor Types	Incidence	Clinical Signs	Diagnosis and Work-up	Treatment and Prognosis
Respiratory tract[3–5,7,31]	Trachea; lungs	An adenosquamous carcinoma of the trachea. Mast cell tumor; mesothelioma No primary lung tumors described, although ferrets are used as a lung cancer model by exposing them to a tobacco carcinogen and thereby inducing lung neoplasia	Uncommon	Progressive dyspnea and tachypnea	Tracheoscopy and CT	No treatment described
Cardiovascular system[3–5]	Vascular endothelium	Hemangioma; hemangiosarcoma; lymphangioma	—	—	—	—
Musculoskeletal system[3–5,7,32–39]	Bones; muscle; joints	Chordoma; chordosarcoma; osteoma; osteosarcoma; chondrosarcoma; intramedullary lumbosacral teratoma; fibrosarcoma; synovial cell sarcoma; leiomyoma; leiomyosarcoma; piloleiomyosarcoma; rhabdomyosarcomas	Chordomas are fairly common tumors arising from notochord remnants The other types of tumors are rare	• Chordoma: irregularly round, whitish gray, firm, clublike swelling at the end of the tail. However, they may arise in any of the vertebra • Chordomas in the cervical and thoracic spine, result in paresis or paralysis caused by spinal cord compression and/or pathologic vertebral fracture • Progressive, unilateral lameness in cases of appendicular tumors	• Radiographs may reveal osteolysis or a swollen joint in case of the synovial cell sarcoma • CT may be useful to determine the extent of the tumor (also for surgical planning) • FNA and cytology • Histopathology	Amputation of the tail tip is curative in chordoma. When other vertebrae are effected, no treatment is available In case of appendicular tumors, amputation of the affected limb is recommended because no metastases are reported

| Nervous system[3-5,7,40] | Brain; spinal cord; peripheral nerves; eyes | Meningioma; granular cell tumor; choroid plexus papilloma; ocular lymphoma; melanocytoma; peripheral nerve sheath tumor (also known as schwannoma), neurofibroma, neurilemmoma and neurofibrosarcoma); ganglioneuroma; spinal cord lymphosarcoma | Uncommon | • Clinical signs depend on the location of the tumor and may include ataxia, seizures, (hemi)paresis/paralysis, and other neurologic deficits
• Peripheral nerve sheath tumors predominantly occur in the face and eyelids | • Use of advanced diagnostic techniques such as CT or MRI is generally required
• Histopathology | In case of peripheral nerve sheath tumors, surgical resection is often not considered because with each attempt the remaining neoplastic cells show increasingly malignant behavior, including more rapid growth and infiltration of adjacent tissue. Similar to other animals, radiation therapy may be considered as palliative treatment but overall prognosis is considered poor |

(continued on next page)

Table 1
(continued)

Organ System	Tissue of Origin	Reported Tumor Types	Incidence	Clinical Signs	Diagnosis and Work-up	Treatment and Prognosis
Endocrine system[3–5,7,41,42]	Adrenal glands; thyroid gland; endocrine pancreas	ACA; pheochromocytoma; insulinoma; thyroid carcinoma; C-cell carcinoma; adrenal neuroblastoma; adenocarcinoma of lachrymal gland origin	Adrenocortical tumors and insulinoma are the most common tumors in ferrets and represent >50% of all neoplasia seen in this species	• ACA: symmetric alopecia; recurrence of sexual behavior after neutering; dysuria may occur in male ferrets. Enlarged mammary glands may be seen in females • Insulinoma: lethargy, stargazing, weakness in the hind limbs, coma, ptyalism, pawing at the mouth, and a glazed look in the eyes	• ACA: ultrasonography, CT (hormone analysis) • Insulinoma: plasma glucose, insulin • Necropsy	• ACA: adrenalectomy was the former treatment of choice. Deslorelin-containing implants are now considered the treatment of choice with an average disease-free period of 16.5 mo • Insulinoma: partial pancreatectomy and medical treatment (diazoxide or prednisolone) result in a mean disease-free period of approximately 1 y. Resection of only the tumor (nodulectomy) is considered to result in a shorter disease-free period

Abbreviations: ACA, adrenocortical adenoma/carcinoma; CBC, complete blood cell count; CT, computed tomography; FNA, fine-needle aspiration; GI, gastrointestinal.

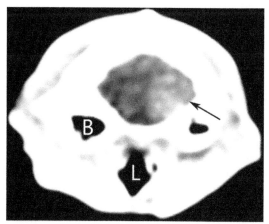

Fig. 1. CT image of ferret skull after administration of intravenous contrast. On the right side of brain the large, space-occupying, contrast-enhancing lesion is seen (*arrow*), which proved to be a choroid plexus papilloma. B, tympanic bulla; L, larynx. (*From* van Zeeland YRA, Schoemaker NJ, Passon-Vastenburg M, et al. Vestibular syndrome due to a choroid plexus papilloma in a ferret. J Am Anim Hosp Assoc 2009;45:97–101)

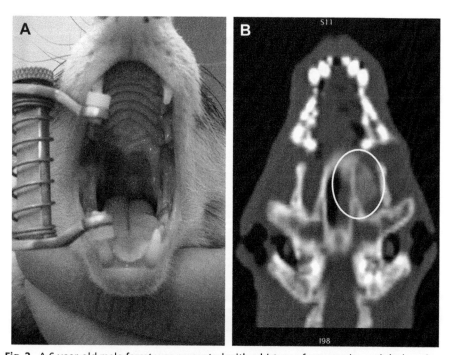

Fig. 2. A 6-year-old male ferret was presented with a history of progressive weight loss since 6 months. Oral inspection revealed a mass on the left side of the soft pallet (*A*). CT imaging (*B*) enabled visualization of the extent of involvement of this oral tumor and revealed that it had resulted in osteolysis of the skull, and thereby an unfavorable prognosis. Histology revealed this tumor to be an adenocarcinoma, likely of salivary gland origin, with regional metastasis and metastasis in the lungs.

have a higher chance of developing hyperadrenocorticism compared with ferrets housed outdoors.[46,47]

A genetic background may also play a role in the cause of this disease. Studies have been performed in search for candidate genes that may play a role in the development of tumor formation in ferrets. Although alterations of specific genes (ie, sfrp1 and Foxl2) have been found in adrenocortical tumors,[48,49] it is still not clear what the pathway is for the development of these tumors.

Clinical signs

The most prominent signs of hyperadrenocorticism in ferrets are symmetric alopecia (**Fig. 3**), a swollen vulva in neutered female ferrets, return of sexual behavior after neutering in male ferrets, and pruritus. The skin is usually not affected, although some excoriations may be seen. In male ferrets, urinary obstruction caused by periprostatic or periurethral cysts and prostatic enlargement may be seen. Occasionally mammary gland enlargement in jills is also seen. There is no sex predilection in the occurrence of this disease. Although signs of hyperadrenocorticism may be seen in ferrets as young as 2 years, more than 80% are more than 5 years of age. Polyuria and polydipsia are reported in ferrets with hyperadrenocorticism. However, these signs may be caused by concurrent kidney disease in these (mostly elderly) ferrets.[50]

Differential diagnosis

The most important differential diagnoses include a nonovariectomized female or the presence of active remnant ovaries. The investigators have also seen a ferret with severe alopecia and pruritus caused by a food allergy.[50] Plasma and urine hormone analysis, in combination with an abdominal ultrasonography, could not find any changes associated with an enlarged, or hyperfunctioning, adrenal gland. Changing the diet in this ferret resolved the alopecia and pruritus. Infectious skin diseases should also be considered in cases of alopecia and pruritus. In these cases, the skin is affected. Seasonal alopecia, a condition that is characterized by a seasonal occurrence of

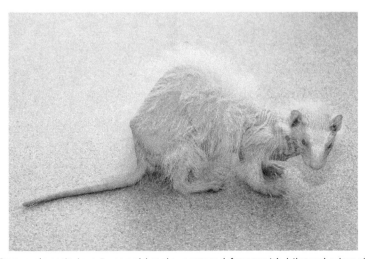

Fig. 3. Severe alopecia in a 5-year-old male, neutered ferret with bilateral adrenal tumors that were seen on ultrasonography. Multiple small crusts can be seen, which were the result of the constant scratching performed by this ferret.

alopecia, with hair loss predominantly occurring on the tail, is also commonly mentioned as a differential diagnosis. Although the cause for this condition is not known, the author suspects that it may be an early sign of hyperadrenocorticism.[50]

Diagnosis

Aside from the clinical signs, abdominal palpation is useful in obtaining the diagnosis of hyperadrenocorticism in ferrets. Palpation of an enlarged adrenal gland helps locate the affected adrenal gland, although the right adrenal gland is more difficult to palpate because of the overlying caudate liver lobe. The most widely reported diagnostic technique is measuring serum/plasma hormone concentrations. The reported hormones that are diagnostic are androstenedione, estradiol, and 17α-hydroxyprogesterone. However, increased levels of 1 or more of these hormones are also seen in intact female ferrets during estrus,[51] and therefore they do not helpful in the differentiation between a ferret with hyperadrenocorticism and one with an active ovarian remnant.

Although in ferrets with adrenocortical disease the urinary corticoid/creatinine ratio (UCCR) is higher than the reference value of 2.1×10^{-6},[52] this ratio is also not useful in the differentiation between a ferret with hyperadrenocorticism and one with an active ovary because the UCCR is also increased in intact ferrets during the breeding season.

An abdominal ultrasonographic examination is the most useful tool to determine whether 1 or both adrenal glands are affected, or whether an ovarian remnant is present. In the past it was considered difficult to correctly identify the adrenal glands ultrasonographically. However, using specific landmarks, the adrenal glands can easily be identified. The left adrenal gland is located ventrolateral to the aorta, at the level of the origin of the cranial mesenteric artery. The right adrenal gland is located more cranial than the left, and is attached to the dorsolateral surface of the caudal vena cava, at the level of the origin of the cranial mesenteric artery, and lies adjacent to the caudomedial aspect of the caudate process of the caudate liver lobe. The adrenal glands of ferrets with hyperadrenocorticism have a significantly increased width (>3.9 mm), a rounded appearance, a heterogeneous structure, an increased echogenicity, and sometimes contain signs of mineralization.[53]

CT has recently been suggested as useful when evaluating the adrenal glands in ferrets. When using this technique, intravenous contrast medium is needed to delineate the adrenal gland better from the caudal vena cava and enable better visualization of the size of this gland.[50]

Treatment

The most commonly used modalities for treating ferrets with hyperadrenocorticism are surgery and/or the use of a long-acting GnRH analogue. The choice of treatment is influenced by many factors. Criteria such as the age of the ferret, presence of concurrent disease (eg, renal failure, lymphoma, and/or cardiomyopathy), risk of surgery (which is higher when the right or both adrenal glands are involved), and/or financial limitations may lead owners to decline surgery. Comparing the average disease-free period following both treatment modalities, treatment with a deslorelin-containing implant has an average disease-free period of 16.5 months (range, 3–30 months), whereas this period is 13.6 months (range, 0–38 months) for surgical intervention.[54]

Surgical treatment

The left adrenal gland can be fairly easily removed, in which only the phrenicoabdominal vein needs to be ligated. Resection of the right adrenal gland is more difficult because of its dorsolateral attachment to the caudal vena cava and close proximity to the liver. Complete resection or partial resection combined with cryosurgery had a less favorable outcome compared with partial resection of the right adrenal gland.[55]

Debulking of the right adrenal gland also did not result in a less favorable survival time compared with complete resection of the left adrenal gland.[55] When both adrenal glands are affected, it has been proposed to remove the entire left adrenal gland and part of the right adrenal gland. This treatment modality led to an addisonian crisis in 5% of these patients.[56] Following surgical removal, disease may recur in approximately 15% of the ferrets because of development of disease in the remaining adrenal gland tissue.[56] In addition, up to 6% of ferrets may die perioperatively.[54,56]

Medical treatment

The depot GnRH agonist deslorelin (Suprelorin-F, Virbac) is the only drug licensed for use in the treatment of hyperadrenocorticism in ferrets. The drug suppresses the release of gonadotropins by continuously releasing deslorelin into the circulation, thereby overriding the pulsatile release of GnRH that is needed for the release of gonadotropins.[47] Because the drug initially results in a (short-lived) release of gonadotropins and potentially associated worsening of clinical signs, the effect is delayed by approximately 2 weeks after placement of the implant. In the experience of the author, the tumor does not decrease in size after placement of the implant. Autonomous production of steroids by the adrenal gland may occur over time, resulting in a loss of efficacy of the implant and recurrence of clinical signs.

Drugs that have been found to be ineffective, or are discourage, in the treatment of hyperadrenocorticism in ferrets include ketoconazole, mitotane (o,p'-DDD) and melatonin. When using melatonin, alleviation of clinical signs is seen, but hormone concentrations did not decrease and the tumors continued to grow.[57] Trilostane, a 3β-hydroxysteroid dehydrogenase (3β-HSD) blocker, has been used anecdotally in ferrets. Although the drug, in theory, is effective in the treatment of hyperadrenocorticism in ferrets (because 3β-HSD is necessary for the synthesis of androstenedione and 17-hydroxyprogesterone), deterioration of clinical signs was seen in a ferrets with hyperadrenocorticism after receiving 5 mg of trilostane by mouth once daily. It is hypothesized that the decrease in 3β-HSD level lead to activation of 17,20-lyase and thus activation (instead of deactivation) of the androgen pathway. This drug is therefore not recommended before understanding the mode of action in ferrets.[50]

Adrenomedullary Tumors

Adrenomedullary tumors (eg, pheochromocytoma and neuroblastoma) are seldom reported, particularly compared with the high incidence of adrenocortical tumors in ferrets.[42] Pheochromocytomas produce excessive amounts of catecholamines and are exclusively seen in the adrenal medulla, whereas a neuroblastoma is a neuroendocrine tumor that can occur in any tissue containing neural crest cells. Only 1 case of a neuroblastoma in the adrenal gland of a ferret has been described,[42] whereas several (presumed) pheochromocytomas have been described. Histologic confirmation of a pheochromocytoma has only been performed in 1 case,[6] whereas the secretion of catecholamines has been confirmed in none.

Insulinoma

Insulinomas are, usually, small (0.5–2 mm) tumors of the pancreatic beta cells (**Fig. 4**) that result in hypoglycemia caused by the excessive production of insulin. Tumor types may be described as hyperplasia, adenoma, or carcinoma. Most are well circumscribed, but infiltration in surrounding tissues may occur. In contrast with dogs, insulinomas in ferrets rarely metastasize.

The distribution of insulinomas is equal among the sexes. With a reported prevalence of 20% to 25% of the diagnosed neoplasms in ferrets, insulinomas are among

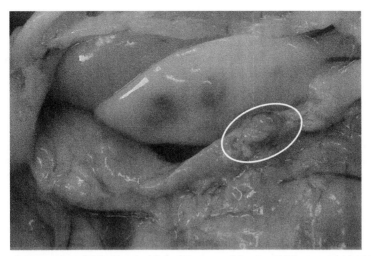

Fig. 4. In the pancreas of this 4-year-old, male castrated ferret, which presented with recurrent signs of stargazing and weakness in the hind legs, an approximately 1-cm mass was present (*circle*), which turned out to be an insulinoma. In general, insulinomas are only 2 to 3 mm in diameter.

the most commonly diagnosed tumors in middle-aged to older ferrets, with a median age of 5 years (range, 2–8 years).[58]

Cause/pathophysiology

The cause of insulinomas in ferrets is currently unknown. It has been suggested that, based on the natural carnivorous diet of mustelids, diets high in carbohydrates may contribute to the development of these tumors. A diet high in protein (42%–55%[a]), high in fat (18%–30%[1]), low in carbohydrates (8%–15%[1]), and low in fiber (1%–3%[1]) has therefore been advised to reduce the incidence.[59] However, no scientific evidence is available to back up any claims on the cause of insulinoma, nor has it been proved that the incidence is reduced when ferrets are fed low-carbohydrate kibble.

Clinical signs

Clinical signs vary from lethargy, stargazing, and weakness in the hind limbs to complete collapse, generalized seizures, and coma. Ptyalism and pawing at the mouth, signs of nausea, may also be seen. In addition, owners may notice a glazed look in the eyes of their ferrets. An important feature in ferrets with an insulinoma is that the clinical signs most likely resolve after the ferret has eaten some food.

Differential diagnosis

The differential diagnosis of hind limb weakness consists of neurologic diseases (eg, trauma, intervertebral disk disease, Aleutian disease), cardiac disease, generalized weakness, and metabolic disorders.[60]

Within the differential diagnosis of hypoglycemia, excessive glucose-consuming conditions, such as rapid multiplying neoplastic cells, severe hepatic disease, severe malnutrition or starvation, sepsis, or iatrogenic insulin overdose should be considered.[58] These conditions can usually be ruled out based on the results of the history, physical examination, and/or diagnostic work-up.

---

[a] On a dry matter basis.

Diagnosis

Blood glucose concentrations lower than 3.3 mmol/L (<60 mg/dL; reference range, 5.0–7.0 mmol/L [90–125 mg/dL]), after withholding food for 4 hours, are highly suggestive of an insulinoma when ferrets display the signs mentioned earlier. In ferrets with blood glucose concentrations between 3.3 and 5.0 mmol/L (60–90 mg/dL), another 2 hours of starving is advised.

The measurement of plasma insulin concentrations is debatable because concentrations within the reference range may be seen. Because insulin plasma concentrations should be low during a hypoglycemic event, insulin concentrations within the reference range should be considered abnormal during a hypoglycemic crisis.[58]

Insulinomas are occasionally visualized by ultrasonography, but are also frequently missed. Diagnostic imaging in the form of radiography or ultrasonography examination is therefore not routinely advised to localize the tumors.

Treatment

The treatment of insulinomas may consist of surgical removal of the neoplasm and/or providing one of the available drugs. Many factors, such as age of the ferret, desire of the owner to have an instant solution, and/or financial restrictions, may play a role in the decision-making process.

Surgical treatment

To fully eliminate the source of excess insulin production, surgical removal is seemingly the best therapeutic option. A partial pancreatectomy has been recommended rather than pancreatic nodulectomy in order to remove as much undetectable islet cell tumor as possible and increase the mean disease-free state after surgery to about 1 year.[61] Recurrence of clinical signs is mainly caused by the occurrence of new insulinomas and not by metastases of the removed tumor. If too much of the pancreas is removed, complications such as diabetes mellitus may occur. It should be stressed that every effort should be taken to avoid this condition from occurring, because the medical management of insulinoma is far easier than that of diabetes mellitus.[50]

Medical treatment

Prednisone and diazoxide are the most commonly used drugs for treating insulinomas. Octreotide, a synthetic long-acting analogue of somatostatin, has also been reported as a treatment option in ferrets, but no clear beneficial effects were seen compared with the other 2 modes of treatment.[58]

Corticosteroids (eg, prednisone, prednisolone, dexamethasone), which induce gluconeogenesis, are frequently used as the drugs of first choice. Ferrets seem to be fairly refractory to developing side effects caused by glucocorticoid administration, and generally respond well to the treatment protocol. However, iatrogenic Cushing disease has been reported in ferrets that have received glucocorticoids for prolonged periods of time.[62] In addition, the gluconeogenic mode of action of glucocorticoids results in an increase of glucose levels, which may be contraindicated in ferrets with insulinomas because of the risk of stimulating the secretion of insulin.

Diazoxide, a drug licensed for the treatment of human patients with insulinoma, inhibits insulin release. Because this drug addresses the cause of the hypoglycemia it is recommended rather than the use of glucocorticoids.[50] Treatment is started at an oral dose of twice-daily 5 mg/kg diazoxide. A gradual increase of the dose may be needed depending on the disappearance or continued presence of clinical signs. Although there is no upper dose of diazoxide, prednisone may be added to the treatment protocol in a concentration of 0.2 to 1 mg/kg by mouth once daily, when the needed diazoxide increases to more than 15 to 20 mg/kg. Medical management based on the aforementioned protocol is usually sufficient to control hypoglycemia for a period of up to 18 months, with some ferrets in the author's clinic even surviving up to 2 years on medical treatment.[50,58]

Recently, the use of constant-rate infusion of glucagon has been described as an emergency treatment of a severely hypoglycemic ferret. A dosage of 15 to 40 ng/kg/min (as extrapolated from data in dogs and cats) proved effective in increasing blood glucose concentrations and alleviating the clinical signs in an elderly ferret that did not respond sufficiently to other types of therapy.[63]

Owners are advised to monitor their ferrets closely for signs of hypoglycemia and feed the ferret immediately if mild signs of hypoglycemia are noted. In the event of a seizure or comatose condition, the owner is advised to give a carbohydrate-rich or protein-rich liquid food to the ferret. This diet may help to temporarily relieve the clinical signs so that the ferret can safely be transported to the veterinary clinic.

Prognosis
In ferrets, the prognosis is better compared with dogs, in which metastases are very common. Although metastases are rare in ferrets, multiple tumors and recurrent signs are common. Recurrent signs are probably caused by the development of new tumors rather than metastases of the earlier tumor.

HEMOLYMPHATIC TUMORS
Lymphoma

Lymphoma is the third most common tumor found in ferrets, and is frequently found in association with adrenocortical tumors and/or insulinomas.[14,29] It is also the most common hemolymphatic tumor. Lymphomas can be diagnosed as early as 9 months of age, and may be localized in all hemolymphatic organs, such as lymph nodes, spleen (**Fig. 5**), liver, and bone marrow. Lymphoma of the skin, also known as mycosis

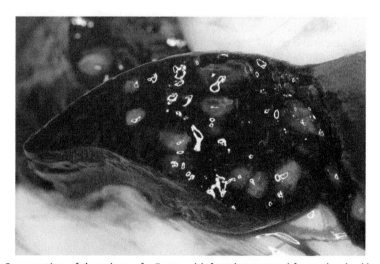

Fig. 5. Cross section of the spleen of a 5-year-old, female neutered ferret that had lost body weight in the past weeks. Splenomegaly was detected on abdominal palpation. On ultrasonography examination the spleen had an irregular aspect. Lymphoma was suspected as cause for the irregular aspect. Although the options of surgical treatment were discussed, the owner elected euthanasia. Histologic examination of the tumor confirmed the suspicion of lymphoma.

fungoides, is also seen in ferrets. An equal distribution among the sexes is seen. A transmission study has shown that at least certain types of lymphoma are transmittable.[64]

Clinical signs
Clinical presentation of ferrets with lymphomas is often nonspecific and may include loss of appetite, weight loss, and peripheral lymph node enlargement. When pleural effusion and mediastinal masses are present, dyspnea, and coughing may be seen.

Diagnosis
Because lymphoma is a tumor from the hemolymphatic system, it is important not only to look at tissue alterations but also at all the hemolymphatic cells. Therefore, a complete blood cell count (CBC) and bone marrow aspiration helps to determine whether the lymphoma is leukemic. Diagnostic imaging characteristics of lymphoma in ferrets are similar to those previously reported in dogs, cats, and humans.[65] Radiographs can be useful in detecting masses in the anterior mediastinum and bony structures.[65,66] CT has an added value when lesions are present in the bony structures.[65] With ultrasonography examination, a more precise diagnosis can be made in both the thoracic as well as the abdominal cavity, in which enlarged lymph nodes, alterations in the spleen and liver, and pleural and abdominal effusions can be visualized. Enlarged lymph nodes are frequently seen during the abdominal ultrasonography examination. Chronic inflammation (eg, *Helicobacter mustelae*) is usually the result of these hyperplastic/reactive lymph nodes. Ultrasonography-guided fine-needle aspiration (**Fig. 6**) biopsies or full-thickness biopsies are useful in differentiating between a reactive lymph node and lymphoma. These biopsies are therefore essential for confirming the diagnosis. Based on the cytologic or histologic findings, lymphoma (in ferrets) can been classified according to the Revised European-American Lymphoma Classification for Domestic Animals by the World Health Organization and/or the National Cancer Institute Working Formulation.[67–69] Based on these classifications, a classification has been described of low, intermediate, and high grade in which, in low-grade cases, predominately diffuse small lymphocytic lymphoma was seen; in the intermediate cases, mixed-cell lymphoma was seen; and in the high-grade cases, diffuse immunoblastic lymphoma was seen.[68] For further differentiation, immunohistochemistry is extremely valuable.

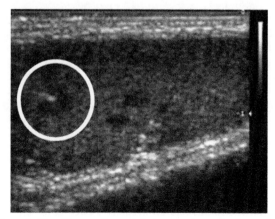

Fig. 6. Fine-needle aspiration biopsy of a nodule in an enlarged spleen of a ferret. The tip of the needle can be seen as the bright white spot in the circle. Cytology revealed this to be lymphoma.

The most commonly used markers are CD3 (cluster of differentiation 3), which is the marker for T-cells, and CD79α is B-cell marker. Both markers have been validated for use in ferrets.[67] In different studies, T-cell lymphoma consistently was shown to be the predominant type of lymphoma seen in ferrets.[14,67,69]

It has been recommended to perform a complete clinical staging of lymphoma to determine the degree of illness affecting the patient, which may help in discussing the prognosis with the owner. Recently, an updated clinical staging system has been proposed[68] in which the higher the stage, the poorer the prognosis:

Stage 1: single anatomic lesion
Stage 2: single lesion with regional lymph node involvement limited to 1 side of the diaphragm
Stage 3: lesions on both sides of the diaphragm, including intra-abdominal or gastrointestinal locations
Stage 4: multiple sites on both sides of the diaphragm are affected with or without the visceral organs
Stage 5: manifestation in the blood and involvement of bone marrow and/or other organ systems

Treatment

Depending on the stage of lymphoma and the wishes of the owner, different protocols can be used for the treatment of lymphoma in ferrets. Surgery (splenectomy, lymph nodectomy) can be performed if only a single anatomic structure is affected (stage 1). In more advanced cases, chemotherapy may be used, for which different protocols have been described for use in ferrets.[1,68,70]

Chemotherapeutic agents that have been used in ferrets are prednisolone, L-asparaginase, chlorambucil, cyclophosphamide, cytarabine, doxorubicin, methotrexate, procarbazine, and vincristine.[68] Chemotherapy can also be used in combination with radiation therapy.

Dosages of chemotherapeutic agents are usually based on body surface area rather than weight, and a recent study determined a reliable method for calculating body surface areas in ferrets based on CT imaging.[71] The investigators concluded that their formula ($9.94 \times$ [body weight]$^{2/3}$) did not differ significantly from the feline-derived formula and would therefore not contribute to a change in the currently used dosages.

The overall mean survival of ferrets with lymphoma has been reported to be 6 months (range, 2 weeks to 19 months).[14] The same investigators report that the mean survival for ferrets with T-cell lymphoma is 5 months (range, 0.5–14.0) and for ferrets with B-cell lymphoma is 8.4 months (range, 2–19 months). Ferrets that received chemotherapy had similar survival rates (4.3 months [range, 0.5–14.0 months] and 8.8 months [range, 2.0–19.0 months] for T-cell lymphoma and B-cell lymphoma, respectively).[14] It is therefore debatable whether chemotherapy provides any added value in the treatment of lymphoma in ferrets. In addition, note that treatment with cyclophosphamide and vincristine is frequently associated with therapy-limiting neutropenia.[14] Glucocorticoids are also frequently used in ferrets with lymphoma. The added value of this treatment is just as debatable as the use of chemotherapy, because the mean survival period also did not increase with the use of this medication.

INTEGUMENTARY TUMORS

Sebaceous epitheliomas (**Fig. 7**) and mast cell tumors (**Fig. 8**) are the most common integumentary tumors seen in ferrets, representing approximately a third of the integumentary tumors each.[20] The other third of the integumentary tumors consist of a wide

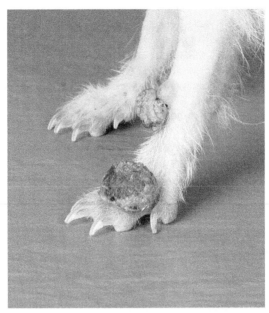

Fig. 7. Close-up of one of multiple skin masses in a 7.5-year-old female, neutered ferret. His-tologic evaluation confirmed this mass to be a sebaceous epithelioma.

variety of types of tumors, such as preputial cell tumors (**Fig. 9**) and cutaneous lym-phoma (**Fig. 10**).

Sebaceous epitheliomas are of basal cell origin and only involve the skin and not the subcutis. Although these tumors both grossly and histologically appear aggressive, with increased mitoses, cellular atypia, and apparent infiltration at inflamed margins, they are all benign and can easily be removed. However, multiple tumors and recur-rence of new tumors are frequently seen.

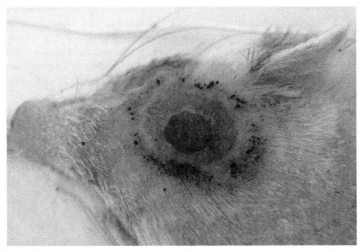

Fig. 8. Mast cell tumor on the head of a 5-year-old, male neutered ferret. The tumor was easily and successfully surgically removed, without any recurrence of the tumor.

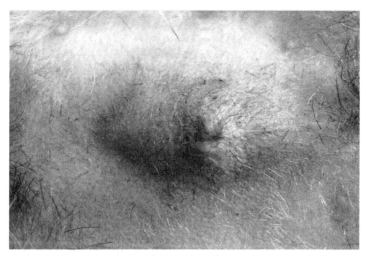

Fig. 9. Apocrine tumor of the preputial gland in a 5-year-old intact male ferret.

Mast cell tumors in ferrets are, like sebaceous epitheliomas, benign tumors. This characteristic is in sharp contrast with mastocytoma in dogs and cats. The overlying skin in these tumors is frequently eroded as a result of self-trauma because of pruritus. The tumors can easily be surgically excised and do not require pretreatment with antihistamines. However, mast cell tumors may reappear at a different site, which should not be seen as an indication of a poor prognosis because these tumors may also be removed without local metastasis.

In contrast with the excellent prognosis of sebaceous epitheliomas and mast cell tumors in ferrets, preputial tumors in ferrets are malignant and invade the surrounding tissues with local metastasis as a frequent result.[13] These tumors are of apocrine gland origin and are seen in middle-aged to geriatric ferrets. A minimal margin of

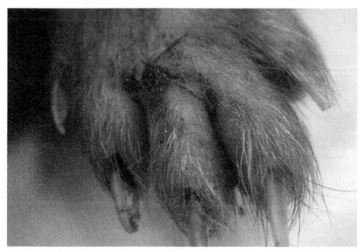

Fig. 10. Swollen and red foot of a 5-year-old, male neutered ferret. Skin biopsies revealed this to be cutaneous lymphoma (not further specified).

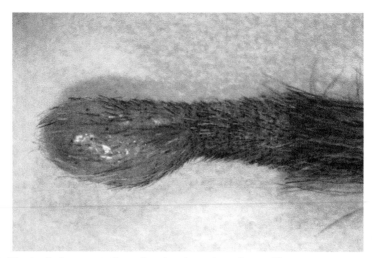

Fig. 11. The typical presentation of a chordoma in a ferret. These tumors can easily be removed when they are present at the tip of the tail.

1 cm is recommended during surgical resection to allow for the best possible postoperative prognosis. However, such a large margin may require (partial) resection of the penis.[13] Radiation therapy has also been used in these tumors, but this was not always successful.[13]

TUMORS IN OTHER SYSTEMS
Chordoma

A tumor that is fairly common in ferrets is chordoma, which is an intraosseous neoplasm originating from mesoderm-derived notochord. Chordomas develop twice as frequently in female ferrets as in male ferrets.[72] The most characteristic aspect of this tumor is the accumulation of mucus in the extracellular myxoid stroma. Almost all of these tumors are considered low grade, slowly growing tumors and are found at the tip of the tail (91%) (**Fig. 11**). Because of their location and their slow rate of development, they are fairly easy to remove, with 1 or 2 extra coccygea being removed as margin. In other species (eg, rats, dogs, cats, humans) chordomas frequently metastasize.[32] Although this is not commonly reported in ferrets, 1 case of suggested cutaneous metastasis has been described,[73] and in a recent case lung metastasis was seen.[33] If the tumor is located further up the spinal column, no therapy is possible.[33] During progression of the disease, pathologic fractures occur, making euthanasia inevitable.

REFERENCES

1. Antinoff A, Hahn K. Ferret oncology: diseases, diagnostics, and therapeutics. Vet Clin North Am Exot Anim 2004;7:579–625.
2. Aizawa K, Liu C, Veeramachaneni S, et al. Development of ferret as a human lung cancer model by injecting4-(N-methyl-N-nitrosamino)-1-(3-pyridyl)-1-butanone (NNK). Lung Cancer 2013;82:390–6.
3. Antinoff N, Williams BH. Neoplasia. In: Quesenberry KE, Carpenter JW, editors. Ferrets, rabbits and rodents: clinical medicine and surgery. 3rd edition. St Louis (MO): Elsevier; 2012. p. 103–21.

4. Fox JG, Muthupalani S, Kiupel M, et al. Neoplastic diseases. In: Fox JG, Marini RP, editors. Biology and diseases of the ferret. 3rd edition. Ames (IA): Wiley Blackwell; 2014. p. 587–626.

5. Miwa Y, Kurosawa A, Ogawa H, et al. Neoplastic diseases in ferrets in Japan: a questionnaire study for 2000 to 2005. J Vet Med Sci 2009;71:397–402.

6. Fox JG, Dangler CA, Snyder SB, et al. C-cell carcinoma (medullary thyroid carcinoma) associated with multiple endocrine neoplasms in a ferret (Mustela putorius furo). Vet Pathol 2000;37:278–82.

7. Lewington JH. General neoplasia. In: Lewington JH, editor. Ferret husbandry, medicine and surgery. 2nd edition. St Louis (MO): Elsevier; 2007. p. 318–45.

8. Martínez A, Martinez J, Burballa A, et al. Spontaneous thecoma in a spayed pet ferret (Mustela putorius furo) with alopecia and swollen vulva. J Exot Pet Med 2011;20:308–12.

9. Batista-Arteaga M, Suárez-Bonnet A, Santana M, et al. Testicular neoplasms (interstitial and Sertoli cell tumours) in a domestic ferret (Mustela putorius furo). Reprod Domest Anim 2011;46:177–80.

10. Hohšteter M, Smolec O, Gudan Kurilj A, et al. Intratesticular benign peripheral nerve sheath tumour in a ferret (Mustela putorius furo). J Small Anim Pract 2012;53:63–6.

11. Inoue S, Yonemaru K, Yanai T, et al. Mixed germ cell-sex cord-stromal tumor with a concurrent interstitial cell tumor in a ferret. J Vet Med Sci 2015;77:225–8.

12. Kammeyer P, Ziege S, Wellhöner S, et al. Testicular leiomyosarcoma and marked alopecia in a cryptorchid ferret (Mustela putorius furo). Tierärztl Prax 2014;42: 406–10.

13. van Zeeland YRA, Lennox A, Quinton JF, et al. Prepuce and partial penile amputation for treatment of preputial gland neoplasia in two ferrets. J Small Anim Pract 2014;55:593–6.

14. Ammersbach M, DeLay J, Caswell JL, et al. Laboratory findings, histopathology, and immunophenotype of lymphoma in domestic ferrets. Vet Pathol 2008;45: 663–73.

15. Gupta A, Gumber S, Schnellbacher R, et al. Malignant B-cell lymphoma with Mott cell differentiation in a ferret (Mustela putorius furo). J Vet Diagn Invest 2010;22: 469–73.

16. Ingrao JC, Eshar D, Vince A, et al. Focal thoracolumbar spinal cord lymphosarcoma in a ferret (Mustela putorius furo). Can Vet J 2014;55:667–71.

17. Bonel-Raposo J, Silveira MF, De Oliveira Gamba C, et al. Sebaceous epithelioma in a ferret (Mustela putorius furo). Braz J Vet Pathol 2008;1:70–2.

18. Fox-Alvarez WA, Moreno AR, Bush J. Diagnosis and successful surgical removal of an aural ceruminous gland adenocarcinoma in a domestic ferret (Mustela putorius furo). J Exot Pet Med 2015;24:350–5.

19. Gardhouse S, Eshar D, Fromstein J, et al. Diagnosis and successful surgical treatment of an unusual inguinal liposarcoma in a pet ferret (Mustela putorius furo). Can Vet J 2013;54:739–42.

20. Kanfer S, Reavill DR. Cutaneous neoplasia in ferrets, rabbits, and guinea pigs. Vet Clin North Am Exot Anim 2013;16:579–98.

21. Mialot M, Prata D, Girard-Luc A, et al. Multiple progressive piloleiomyomas in a ferret (Mustela putorius furo): a case report. Vet Dermatol 2010;22:100–3.

22. Rodrigues A, Gates L, Payne HR, et al. Multicentric squamous cell carcinoma in situ associated with papillomavirus in a ferret. Vet Pathol 2010;47:964–8.

23. van Zeeland YRA, Hernandez-Divers SJ, Blasier MW, et al. Carpal myxosarcoma and forelimb amputation in a ferret (*Mustela putorius furo*). Vet Rec 2006;159: 783–5.

24. Castillo-Alcala F, Mans C, Squires Bos A, et al. Clinical and pathologic features of an adenomatous polyp of the colon in a domestic ferret (*Mustela putorius furo*). Can Vet J 2010;51:1261–4.

25. Girard-Luc A, Prata D, Huet H, et al. A KIT-positive gastrointestinal stromal tumor in a ferret (*Mustela putorius furo*). J Vet Diagn Invest 2009;21:915–7.

26. Jones Y, Wise A, Maes R, et al. Peliod hepatocellular carcinoma in a domesticated ferret (*Mustela putorius furo*). J Vet Diagn Invest 2006;18:228–31.

27. Petterino C, Bedin M, Vascellari M, et al. An intra-abdominal malignant mesenchymoma associated with nonabsorbable sutures in a ferret (*Mustela putorius furo*). J Vet Diagn Invest 2010;22:327–31.

28. Rhody JL, Williams BH. Exocrine pancreatic adenocarcinoma and associated extrahepatic biliary obstruction in a ferret. J Exot Pet Med 2013;22:206–11.

29. Sinclair KM, Eckstrand C, Moore PF, et al. Epitheliotropic gastrointestinal T-cell lymphoma with concurrent insulinoma and adrenocortical carcinoma in a domestic ferret (*Mustela putorius furo*). J Exot Pet Med 2016;25:34–43.

30. Kawaguchi H, Miyoshi N, Souda M, et al. Renal adenocarcinoma in a ferret. Vet Pathol 2006;43:353–6.

31. Petritz OA, Antinoff N, Pfent C, et al. Adenosquamous carcinoma of the trachea in a domestic ferret (*Mustela putorius furo*). J Exot Pet Med 2013;22:287–92.

32. Cho E-S, Kim J-Y, Ryu S-Y, et al. Chordoma in the tail of a ferret. Lab Anim Res 2011;27:53–7.

33. Frohlich JR, Donovan TA. Cervical chordoma in a domestic ferret (*Mustela putorius furo*) with pulmonary metastasis. J Vet Diagn Invest 2015;27:656–9.

34. Johnson JG III, Brandão J, Fowlkes N, et al. Calvarial osteoma with cranial vault invasion of the skull of a ferret (*Mustela putorius furo*). J Exot Pet Med 2014;23: 266–9.

35. Keller DL, Schneider LK, Chamberlin T, et al. Intramedullary lumbosacral teratoma in a domestic ferret (*Mustela putorius furo*). J Vet Diagn Invest 2012;24: 621–4.

36. Maguire R, Reavill DR, Maguire P, et al. Chondrosarcoma associated with the appendicular skeleton of 2 domestic ferrets. J Exot Pet Med 2014;23:165–71.

37. Ohta G, Kobayshi M, Yanai T, et al. A case of fibrosarcoma on the perivertebral surface of a ferret with hind limb paralysis. Exp Anim 2008;57:397–400.

38. Pezzolato M, Varello K, Mascarino D, et al. Intra-Abdominal leiomyosarcoma in a ferret (*Mustela putorius furo*): histopathological and immunohistochemical characterization. J Vet Med Sci 2008;70:513–5.

39. Perpiñán D, Bargalló F, Ramis A, et al. Thoracic vertebral osteoma in a domestic ferret (*Mustela putorius furo*). J Exot Pet Med 2008;17:144–7.

40. van Zeeland YRA, Schoemaker NJ, Passon-Vastenburg MHAC, et al. Vestibular syndrome due to the presence of a choroid plexus papilloma in a ferret. J Am Anim Hosp Assoc 2009;45:97–101.

41. McBride M, Mosunic CB, Barron GHW, et al. Successful treatment of a retrobulbar adenocarcinoma in a ferret (*Mustela putorius furo*). Vet Rec 2009;165:206–8.

42. Miwa Y, Uchida K, Nakayama H, et al. Neuroblastoma of the adrenal gland in a ferret. J Vet Med Sci 2010;72:1229–32.

43. Vandermeulen E, Peremans K. Scintigraphic diagnosis and 131I treatment of hyperthyroidism in a ferret (*Mustela putorius furo*). Proceedings of the ECVDI annual conference Cascais Portugal; 2013. Vet Radiol Ultrasound 2014;55:675.

44. Weiss CA, Scott MV. Clinical aspects and surgical treatment of hyperadrenocorticism in the domestic ferret: 94 cases (1994-1996). J Am Anim Hosp Assoc 1997; 33:487–93.

45. Schoemaker NJ, Teerds KJ, Mol JA, et al. The role of luteinizing hormone in the pathogenesis of hyperadrenocorticism in neutered ferrets. Mol Cell Endocrinol 2002;197:117–25.

46. Wagner RA, Bailey EM, Schneider JF, et al. Leuprolide acetate treatment of adrenocortical disease in ferrets. J Am Vet Med Assoc 2001;218:1272–4.

47. Wagner RA, Piché CA, Jöchle W, et al. Clinical and endocrine responses to treatment with deslorelin acetate implants in ferrets with adrenocortical disease. Am J Vet Res 2005;66:910–4.

48. de Jong MK, Schoemaker NJ, Mol JA. Expression of *Sfrp1* and activation of the Wnt pathway in the adrenal glands of healthy ferrets and neutered ferrets with hyperadrenocorticism. Vet J 2013;196:176–80.

49. Schillebeeckx M, Pihlajoki M, Gretzinger E, et al. Novel markers of gonadectomy-induced adrenocortical neoplasia in the mouse and ferret. Mol Cell Endocrinol 2015;399:122–30.

50. Schoemaker NJ, van Zeeland YRA. Endocrine diseases in ferrets. Eur J Companion Anim Pract 2013;23:19–30.

51. Quesenberry KE, Rosenthal KL. Endocrine diseases. In: Quesenberry KE, Carpenter JW, editors. Ferrets, rabbits and rodents; clinical medicine and surgery. 2nd edition. St Louis (MO): WB Saunders; 2003. p. 79–90.

52. Schoemaker NJ, Wolfswinkel J, Mol JA, et al. Urinary excretion of glucocorticoids in the diagnosis of hyperadrenocorticism in ferrets. Domest Anim Endocrinol 2004;27:13–24.

53. Kuijten AM, Schoemaker NJ, Voorhout G. Ultrasonographic visualization of the adrenal glands of healthy and hyperadrenocorticoid ferrets. J Am Anim Hosp Assoc 2007;43:78–84.

54. Lennox AM, Wagner RA. Comparison of 4.7-mg deslorelin implants and surgery for the treatment of adrenocortical disease in ferrets. J Exot Pet Med 2012;21: 332–5.

55. Swiderski JK, Seim HB III, MacPhail CM, et al. Long-term outcome of domestic ferrets treated surgically for hyperadrenocorticism: 130 cases (1995–2004). J Am Vet Med Assoc 2008;232:1338–43.

56. Weiss CA, Williams BH, Scott JB, et al. Surgical treatment and long-term outcome of ferrets with bilateral adrenal tumors or adrenal hyperplasia: 56 cases (1994-1997). J Am Vet Med Assoc 1999;215:820–3.

57. Ramer JC, Benson KG, Morrisey JK, et al. Effects of melatonin administration on the clinical course of adrenocortical disease in domestic ferrets. J Am Vet Med Assoc 2006;229:1743–8.

58. Rosenthal KL, Wyre NR. Endocrine diseases. In: Quesenberry KE, Carpenter JW, editors. Ferrets, rabbits and rodents: clinical medicine and surgery. 3rd edition. St Louis (MO): WB Saunders; 2012. p. 86–102.

59. Finkler MR. A nutritional approach to the prevention of insulinomas in the pet ferret. Exot Mam Med Surg 2004;2:1–5.

60. Antinoff N, Giovanella CJ. Musculoskeletal and neurologic diseases. In: Quesenberry KE, Carpenter JW, editors. Ferrets, rabbits and rodents: clinical medicine and surgery. 3rd edition. St Louis (MO): Elsevier; 2012. p. 132–40.

61. Weiss CA, Williams BH, Scott MV. Insulinoma in the ferret: clinical findings and treatment comparison of 66 cases. J Am Anim Hosp Assoc 1998;34:471–5.

62. Chen S. Advanced diagnostic approaches and current medical management of insulinomas and adrenocortical disease in ferrets (*Mustela putorius furo*). Vet Clin North Am Exot Anim 2010;13:439–52.

63. Bennett KR, Gaunt MC, Parker DL. Constant rate infusion of glucagon as an emergency treatment for hypoglycemia in a domestic ferret (*Mustela putorius furo*). J Am Vet Med Assoc 2015;246:451–4.

64. Erdman SE, Reimann KA, Moore FM, et al. Transmission of a chronic lymphoproliferative syndrome in ferrets. Lab Invest 1995;72:539–46.

65. Suran JN, Wyre NR. Imaging findings in 14 domestic ferrets (*Mustela putorius furo*) with lymphoma. Vet Radiol Ultrasound 2013;5(5):522–31.

66. Eshar D, Wyre NR, Griessmayr P, et al. Diagnosis and treatment of myeloosteolytic plasmablastic lymphoma of the femur in a domestic ferret. J Am Vet Med Assoc 2010;237:407–14.

67. Hammer AS, Williams B, Dietz HH. High-throughput immunophenotyping of 43 ferret lymphomas using tissue microarray technology. Vet Pathol 2007;44:196–203.

68. Mayer J, Susan E, Erdman SE, et al. Diseases of the hematopoietic system. In: Fox JG, Marini RP, editors. Biology and diseases of the ferret. 3rd edition. Ames (IA): Wiley Blackwell; 2014. p. 311–34.

69. Onuma M, Kondo H, Ono S, et al. Cytomorphological and immunohistochemical features of lymphoma in ferrets. J Vet Med Sci 2008;70(9):893–8.

70. Fisher PG, Lennox A. Therapeutic options for ferret lymphoma: a review. Exot Mam Med Surg 2003;1(2):1–5.

71. Jones KL, Granger LA, Kearney MT, et al. Evaluation of a ferret-specific formula for determining body surface area to improve chemotherapeutic dosing. Am J Vet Res 2015;76:142–8.

72. Dunn DG, Harris RK, Meis JM, et al. A histomorphologic and immunohistochemical study of chordoma in twenty ferrets (*Mustela putorius furo*). Vet Pathol 1991;28:467–73.

73. Munday JS, Brown CA, Richey LJ. Suspected metastatic coccygeal chordoma in a ferret (*Mustela putorius furo*). J Vet Diagn Invest 2004;16:454–8.

Principles and Applications of Medical Oncology in Exotic Animals

Tara Myers Harrison, DVM, MPVM, DACZM, DACVPM[a],*,
Barbara E. Kitchell, DVM, PhD, DACVIM (Internal Medicine and Oncology)[b]

KEYWORDS

• Neoplasia • Chemotherapeutics • Exotic • Wildlife

KEY POINTS

• Chemotherapy can be used in exotic and zoologic animal species.
• Chemotherapy, in exotic and zoologic species, can be performed successfully through oral, subcutaneous, intramuscular, and intravenous routes.
• The use of a vascular access port can make intravenous administration of chemotherapy possible in exotic and zoologic species of animals.
• Continued research and evaluation of chemotherapeutics in exotic and zoologic animal species will improve treatments of these animals.

INTRODUCTION

Neoplasia and successful therapy for neoplasia has been reported in fish, birds, reptiles, small mammals, primates, and megavertebrates.[1–6] This article introduces medications and therapeutic approaches being used in a variety of exotic animal species (**Table 1**). These animals range in size from grams to thousands of pounds. Discussion of administration techniques will also be introduced.

Medical treatment of cancer is still largely used as an adjunctive or palliative treatment. However, there are therapies that can produce remission for months to years, depending on the animal, tumor type, and stage of disease. The acceptance of many exotic species into the human family unit has contributed to owners who are seeking out and are willing to dedicate the financial and emotional resources for improved medical care and therapeutics for their pets.

The authors have nothing to disclose.
[a] Department of Clinical Sciences, North Carolina State University College of Veterinary Medicine, 1060 William Moore Drive, Raleigh, NC 27607, USA; [b] Department of Oncology, VCA Veterinary Care Referral Center, 9901 Montgomery Boulevard, Albuquerque, NM 87111, USA
* Corresponding author.
E-mail address: tara_harrison@ncsu.edu

Table 1
Chemotherapeutics given to exotic animals by class

Animal	Chemotherapeutic	Neoplasia Type	Dose	Route	Side Effect Noted	Reference
Reptiles						
Bearded dragon	Cytarabine	Leukemia	100 mg/m^2	Intravenous	Died during therapy but was at advanced stage	27
Green iguana	Vincristine	Lymphoma	0.008 mg/kg	Intravenous	None	15
Green iguana	Cyclophosphamide	Lymphoma	3 mg/kg	Intravenous	None	15
Green iguana	Doxorubicin	Lymphoma	0.26 mg/kg	Intravenous	None	15
Green iguana	Prednisone	Lymphoma	2 mg/kg, then 1 mg/kg	Oral	None	15
Green sea turtle	Bleomycin	Fibropapilloma	1 u/cm^3	Intralesional	None	42
Yellow-bellied slider	Bleomycin	Squamous cell carcinoma	1 mg	Intralesional	None	41
Birds						
African penguin	Cisplatin	Squamous cell carcinoma	0.2–0.9 mg/kg	Intralesional	None, did have recurrence	47
Bald eagle	Cisplatin	Squamous cell carcinoma	0.8 mg	Intralesional	None	NA
Black swan	Chlorambucil	Lymphocytic leukemia	2 mg	Oral	None; however, minimal response to therapy	11
Black swan	Lomustine	Lymphocytic leukemia	60 mg/m^2	Oral	None; however, minimal response to therapy	11
Black swan	Prednisone	Lymphocytic leukemia	0.5 mg/kg	Oral	None; however, minimal response to therapy	11

Black swan	L-asparaginase	Lymphocytic leukemia	400 IU/kg	Subcutaneous	None; however, minimal response to therapy and minor tumor ulceration	11
Blue-fronted Amazon	Bleomycin	Xanthoma	0.7 mg/kg	Intralesional	None	NA
Budgerigar	Carboplatin	Renal adenocarcinoma	5 mg/kg	Intravenous	None; however, mass regrew within 3 mo while being treated	55
Budgerigar	Carboplatin	Pharmacokinetic study	5 mg/kg	Intravenous	None reported	57
Chicken	Carboplatin	Pharmacokinetic study	5 mg/kg	Intravenous	None reported	57
Double-yellow headed Amazon parrot	Chlorambucil	Lymphocytic leukemia	2 mg/kg	Oral	No response to treatment	23
Duck	Carboplatin	Pharmacokinetic study	5 mg/kg	Intravenous	None reported	57
Goose	Cisplatin	Xanthoma	20 mg	Intralesional	None, no response to treatment	46
Green-winged macaw	Chlorambucil	Chronic lymphocytic leukemia	1 mg/kg	Oral	Thrombocytopenia	14
Green-winged macaw	Prednisone	Chronic lymphocytic leukemia	1 mg/kg	Oral	None; however, may not have affected neoplasia	14
Green-winged macaw	Cyclophosphamide	Chronic lymphocytic leukemia	5 mg/kg	Oral	None; however, may not have affected neoplasia	14
Great horned owl	Chlorambucil	Lymphoma	2 mg/kg	Oral	No response to treatment	18
Java sparrow	Chlorambucil	Lymphoma	2 mg/kg	Oral	Anorexia, did not seem to affect tumor growth	22
Kori bustard	Cyclophosphamide	Myxosarcoma	10 mg/m^2	Oral	None	13

(continued on next page)

Table 1
(continued)

Animal	Chemotherapeutic	Neoplasia Type	Dose	Route	Side Effect Noted	Reference
Kori bustard	Carboplatin	Myxosarcoma	12, 4.6 mg beads	Surgical implantation	No response to treatment	13
Kori bustard	Meloxicam	Myxosarcoma	0.1 mg/kg	Oral	None	13
Mallard duck	Carboplatin	Sertoli cell tumor	15 mg/kg	Intravenous	Heteropenia, neoplasm decreased in size; however, returned 12 mo later	54
Pigeon	Carboplatin	Pharmacokinetic study	5 mg/kg	Intravenous	None reported	57
Sulfur-crested cockatoo	Carboplatin	Pharmacokinetic study	5 mg/kg	Intravenous and intraosseous	Mild gastrointestinal signs	56
Sulfur-crested cockatoo	Doxorubicin	Pharmacokinetic study	2 mg/kg	Intravenous	Mild, transient inappetence	36
Umbrella cockatoo	Chlorambucil	Lymphoma	2 mg/kg	Oral	Anemia	20
Umbrella cockatoo	Vincristine	Lymphoma	0.1 mg/kg	Intravenous	Anemia	20
Mammals						
African hedgehog	Piroxicam	Renal	0.3 mg/kg	Oral	None; however, likely minimal response to treatment	NA
African lion	Lomustine	Lymphoma	61 mg/m^2	Oral	None	3
African lion	Doxorubicin	Lymphoma	205 mg	Intravenous	None	3
African lion	Prednisone	Lymphoma	115 mg	Oral	Gastric ulceration at 504 d	3
Binturong	Toceranib	Renal adenocarcinoma	1.4–2 mg/kg	Oral	Initial anorexia after start of treatment, then it resolved; no response to treatment	67

Animal	Cancer type	Drug	Dose	Route	Response	Reference
Dhole	Lymphocytic leukemia	Melphalan	4.41 mg/m²	Oral	None, animal euthanized shortly after starting treatment	25
Ferret 1	Lymphoma	Chlorambucil	20 mg/m²	Oral	Not complete remission, survived 10 mo	19
Ferret 1	Lymphoma	Asparaginase	5000 IU	Intraperitoneal	Not complete remission, survived 10 mo	19
Ferret 1	Lymphoma	Vincristine	0.75 mg/m²	Intravenous	Not complete remission, survived 10 mo	19
Ferret 1	Lymphoma	Doxorubicin	2.8 mg/kg	Intravenous	Not complete remission, survived 10 mo	19
Ferret 1	Lymphoma	Cyclophosphamide	80 mg/m²	Oral	Not complete remission, survived 10 mo	19
Ferret 1	Lymphoma	Methotrexate	0.5 mg/kg	Intravenous	Not complete remission, survived 10 mo	19
Ferret 1	Lymphoma	Chlorambucil	20 mg/m²	Oral	Not complete remission, survived 10 mo	19
Ferret 2	Multiple myeloma	Cyclophosphamide	175 mg/m², then 10 mg/m²	Oral	Anorexia; however, minimal response to treatment	NA
Ferret 2	Multiple myeloma	Prednisone	30 mg/m² tapering dose	Oral	Anorexia; however, minimal response to treatment	NA
Ferret 3	Lymphoma	Lomustine	50 mg/m²	Oral	Unknown at this time	NA
Fishing cat	Transitional cell carcinoma	Carboplatin	175 mg/m²	Intravenous	Some response to treatment	58
Fishing cat	Transitional cell carcinoma	Piroxicam	0.3 mg/kg	Oral	Some response to treatment	58
Greater hedgehog tenrec	Squamous cell carcinoma	Bleomycin	15 IU/m²	Intralesional	None	NA

(continued on next page)

Table 1
(continued)

Animal	Chemotherapeutic	Neoplasia Type	Dose	Route	Side Effect Noted	Reference
Gray wolf	Doxorubicin	Myxosarcoma	30 mg	Intravenous	Mild anorexia, mild nausea	NA
Gray wolf	Piroxicam	Myxosarcoma	10 mg	Oral	None	NA
Ground cuscus	Lomustine	Lymphoma	10 mg	Oral	None	9
Guinea pig	Prednisolone	Peripheral nodal lymphoma	0.5 mg/kg	Oral	None	NA
Guinea pig	Vincristine	Peripheral nodal lymphoma	0.025 mg/kg	Intravenous	Mild ileus, decreased appetite	NA
Guinea pig	Cyclophosphamide	Peripheral nodal lymphoma	60 mg/kg	Oral	Mild leukocytosis and thrombocytopenia	NA
Guinea pig	Doxorubicin	Peripheral nodal lymphoma	0.75 mg/kg	Intravenous	Mild leukocytosis, thrombocytopenia	NA
Guinea pig	Asparaginase	Peripheral nodal lymphoma	890 units	Subcutaneous	None	NA
Guinea pig	Lomustine	Peripheral nodal lymphoma	8 mg	Oral	None	NA
Mongoose lemur	Carboplatin	Hepatocellular carcinoma	10 mg/kg	Intravenous	None	NA
Mongoose lemur	Gemcitabine	Hepatocellular carcinoma	2 mg/kg	Intravenous	None	NA
Orangutan	Rituximab	Lymphoma	375 mg/m^2	Intravenous	Pyrexia, moderate anorexia, moderate lethargy; 3 treatments, then terminated	16

Orangutan	Cyclophosphamide	Lymphoma	750 mg/m^2	Intravenous	Pyrexia, moderate anorexia, moderate lethargy; 3 treatments, then terminated	16
Orangutan	Doxorubicin	Lymphoma	37.5 mg/m^2	Intravenous	Pyrexia, moderate anorexia, moderate lethargy; 3 treatments, then terminated	16
Orangutan	Vincristine	Lymphoma	1.4 mg/m^2	Intravenous	Pyrexia, moderate anorexia, moderate lethargy; 3 treatments, then terminated	16
Orangutan	Prednisone	Lymphoma	60 mg/m^2	Oral	Pyrexia, moderate anorexia, moderate lethargy; 3 treatments, then terminated	16
Puma	Vincristine	Squamous cell carcinoma	0.5 mg/m^2	Intravenous	Vomiting, weight loss, diarrhea, no tumor regression	44
Puma	Vincristine	Squamous cell carcinoma	0.2 mg	Intralesional	None, tumor completely regressed	44
Rabbit 1	Prednisolone	Confirmed thymoma	0.5 mg/kg	Oral	None, mass reduced in size	NA
Rabbit 2	Prednisolone	Lymphocytic leukemia	0.5 mg/kg	Oral	None, lymphocytosis resolved	NA
Rabbit 3	Carboplatin	Thymic carcinoma	150 mg/m^2	Intravenous	None; however, minimal response to treatment	NA

(continued on next page)

Table 1
(continued)

Animal	Chemotherapeutic	Neoplasia Type	Dose	Route	Side Effect Noted	Reference
Rabbit 4	Carboplatin	Salivary adenocarcinoma	150 mg/m^2	Intravenous	None; however, minimal response to treatment	NA
Rabbit 4	Vinorelbine	Salivary adenocarcinoma	9 mg/m^2	Intravenous	None; however, minimal response to treatment	NA
Rabbit 4	Doxorubicin	Salivary adenocarcinoma	1 mg/kg	Intravenous	None; however, minimal response to treatment	NA
Rabbit 5	Gemcitabine	Adenocarcinoma	2 mg/kg	Intravenous	None; however, minimal response to treatment	NA
Rabbit 6	Carboplatin	Osteosarcoma	150 mg/m^2	Intravenous	None; however, minimal response to treatment	NA
Raccoon	Doxorubicin	Thyroid neoplasia	1 mg/kg	Intravenous	Pancytopenia, anorexia	38
Raccoon	Piroxicam	Thyroid neoplasia	0.11 mg/kg	Oral	None	38
Southern black rhinoceros	Cytarabine	Lymphoblastic leukemia	1000 mg	Intravenous	Progressive dyspnea	28
Southern black rhinoceros	Prednisone	Lymphoblastic leukemia	500 mg	Oral	None	28
Southern black rhinoceros	Cyclophosphamide	Lymphoblastic leukemia	1000 mg	Intravenous	Transient results for treatment	28
Southern black rhinoceros	Vincristine	Lymphoblastic leukemia	3 mg	Intravenous	Lymphopenia, anemia	28
Southern black rhinoceros	Doxorubicin	Lymphoblastic leukemia	200 mg	Intravenous	Cardiotoxicity	28

Species	Drug	Disease	Dose	Route	Response	Ref
Spotted hyena	Chlorambucil	Leukemia	0.16 mg/kg	Oral	Suspected bone marrow toxicity	21
Spotted hyena	Chlorambucil	Leukemia	0.1 mg/kg	Oral	None, died of lymphoma 2 y later with lymphocytosis and hemoabdomen	21
Spotted hyena	Prednisone	Leukemia	1 mg/kg	Oral	None, died of lymphoma 2 y later with lymphocytosis and hemoabdomen	21
Spotted hyena	Asparaginase	Leukemia	167 IU/kg	Intramuscular	None, died of lymphoma 2 y later	21
Tasmanian devil	Lomustine	Lymphoma	20 mg/kg	Oral	None; however, did not affect growth	10
Tasmanian Devil	Carboplatin	Devil facial tumor disease	20 mg/kg	Intravenous	No response to treatment, dose-limiting responses were anorexia, weight loss	37
Tasmanian devil	Doxorubicin	Devil facial tumor disease	1 mg/kg	Intravenous	No response to treatment, dose-limiting responses were neutropenia, anorexia, weight loss	37
Tasmanian devil	Vincristine	Devil facial tumor disease	0.015 mg/kg	Intravenous	No response to treatment, dose-limiting effects anorexia, vomiting, diarrhea, neutropenia	45

Most of the drugs described here have not been used widely to treat exotic species, thus this article describes both the veterinary literature and personal experience in providing these observations. Further, none of the medications included in the following discussions have license indications for the species under treatment and the use of these agents should be undertaken only with owner-informed consent in the case of companion exotic animals.

In most cases, undergoing chemotherapy treatment of an animal should involve a close working relationship with a veterinary oncologist. Veterinary oncologists can help determine which chemotherapy agents may be best to treat cancer in the patient. Although not all oncologists are well versed in individual animal variations for exotic or zoologic animals, there are some oncologists who have expertise in this area and can work with a local oncologist to determine a treatment plan. Further, the process of acquiring, preparing, and administering many of these medications should be only undertaken by a trained oncologist, or someone working directly with an oncologist, due to human health and safety risks from exposure to genotoxic medications.

CHEMOTHERAPEUTIC ROUTES OF ADMINISTRATION
Oral Therapies

Oral therapies are particularly useful in treatment of exotic species because they may be hidden in food or treats to limit excessive handling of patients. Many agents used in human cancer therapy protocols are available in oral formulations that can be compounded into appropriately sized doses for exotic species. Some of these medications need to be swallowed whole and cannot be crushed; therefore, some of these medications may be unavailable for very small patients.

Intravenous Therapies

Many chemotherapy protocols have intravenous treatment components and this can be difficult in exotic species. Administration of a single intravenous dose can usually be accomplished a few times through the use of sedation or general anesthesia; however, the risk to the patient and the challenge of maintaining venous access can make frequent or repeated dosing difficult or impossible. Repeated intravenous chemotherapy can be accomplished through the use of vascular access ports (VAPs). These medical devices are available in sizes as small as 2 French, which is appropriate for a typical laboratory mouse. These ports can be surgically implanted, most commonly in a jugular vein, and have intravenous catheter components that are placed at the level of the heart. The jugular vein is permanently occluded proximal to the port catheter access, so that the only venous access is through the port catheter that delivers drugs just proximal to the heart. The injection bell is generally located near or between the scapulae (**Figs. 1–8**). To collect blood from a VAP, a syringe that has a volume just greater than the quantity held within the catheter is used to remove the heparin lock portion in the catheter. After removal of the heparinized saline, a blood sample or treatment can be performed. The procedure is concluded by replacement of the heparin lock with an amount adequate to fill the length of the catheter.

VAPs are ideal for use in exotic or zoologic animals due to having venous access readily available throughout the course of chemotherapy. These ports, when heparin locked after each use, can last throughout the animal's therapy. The ports provide access to check blood samples as well as for administration of medication. In small animals, having a site readily available for blood collection and medicine administration avoids the challenge of potentially placing a catheter and drawing blood weekly. In dangerous animals that can be conditioned for subcutaneous or intramuscular

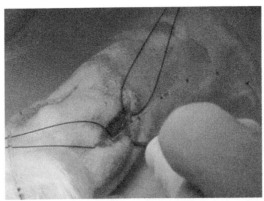

Fig. 1. Surgical implantation of a VAP catheter in the jugular vein of a domestic ferret (*Mustela putorius furo*).

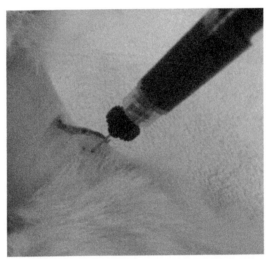

Fig. 2. Use of a VAP to collect a blood sample from a domestic ferret (*M putorius furo*).

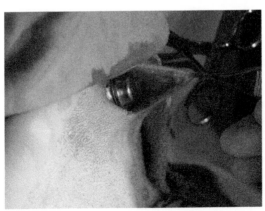

Fig. 3. Vascular access injection port being surgically implanted in a gray wolf (*C lupus*).

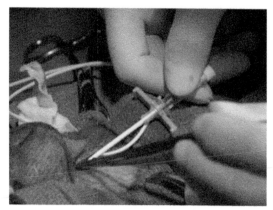

Fig. 4. Inserting a VAP with the use of a peel-away needle introducer into a gray wolf (*C lupus*).

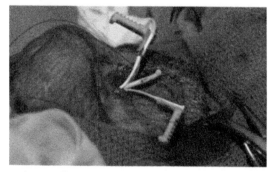

Fig. 5. Peeling away the needle introducer and inserting the catheter for a VAP in a gray wolf (*C lupus*).

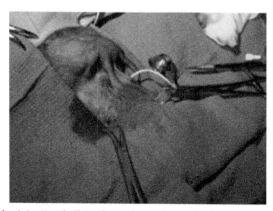

Fig. 6. Inserting the injection bell to the catheter for a VAP in a gray wolf (*C lupus*).

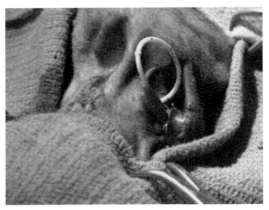

Fig. 7. Surgically implanting the injection port in a gray wolf (*C lupus*) for a VAP.

access, the VAP provides a method to collect blood and administer intravenous medication without anesthesia. Very small VAPS are prone to intracatheter clotting if they are not adequately heparin locked after treatment, so there is the potential for the catheter to become nonfunctional. VAPS are typically left in place in the animal for the rest of its life, similar to other medically implanted devices. Removal of VAPS could potentially cause clots that may have adhered to the port to dislodge and cause embolisms (Tara Harrison, personal communication, 2008).

Intralesional Therapies

Intralesional chemotherapy involves injecting chemotherapy directly into tumor masses (**Fig. 9**). This obviates intravenous access, although the animals require

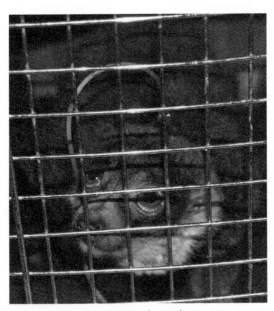

Fig. 8. Use of a VAP to administer intravenous chemotherapy to a mongoose lemur (*E mongoz*) without manual restraint or the use of anesthesia.

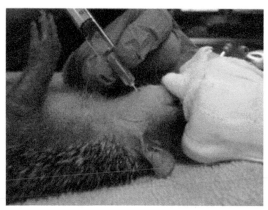

Fig. 9. Injecting bleomycin intralesionally in a squamous cell carcinoma in a greater hedgehog tenrec (*S setosus*).

heavy sedation or anesthesia for safe administration through this route. This method is typically used for single masses, or masses that are too large to surgically remove.

CHEMOTHERAPEUTIC AGENTS
Nitrosourea

Lomustine, is an alkylating agent in the nitrosourea class that causes DNA crosslinking.[7] It is highly lipid soluble and can enter cells through passive diffusion. Lomustine is metabolized by the liver but also excreted through the urinary system.[7] Lomustine is available in oral and injectable forms and has a long intertreatment interval (21–28 days). Lomustine has been used in human medicine primarily to treat brain tumors and Hodgkin lymphoma, and has been used in exotic and zoologic medicine to treat lymphoma, mast cell tumors, and histiocytic sarcoma.[7,8] Adverse effects of this medication in humans include myelosuppression, nausea and vomiting, anorexia, pulmonary toxicity, renal toxicity, and sores in the oral cavity. Hepatotoxicity has also been reported in humans, dogs, cats, and rats.[7] Lomustine use described in exotic animals has included therapy for cutaneous lymphoma in a ground cuscus (*Phalanger gymnotis*) with a clinical remission that lasted 255 days.[9] An African lion (*Panthera leo*) was treated with lomustine as part of a chemotherapy protocol and survived 504 days.[3] A Tasmanian devil (*Sarcophilus harrisii*) was treated with oral lomustine for a cutaneous T-cell lymphoma. The medication did not seem to slow the growth of the neoplasm in this individual, yet no adverse effects were reported.[10] A black swan (*Cygnus atratus*) was treated with lomustine, prednisone, chlorambucil, asparaginase, and radiation therapy for a chronic T-cell lymphocytic leukemia.[11] There were minimal responses to chemotherapy but the bird tolerated all therapies well with no adverse effects reported.

Alkylating Agents

Drugs classed as alkylating agents have a primary mechanism of action that involves covalent binding of alkyl groups to cellular macromolecules.[7] Alkylators target the DNA to generate interstrand or intrastrand crosslinks or adducts, which result in chromosome strand breaks and interference with the function of both DNA and RNA polymerases.[7]

Cyclophosphamide is a nitrogen mustard alkylating agent that is activated primarily in the liver.[7] It is used in human oncology to treat lymphomas, neuroblastoma, multiple myeloma, leukemias, and some solid tumors, and in veterinary medicine to treat lymphoma, primarily as part of a multiagent protocol.[7,12] Adverse effects in humans can be severe and include induction of acute myeloid leukemia, bladder cancer, sterile hemorrhagic cystitis, anaphylaxis, and pulmonary conditions, including pulmonary fibrosis.[12] Cyclophosphamide has been used in a kori bustard (*Ardeotis kori*) as part of a metronomic (continuous low dose) protocol to treat a large subcutaneous myxosarcoma.[13] Prior treatment had included intratumoral implantation of carboplatin-impregnated beads, which did not prevent tumor regrowth. Metronomic (continuous low dose) therapy with cyclophosphamide and meloxicam for 17 weeks resulted in tumor regression. The myxosarcoma returned when therapy was discontinued, so chemotherapy was reinitiated and continued for the duration of the bird's reported life. Treatment with cyclophosphamide was used in combination with prednisone in a green-winged macaw (*Ara chloroptera*) to control T-cell chronic lymphocytic leukemia.[14] This protocol was used for 29 weeks and the bird exhibited a good quality of life with clinical remission but died shortly after the medication was discontinued. Cyclophosphamide and prednisolone were used in a ferret with multiple myeloma. An initial high dose of cyclophosphamide was given as a loading dose, followed by metronomic therapy. The ferret developed anorexia a week and a half after treatment initiation and was euthanized at 2 weeks after diagnosis (Tara Myers Harrison, personal communication, 2016). Cyclophosphamide was used in a combination therapy as an intravenous agent in a green iguana with lymphoma through the use of a VAP in conjunction with a modified cyclophosphamide, hydroxydaunomycin (doxorubicin), Oncovin (vincristine), and prednisone (CHOP) protocol and radiation therapy.[15] There was a decrease in lymphocyte counts so the cyclophosphamide was changed to an every 2-week administration at day 161. On day 525, due to an increase in lymphocyte count, this medication was discontinued and doxorubicin was added.[15] A diffuse B-cell lymphoma was treated in an orangutan with intravenous cyclophosphamide in combination with rituximab, doxorubicin, and vincristine.[16]

Chlorambucil is a nitrogen mustard derivative that enters cells through passive diffusion and has a direct bifunctional alkylating ability that allows for its cytotoxic activity.[7] Chlorambucil has been used in human medicine for treatment of chronic lymphocytic leukemia, Hodgkin lymphoma, and non-Hodgkin lymphoma, and in domestic animals to treat lymphoma and chronic lymphocytic leukemia.[7,17] Adverse effects noted in humans include nausea, diarrhea, bone marrow failure, hepatotoxicity, interstitial pneumonia, pulmonary fibrosis, and allergic reactions.[17] In exotic animals, chlorambucil has been used as a long-term therapy in multiple species.[11,14,18–21] It was given over 28 weeks to a Java sparrow (*Lonchura oryzivora*) for treatment of thymic lymphoma. The thymic mass decreased 60% in size over the first 3 weeks.[22] The bird became ill at week 19 and the medication was withheld for 2 weeks, then restarted for 6 weeks during which the mass remained the same size. The owner at this time elected to stop this treatment and changed to prednisolone therapy.[22] Chlorambucil therapy was attempted in a double yellow-headed Amazon parrot (*Amazona ochrocephala oratrix*) for treatment of a T-cell lymphocytic leukemia but no response was evident after 40 days of treatment.[23] An umbrella cockatoo (*Cacatua alba*) was treated for B-cell lymphoma with chlorambucil and vincristine for 17 weeks and achieved an 8-year remission.[20] A green-winged macaw with chronic lymphocytic leukemia was treated for 6 weeks, in combination with prednisone; however, chlorambucil was discontinued due to thrombocytopenia.[14] A great horned owl (*Bubo virginianus*) was treated with chlorambucil for disseminated, presumed T-cell lymphoma for 3 weeks with no success.[18] Chlorambucil was used in combination therapy, as previously mentioned, for treatment of a chronic T-cell lymphocytic leukemia in a black swan with minimal efficacy but no adverse effects.[11] Chlorambucil was reported as part of a therapeutic protocol in a ferret with lymphoma that was treated for 10 months.[19] Additionally, a spotted hyena (Crocuta crocuta) with chronic T-cell lymphocytic leukemia was successfully treated with chlorambucil for 2 years. During this course of therapy, a higher dose of chlorambucil was thought to cause thrombocytopenia, so the dose was decreased and maintained until the animal was euthanized due to hemoabdomen and lymphocytosis.[21]

Melphalan is actively transported into cells by amino acid transporters. Melphalan is similar in structure and function to chlorambucil.[7] This medication does not require metabolic activation.[7,24] This agent is a nitrogen mustard alkylating agent that has been used in human medicine for treatment of ovarian carcinoma, multiple myeloma, neuroblastoma, rhabdomyosarcoma, breast cancer, and Hodgkin lymphoma, and in veterinary medicine primary for treatment of myeloma.[7,24] Some adverse effects in humans and animals include nausea, vomiting, myelosuppression, leucopenia, thrombocytopenia, and hypersensitivity.[7,24] Use of this medication is not reported commonly in exotic animals, although a single dose was administered to a captive dhole (Cuon alpinus) for treatment of lymphocytic leukemia.[25]

Antimetabolites

These medications primarily inhibit cell growth and division. This includes gemcitabine, which has been rarely used in exotic animal species other than as part of a combination protocol in a mongoose lemur (Tara Harrison, personal communication, 2012).

Cytarabine (cytosine arabinoside), an antimetabolite antineoplastic agent, acts as an analogue to deoxycytidine and is phosphorylated in cells to generate arabinosylcytosine triphosphate, which then acts as a competitive inhibitor of DNA polymerase alpha.[7] It is also incorporated into DNA, which allows for its primary mechanism of action to be cytotoxicity due to DNA chain termination during DNA synthesis.[7] This agent has been used in human medicine to treat acute or chronic lymphocytic leukemia, leukemia in the central nervous system, meningeal leukemia, and Hodgkin or non-Hodgkin leukemia.[26] It has been used in veterinary medicine primarily to treat lymphomas that have potential central nervous system involvement.[7] Adverse effects in human patients include fever, rash, myelosuppression, hepatic dysfunction, and thrombophlebitis.[26] This medication has been used to treat a bearded dragon for advanced leukemia. The animal died 44 hours into treatment likely due to disseminated intravascular coagulation with metastases in the heart, skeletal muscle, gastrointestinal tract, liver, kidney, lung, and cloacal tissue.[27] There was no evidence of any toxicity due to the medication in the kidneys or other organs. The investigators suspected this animal died due to advanced disease rather than a reaction to the medication.[27] Cytarabine was used in a southern black rhinoceros in combination with prednisone, cyclophosphamide, vincristine, and doxorubicin to treat lymphoblastic leukemia.[28] Progressive dyspnea was noted that may have been due to advanced disease.

ANTITUMOR ANTIBIOTICS OR TOPOISOMERASE INHIBITORS

Doxorubicin is an anthracycline antibiotic classified as a topoisomerase inhibitor drug. Doxorubicin is a commonly used intravenous antineoplastic agent in human and veterinary medicine.[7] It inhibits DNA and RNA polymerases and topoisomerase II activity.

Doxorubicin acts through alkylation of DNA, DNA intercalation, reactive oxygen generation, perturbation of cellular calcium homeostasis, inhibition of thioredoxin reductase, and interaction with plasma membrane components.[7] Doxorubicin has been used in human medicine as a treatment of many cancer types, including hepatic, renal, breast, endometrial, ovarian, and thyroid cancers, as well as transitional cell carcinoma.[29–34] Doxorubicin adverse effects in humans include severe tissue injury and necrosis in cases of extravasation, myocardial toxicity, myelosuppression, and hypersensitivity reactions.[35] Side effects in veterinary medicine include dose-limiting toxicities, infusion-rate–dependent hypersensitivity, myelosuppression, gastrointestinal toxicity, cumulative dose-related cardiotoxicity, and renal tubular damage in cats.[7] Doxorubicin is a tissue vesicant and can cause serious damage if delivered extravascularly in animals as in human patients.[7] The pharmacokinetics of doxorubicin have been studied in sulfur-crested cockatoos (Cacatua galerita), with mild transient inappetence as the primary adverse effect.[36] As previously mentioned, lymphoma was treated with doxorubicin and other therapies in a green iguana, ferret, and an orangutan.[15,16,19] Doxorubicin has been used in combination with lomustine, prednisone, and prednisolone to treat an African lion (P leo) diagnosed with T-cell lymphoma.[3] There were no adverse effects attributed to doxorubicin. Doxorubicin was used to treat myxosarcoma of the urinary bladder with the use of a VAP for drug delivery in a gray wolf (Canis lupus) (see Figs. 3–7). The wolf had periods of nausea and mild anorexia after doxorubicin treatment (Tara Myers Harrison, personal communication, 2008). Doxorubicin and other therapies were used in a rabbit with nonresectable invasive salivary adenocarcinoma with no adverse effects (Barbara E. Kitchell, personal communication, 2015). Doxorubicin was used in combination with carboplatin at increasing levels to attempt to treat facial tumor disease in Tasmanian devils (S harrisii).[37] There was no response to treatment, and neutropenia, anorexia, and weight loss were noted to be dose-limiting adverse effects. A raccoon (Procyon lotor) with a thyroid neoplasia was treated with doxorubicin through a VAP. The animal developed pancytopenia and anorexia and was euthanized due to this complication.[38] The only other reported adverse effect attributed to doxorubicin in an exotic animal literature was congestive heart failure in a juvenile black rhinoceros (Diceros bicornis minor) treated for lymphoblastic leukemia. Heart failure was presumed to be secondary to doxorubicin cardiotoxicity, due to potential sensitivity to tissue damage from free hydroxyl radicals.[28]

ANTITUMOR ANTIBIOTICS

Bleomycin is an antitumor agent used in human and veterinary medicine.[39] Human oncologic indications for bleomycin treatment include direct injection into viral papillomas (warts), and systemic treatment of hemangiomas, cutaneous squamous cell carcinoma, Hodgkin and non-Hodgkin lymphoma, testicular carcinoma, and malignant pleural effusion.[39] Adverse effects of systemic administration in humans include pneumonitis leading to pulmonary fibrosis, which is considered an idiosyncratic reaction.[40] Bleomycin was used intralesionally to treat squamous cell carcinoma in a yellow-bellied slider (Trachemys scripta scripta) in combination with electrochemotherapy. The animal tolerated treatment well and had no evidence of neoplasia 12 months after completion of the treatment protocol.[41] Electrochemotherapy with bleomycin has also been used to treat fibropapillomas in a green sea turtle (Chelonia mydas) with no signs of recurrence after 1 year.[42] Bleomycin has been used to treat advanced stage squamous cell carcinoma in a greater hedgehog tenrec (Setifer setosus) (Tara Myers Harrison, personal communication, 2015) (see Fig. 9). There was no evidence of bleomycin-induced adverse effects but the patient was euthanized 1 month after treatment. A blue-fronted Amazon parrot (*Amazona aestiva*) was treated intralesionally with bleomycin for a xanthoma. There are reports of bleomycin being successful in treatment of human papillomas, so this agent was attempted as a therapy for the xanthomas because surgical removal was not possible due to the large and extensive size of the masses. There was minimal response to treatment and minor ulceration of the tumor over 2 months. There was no evidence of systemic adverse effects (Tara Myers Harrison, personal communication, 2016).

VINCA ALKALOIDS

Vinca alkaloids function by binding to a site that is distinct on alpha and beta tubulin, thereby inhibiting microtubule assembly. This disrupts the mitotic spindle apparatus and results in metaphase arrest and cytotoxicity.[7]

Vincristine has been used in human medicine to treat acute leukemias, central nervous system tumors, multiple myeloma, Hodgkin and non-Hodgkin lymphoma, ovarian cancer, small cell lung cancer, and thymoma.[43] Adverse effects in human patients include edema, hypotension or hypertension, ataxia, coma, paralysis, fever, neurotoxicity, seizure, anorexia, constipation, diarrhea, hemolytic uremic syndrome, dyspnea, and allergic reactions.[43] Vincristine is primarily used in veterinary medicine for the treatment of lymphoma and for inducing platelet release in immune-mediated thrombocytopenia.[7] Vincristine is a tissue vesicant if it is delivered into the extravascular space. Vincristine should only be delivered through an indwelling intravenous catheter or a clean intravenous injection.[7] An umbrella cockatoo was treated with vincristine and chlorambucil for cutaneous B-cell lymphoma and remained in remission for 8 years.[20] Vincristine was used for lymphoma treatment, using a VAP, in a green iguana in combination with radiation therapy, doxorubicin, cyclophosphamide, and prednisone.[15] Vincristine is commonly used as an intravenous therapy, especially with VAP placement, to treat lymphoma in a ferret.[19] A puma (*Puma concolor*) was treated for squamous cell carcinoma with intravenous vincristine but the medication caused vomiting, diarrhea, and weight loss, and had no effect on the neoplasm. Intralesional use of vincristine was effective.[44] A diffuse B-cell lymphoma was treated in an orangutan (*Pongo pygmaeus*) with 3 cycles of intravenous rituximab (a monoclonal antibody directed against the human B-cell marker CD20), cyclophosphamide, doxorubicin, and vincristine and oral prednisone. The animal maintained clinical remission for 25 months.[16] Adverse effects noted in the orangutan included fever, moderate anorexia, and moderate lethargy. Acute lymphoblastic leukemia in a juvenile southern black rhinoceros (*D bicornis minor*) was treated with combination chemotherapy that included vincristine, and remission was achieved at a 19-day recheck; however, the animal passed away due to a presumed cardiac toxicity from doxorubicin.[28] Vincristine was used at increasing dosages to evaluate treatment of devil facial tumor disease in Tasmanian devils (*S harrisii*).[45] Despite the biological similarities of this communicable neoplastic disease to canine transmissible venereal tumor, in which vincristine is the standard of care agent, there was no response to vincristine treatment in Tasmanian devils. Dose-limiting adverse effects were noted to be anorexia, vomiting, diarrhea, and neutropenia.

PLATINUMS

Platinum medications act through covalent binding to DNA through displacement reactions.[7] This forms intrastrand crosslinks, which correlates with cytotoxicity.[7]

Cisplatin is an analogue of carboplatin and thus acts as a DNA crosslinking agent. Cisplatin has been used as an intravenous infusion in human medicine to treat bladder cancer, ovarian cancer, and testicular cancer. Adverse effects in humans can include cumulative renal toxicity, ototoxicity, myelosuppression, severe and sometimes prolonged nausea and vomiting, vascular toxicities, peripheral neuropathy, blindness, hepatotoxicity, and hypersensitivity reactions. Cisplatin is contraindicated in domestic cats.[7] Cisplatin has been primarily used to treat osteosarcoma in dogs but has also been occasionally used for a variety of other tumor types.[7] Cisplatin has been used intralesionally in the treatment of squamous cell carcinoma in a bald eagle's (*Haliaeetus leucocephalus*) patagium. There were no adverse effects of treatment and the neoplasm completely resolved (Tara Myers Harrison, personal communication, 2011). Two treatments of intralesional cisplatin were attempted in a goose (*Anser anser*) for a xanthoma type of neoplasm. Although treatment was not successful, there were no adverse effects of the therapy.[46] An African penguin (*Spheniscus demersus*) was treated for choanal squamous cell carcinoma with intralesional cisplatin and cryotherapy with liquid nitrogen. The penguin was disease free for 9 months, after which squamous cell carcinoma recurred.[47]

Intralesional carboplatin was also used, as previously mentioned, through carboplatin-impregnated beads in a kori bustard.[13] Intralesional vincristine was used, as previously mentioned, to treat a puma.[44]

Carboplatin acts in a manner analogous to an alkylating agent by virtue of its ability to induce crosslinks within the DNA structure. Carboplatin has been used in human medicine to treat breast cancer, lung cancer, cervical cancer, prostate cancer, melanoma, and oropharyngeal cancer.[48–52] Adverse effects in humans include vomiting, bone marrow reactions and hypersensitivity reactions.[53] Carboplatin has been used for management of osteosarcomas, carcinomas, and sarcomas. The dose-limiting toxicity is myelosuppression in domestic animals.[7] Carboplatin was used in the treatment of a mallard duck (*Anas platyrhynchos*) with a Sertoli cell tumor. Carboplatin was considered effective in causing clinical improvement and in reducing the size of the neoplasm as interpreted through radiographic monitoring.[54] Heteropenia was noted after the carboplatin treatments.[54] The duck was maintained on itraconazole throughout treatment without developing aspergillosis.[54] A budgerigar (*Melopsittacus undulatus*) with renal adenocarcinoma was treated with monthly carboplatin injections, and initially improved; however, after 3 months, the bird's health declined and the mass regrew.[55] Carboplatin therapy has been used to treat a kori bustard with a myxosarcoma through the use of carboplatin-impregnated calcium-based matrix beads, as previously mentioned.[13] Pharmacokinetics of carboplatin were evaluated in sulfur-crested cockatoos; these birds had no adverse effects at the doses prescribed.[56,57] Carboplatin has been used as a treatment of transitional cell carcinoma in fishing cats (*Prionailurus viverrinus*), in combination with piroxicam, with no adverse effects.[58] A mongoose lemur (*Eulemur mongoz*) was treated intravenously with carboplatin in combination with gemcitabine via a VAP for 6 sessions for hepatocellular carcinoma (see **Fig. 8**). The animal remained in remission for 6 months, at which point the neoplasm recurred (Tara Myers Harrison, personal communication, 2012). Carboplatin was used in increasing amounts to attempt to treat devil facial tumor disease in Tasmanian devils (*S harrisii*) in combination with doxorubicin.[37] There was no response to treatment, and anorexia and weight loss were noted to be dose-limiting adverse effects. A rabbit with thymic carcinoma was treated with carboplatin with minimal response to treatment based on radiographs but with no noted adverse effects (Barbara E. Kitchell, personal communication, 2015). A rabbit with invasive, nonresectable salivary adenocarcinoma was treated with carboplatin, doxorubicin, and vinorelbine with minimal measurable tumor regression but with no adverse effects (Barbara E. Kitchell, personal communication, 2015). A rabbit with pulmonary metastasis of distal femoral osteosarcoma was treated with carboplatin after rear limb amputation with minimal response, based on radiographs, but with no adverse effects (Barbara E. Kitchell, personal communication, 2015).

L-ASPARAGINASE

Asparaginase is an agent derived from *Escherichia coli* that contains the enzyme L-asparagine amidohydrolase. Asparaginase inhibits protein synthesis in tumor cells, which causes apoptosis of those cells.[7] Asparaginase has been used in human medicine almost exclusively to induce rapid remission in pediatric acute lymphoblastic leukemia patients.[59,60] Adverse effects in humans include stroke, potentially fatal acute peritonitis, nausea, vomiting, coagulopathies, decreased clotting factors, hepatotoxicity, septicemia, renal failure, and pyrexia.[60] Asparaginase has been used to treat lymphoproliferative disorders in domestic animals.[7] Hypersensitivity reactions have been noted in domestic animals, which may increase in risk with repeated dosing. Hypersensitivity reactions can be managed with dexamethasone and diphenhydramine.[7] Asparaginase has been documented in a ferret lymphoma treatment protocol and seems to add no adverse effects.[19] Asparaginase has also been used intramuscularly in a multidrug protocol for T-cell lymphocytic leukemia in a spotted hyena.[21] Asparaginase was used subcutaneously, in combination with a protocol previously mentioned, for the treatment of a chronic T-cell lymphocytic leukemia in a black swan with no adverse effects.[11]

CORTICOSTEROIDS

Prednisone and prednisolone are corticosteroids frequently used as adjunct therapy in combination with many of the aforementioned medications in a variety of chemotherapeutic protocols. The use of corticosteroids may have a direct anticancer effect for lymphomas and mast cell tumors, and may provide palliative appetite and anti-inflammatory support in other disease settings. Adverse effects of corticosteroids can include clinical signs of hyperadrenocorticism, polyuria, polydipsia, weight gain, dull hair coat, gastrointestinal ulceration, elevated liver enzymes, and pancreatitis.[61] There are some concerns regarding use of steroid therapy in avian patients due to some cases of long-term steroid therapy for chronic conditions that coincided with aspergillosis infection or potential immune suppression.[62,63] There are also reports of concerns for immunosuppression with steroid therapy in rabbits.[64] Some owners have elected to treat small mammal lymphomas solely with prednisone or prednisolone; however, there is a concern that prolonged pretreatment with corticosteroids can result in increased levels of chemotherapy drug resistance.[65] A rabbit diagnosed with thymoma was successfully treated with prednisone over 8 months, monitored radiographically monthly for 3 months, then 2 months later, and then 3 months later, at which time the rabbit was euthanized (Tara Myers Harrison, personal communication, 2015). Prednisone has been used in combination therapy for a black swan with lymphocytic leukemia, as previously mentioned, without any adverse effects.[11] The black swan received concurrent itraconazole to prevent secondary aspergillosis infection.[11] There was no report of any resulting aspergillosis infection. A green-winged macaw was treated with long-term prednisone, as previously mentioned, with no adverse effects. Unfortunately, corticosteroids did not limit metastases.[14] This bird was also simultaneously treated with enrofloxacin and itraconazole to minimize secondary infections.[14] Prednisone was used in a multidrug protocol for management of lymphoma in a green iguana (*Iguana iguana*) for 2.5 years with no adverse effect noted.[15] The iguana was treated with enrofloxacin for 30 days after the initiation of therapy and placement of a VAP.[15] Additionally, this animal received meloxicam for a short time after surgery concurrently with prednisone with no adverse effects.[15] Prednisone was used in combination with several other chemotherapeutics in a juvenile southern black rhinoceros with acute lymphoblastic leukemia.[28] This animal was concurrently treated with ampicillin due to the deteriorated condition of the animal during therapy.[28] Prednisone was also paired with chlorambucil to treat T-cell lymphocytic leukemia in a spotted hyena with no supplemental antibiotics.[21] Prednisone, and later prednisolone, was used for treatment of T-cell lymphoma in an African lion, as previously mentioned.[3] The lion was not treated with any antibiotics at the time of the chemotherapy protocol. Prednisolone was paired with cyclophosphamide in a ferret with multiple myeloma, as previously mentioned (Tara Myers Harrison, personal communication, 2016).

OTHERS

Toceranib (Palladia), is a receptor tyrosine kinase inhibitor that is licensed for treatment of canine mast cell neoplasia.[66] However, it has been used to treat a variety of tumors due to its ability to block signaling through vascular endothelial growth factor receptors, thereby inhibiting neoangiogenesis in a broad range of tumors. Toceranib is known to be ulcerogenic in dogs. Adverse effects of toceranib reported in domestic dogs can be as severe as gastrointestinal perforation but may also include vomiting, lethargy, lameness, weight loss, dehydration, hematochezia, pruritus, nausea, localized edema, conjunctivitis, and pyrexia. Recently, this medication has been used to treat a binturong (*Arctictis binturong*) with renal adenocarcinoma.[67] Toceranib did not seem to significantly prolong the life of the animal but there were no adverse effects.

Piroxicam, a nonselective cyclooxygenase (COX) inhibitor, has been used with modest efficacy reported in treating canine transitional cell carcinoma, squamous cell carcinoma, soft tissue sarcoma, and melanoma. There are reports of remissions induced by piroxicam alone in certain tumors. Adverse effects in domestic animals include gastrointestinal ulceration, renal papillary necrosis, and peritonitis.[68] A 2.5-year-old African pygmy hedgehog (*Atelerix albiventris*) was treated with piroxicam for a poorly differentiated renal neoplasm (Tara Myers Harrison, personal communication, 2016). There were no adverse effects noticed during 3-week of treatment of this animal. The neoplasm grew throughout treatment and the animal was euthanized for another reason. Piroxicam was used in combination with carboplatin to treat transitional cell carcinoma in fishing cats, with no observed adverse effects.[58] A gray wolf was given piroxicam in combination with doxorubicin for treatment of a myxosarcoma of the urinary bladder (Tara Myers Harrison, personal communication, 2008). The wolf survived 8 months and was euthanized due to another cause. A raccoon was treated with piroxicam initially and later in combination with doxorubicin for thyroid carcinoma.[38] There were no adverse effects noted from the piroxicam.

COMBINATION THERAPIES

Established combination chemotherapy protocols have been used primarily in the treatment of lymphomas in exotic species. Various protocols have been described in the veterinary literature, including (1) CHOP protocol, used in ferrets (Tara Myers Harrison, personal communication, 2016), a green iguana,[15] and a guinea pig (Tara

Myers Harrison, personal communication, 2015); (2) the Wisconsin-Madison protocol version of the CHOP protocol used to treat lymphoma in ferrets; and (3) the Tufts protocol of prednisone, L-asparaginase, cyclophosphamide, cytarabine, methotrexate, chlorambucil and procarbazine (ACOPA), used to treat ferret lymphoma.[15,65]

TREATMENT RESISTANCE AND ADVERSE EVENTS COMPLICATIONS

In the cases of the exotic animals reviewed in this article, it is challenging to interpret resistance or lack of response to therapy because species-specific pharmacokinetics are largely unavailable. Thus apparent drug resistance could arise from underdosing. Complications observed after chemotherapy treatment included similar adverse effects to those seen when the drugs are used to treat human, canine, or feline patients (see **Table 1**).

EVALUATION OF OUTCOME AND LONG-TERM TREATMENT RECOMMENDATION

The frequency of treatments largely determines the frequency of evaluation for response to therapy. For most treatments, when chemotherapy is used alone, a remission is expected rather than a cure. The length of survival can range from days to months and years, depending on the histologic type and dissemination stage of the neoplasm when treatment is initiated.

In addition to observing for response to treatment, the clinician should monitor for evidence of toxicity secondary to chemotherapy. Common adverse effects can include gastrointestinal signs or myelosuppression. Regular complete blood counts are recommended during chemotherapy. As a general rule, a level of neutrophils greater than 2000 cells/µL is considered safe to allow a subsequent chemotherapy dose.[7] A platelet count adequate to prevent spontaneous hemorrhage is also necessary before the administration of additional drugs (typically>50,000 platelets/µL, depending on the species).[7] In small animals, the nadir for white blood cells and platelets often falls at approximately 7 to 10 days, depending on the medication, so monitoring 1 week after chemotherapy treatment is the standard time frame. However, white blood cell and platelet nadirs have not been adequately evaluated in exotic species. For renally cleared drugs, such as the alkylating agents and platinum compounds, assessing sera urea nitrogen (BUN) and creatinine values before subsequent chemotherapy dosing can prevent excessive toxicity. Similarly, hepatotoxic drugs, such as lomustine, require assessment of liver transaminase levels before additional chemotherapy dosing. Additional hematologic and biochemical assessment should be performed following cessation of treatment.

Other monitoring can include repeated radiographs, ultrasound examination, MRI, or computed tomography scans, which are often performed during and after treatments.

Other diagnostics can be repeated monthly, or as determined necessary by the clinician and the specific toxicity profile of the administered chemotherapeutics. Repeated imaging could be performed at 1 month, 3 months, 6 months, and then every 6 months thereafter.

ACKNOWLEDGMENTS

The authors would like to thank Drs Marlene Hauck, Erin Brewer, and Erika Rost for their assistance. We would like to extend an extra thanks to Dr Bethany Walters for her assistance.

REFERENCES

1. Antinoff N, Hahn K. Ferret oncology: diseases, diagnostics, and therapeutics. Vet Clin North Am Exot Anim Pract 2004;7(3):579–625.
2. Chen S. Advanced diagnostic approaches and current medical management of insulinomas and adrenocortical disease in ferrets (*Mustela putorius furo*). Vet Clin North Am Exot Anim Pract 2010;13(3):439–52.
3. Harrison TM, Sikarskie J, Kitchell B, et al. Treatment of malignant lymphoma in an African lion (*Panthera leo*). J Zoo Wildl Med 2007;38(2):333–6.
4. Kent MS. The use of chemotherapy in exotic animals. Vet Clin North Am Exot Anim Pract 2004;7(3):807–20.
5. Done LB, Deem SL, Fiorello CV. Surgical and medical management of a uterine spindle cell tumor in an African hedgehog (*Atelerix albiventris*). J Zoo Wildl Med 2007;38(4):601–3.
6. Willens S, Dunn JL, Frasca S Jr. Fibrosarcoma of the brood pouch in an aquarium-reared lined seahorse (*Hippocampus erectus*). J Zoo Wildl Med 2004;35(1):107–9.
7. Withrow SJ, Vail DM, Page RL, editors. Small animal clinical oncology, vol, 5th edition. St Louis (MO): Saunders; 2013.
8. Lomustine [package insert]. Princeton, NJ: Bristol Myers. 2013.
9. Goodnight AL, Couto CG, Green E, et al. Chemotherapy and radiotherapy for treatment of cutaneous lymphoma in a ground cuscus (*Phalanger gymnotis*). J Zoo Wildl Med 2008;39(3):472–5.
10. Scheelings TF, Dobson EC, Hooper C. Cutaneous T-cell lymphoma in two captive Tasmanian devils (*Sarcophilus harrisii*). J Zoo Wildl Med 2014;45(2):367–71.
11. Sinclair KM, Hawkins MG, Wright L, et al. Chronic T-cell lymphocytic leukemia in a black swan (*Cygnus atratus*): diagnosis, treatment, and pathology. J Avian Med Surg 2015;29(4):326–35.
12. Cyclophosphamide [package insert]. Princeton, NJ: Bristol Myers. 2013.
13. Sander SJ, Hope KL, McNeill CJ, et al. Metronomic chemotherapy for myxosarcoma treatment in a kori bustard (*Ardeotis kori*). J Avian Med Surg 2015;29(3): 210–5.
14. Hammond EE, Guzman DS, Garner MM, et al. Long-term treatment of chronic lymphocytic leukemia in a green-winged macaw (*Ara chloroptera*). J Avian Med Surg 2010;24(4):330–8.
15. Folland DW, Johnston MS, Thamm DH, et al. Diagnosis and management of lymphoma in a green iguana (*Iguana iguana*). J Am Vet Med Assoc 2011;239(7): 985–91.
16. Ikpatt OF, Reavill D, Chatfield J, et al. Diagnosis and treatment of diffuse large B-cell lymphoma in an orangutan (*Pongo pygmaeus*). J Zoo Wildl Med 2014; 45(4):935–40.
17. Chlorambucil [package insert]. Triangle Park, NC: Glaxo Smith Kline. 2006.
18. Malka S, Crabbs T, Mitchell EB, et al. Disseminated lymphoma of presumptive T-cell origin in a great horned owl (*Bubo virginianus*). J Avian Med Surg 2008; 22(3):226–33.
19. Rassnick KM, Gould WJ 3rd, Flanders JA. Use of a vascular access system for administration of chemotherapeutic agents to a ferret with lymphoma. J Am Vet Med Assoc 1995;206(4):500–4.
20. Rivera S, McClearen JR, Reavill DR. Treatment of nonepitheliotropic cutaneous B-cell lymphoma in an umbrella cockatoo (*Cacatua alba*). J Avian Med Surg 2009;23(4):294–302.

21. Singleton CL, Wack RF, Zabka TS, et al. Diagnosis and treatment of chronic T-lymphocytic leukemia in a spotted hyena (*Crocuta crocuta*). J Zoo Wildl Med 2007; 38(3):488–91.

22. Yu PH, Chi CH. Long-term management of thymic lymphoma in a java sparrow (*Lonchura oryzivora*). J Avian Med Surg 2015;29(1):51–4.

23. Osofsky A, Hawkins MG, Foreman O, et al. T-cell lymphocytic leukemia in a double yellow-headed Amazon parrot (*Amazona ochrocephala oratrix*). J Avian Med Surg 2011;25(4):286–94.

24. Melphalan [package insert]. Research Triangle Park, NC: Glaxo Smith Kline. 2010.

25. Scala C, Ortiz K, Nicolier A, et al. Lymphocytic leukemia in a captive dhole (*Cuon alpinus*). J Zoo Wildl Med 2013;44(1):204–7.

26. Cytarabine [package insert]. Kalamazoo, MI: Upjohn Company. 2014.

27. Jankowski G, Sirninger J, Borne J, et al. Chemotherapeutic treatment for leukemia in a bearded dragon (*Pogona vitticeps*). J Zoo Wildl Med 2011;42(2):322–5.

28. Radcliffe RW, Paglia DE, Couto CG. Acute lymphoblastic leukemia in a juvenile southern black rhinoceros (*Diceros bicornis minor*). J Zoo Wildl Med 2000; 31(1):71–6.

29. Espelin CW, Leonard SC, Geretti E, et al. Dual HER2 targeting with trastuzumab and liposome-encapsulated doxorubicin (MM-302) demonstrates synergistic antitumor activity in breast and gastric cancer. Cancer Res 2016;76(6):1517–27.

30. AlGhamdi S, Leoncikas V, Plant KE, et al. Synergistic interaction between lipid-loading and doxorubicin exposure in Huh7 hepatoma cells results in enhanced cytotoxicity and cellular oxidative stress: implications for acute and chronic care of obese cancer patients. Toxicol Res 2015;4(6):1479–87.

31. Chou R, Selph S, Buckley D, et al, AHRQ Comparative Effectiveness Reviews. Treatment of nonmetastatic muscle-invasive bladder cancer. Rockville (MD): Agency for Healthcare Research and Quality (US); 2015.

32. Tempfer CB, Rezniczek GA, Ende P, et al. Pressurized Intraperitoneal aerosol chemotherapy with cisplatin and doxorubicin in women with peritoneal carcinomatosis: a cohort study. Anticancer Res 2015;35(12):6723–9.

33. Tahir S. Real-life experience using trabectedin plus pegylated liposomal doxorubicin combination to treat patients with relapsed ovarian cancer. EJC Suppl 2014; 12(2):17–20.

34. Pouessel D, Chevret S, Rolland F, et al. Standard or accelerated methotrexate, vinblastine, doxorubicin and cisplatin as neoadjuvant chemotherapy for locally advanced urothelial bladder cancer: Does dose intensity matter? Eur J Cancer 2015;54:69–74.

35. Doxorubicin [package insert]. Horsham, PA: Janssen Products, LP. 2012.

36. Gilbert CM, Filippich LJ, Charles BG. Doxorubicin pharmacokinetics following a single-dose infusion to sulphur-crested cockatoos (*Cacatua galerita*). Aust Vet J 2004;82(12):769–72.

37. Phalen DN, Frimberger AE, Peck S, et al. Doxorubicin and carboplatin trials in Tasmanian devils (*Sarcophilus harrisii*) with Tasmanian devil facial tumor disease. Vet J 2015;206(3):312–6.

38. McCain SL, Allender MC, Bohling M, et al. Thyroid neoplasia in captive raccoons (*Procyon lotor*). J Zoo Wildl Med 2010;41(1):121–7.

39. Saitta P, Krishnamurthy K, Brown LH. Bleomycin in dermatology: a review of intralesional applications. Dermatol Surg 2008;34:1299–313.

40. Bleomycin [package insert]. Irving, CA: Teva Parenteral Medicines. 2013.

41. Lanza A, Baldi A, Spugnini EP. Surgery and electrochemotherapy for the treatment of cutaneous squamous cell carcinoma in a yellow-bellied slider (*Trachemys scripta scripta*). J Am Vet Med Assoc 2015;246(4):455–7.

42. Brunner CH, Dutra G, Silva CB, et al. Electrochemotherapy for the treatment of fibropapillomas in Chelonia mydas. J Zoo Wildl Med 2014;45(2):213–8.

43. Vincristine [package insert]. Newbury, Brookshire, UK: Genus Pharmaceuticals. 2006.

44. Sandoval BJ, Amat AC, Sabri J, et al. Intralesional vincristine use for treatment of squamous cell carcinoma in a puma (*Puma concolor*). J Zoo Wildl Med 2013; 44(4):1059–62.

45. Phalen DN, Frimberger A, Pyecroft S, et al. Vincristine chemotherapy trials and pharmacokinetics in tasmanian devils with tasmanian devil facial tumor disease. PLoS One 2013;8(6):e65133.

46. Jaensch SM, Butler R, O'Hara A, et al. Atypical multiple, papilliform, xanthomatous, cutaneous neoplasia in a goose (*Anser anser*). Aust Vet J 2002;80(5): 277–80.

47. Ferrell ST, Marlar AB, Garner M, et al. Intralesional cisplatin chemotherapy and topical cryotherapy for the control of choanal squamous cell carcinoma in an African penguin (*Spheniscus demersus*). J Zoo Wildl Med 2006;37(4):539–41.

48. Musaev A, Guzel AB, Khatib G, et al. Assessment of primary radical hysterectomy and neoadjuvant chemotherapy followed by radical hysterectomy in Stage IB2, IIA bulky cervical cancer. Eur J Gynaecol Oncol 2015;36(5):579–84.

49. Sunada T, Kobayashi T, Shibasaki N, et al. A case of rapidly progressive metastatic castration-resistant prostate cancer: durable control by early induction of carboplatin and paclitaxel. Hinyokika Kiyo 2015;61(9):369–73 [in Japanese].

50. Wang Q, Yang L, Xu F, et al. Changes of lymphocyte subgroups in non-small cell lung cancer patients before and during chemotherapy. Clin Lab 2015;61(10): 1343–51.

51. Wilson MA, Schuchter LM. Chemotherapy for melanoma. Cancer Treat Res 2016; 167:209–29.

52. Yardley DA, Brufsky A, Coleman RE, et al. Phase II/III weekly nab-paclitaxel plus gemcitabine or carboplatin versus gemcitabine/carboplatin as first-line treatment of patients with metastatic triple-negative breast cancer (the tnAcity study): study protocol for a randomized controlled trial. Trials 2015;16(1):575.

53. Carboplatin [package insert]. Princeton, NJ: Bristol-Myers Squibb. 2010.

54. Childs-Sanford SE, Rassnick KM, Alcaraz A. Carboplatin for treatment of a Sertoli cell tumor in a mallard (*Anas platyrhynchos*). Vet Comp Oncol 2006;4(1):51–6.

55. Macwhirter P, Pyke D, Wayne J. Use of carboplatin in the treatment of renal adenocarcinoma in a budgerigar. Exotic DVM 2002;4:11–2.

56. Filippich LJ, Charles BG, Sutton RH, et al. Carboplatin pharmacokinetics following a single-dose infusion in sulphur-crested cockatoos (*Cacatua galerita*). Aust Vet J 2004;82(6):366–9.

57. Antonissen G, Devreese M, De Baere S, et al. Comparative pharmacokinetics and allometric scaling of carboplatin in different avian species. PLoS One 2015;10(7):e0134177.

58. Sutherland-Smith M, Harvey C, Campbell M, et al. Transitional cell carcinomas in four fishing cats (*Prionailurus viverrinus*). J Zoo Wildl Med 2004;35(3):370–80.

59. Hunault-Berger M, Leguay T, Huguet F, et al. A Phase 2 study of L-asparaginase encapsulated in erythrocytes in elderly patients with Philadelphia chromosome negative acute lymphoblastic leukemia: The GRASPALL/GRAALL-SA2-2008 study. Am J Hematol 2015;90(9):811–8.

60. Asparaginase [package insert]. West Point, PA: Merck and Co., Inc. 2000.
61. Prednisolone [package insert]. Columbus, OH: Roxane Laboratories, Inc. 2008.
62. Verstappen FALM, Dorrestein GM. Aspergillosis in Amazon parrots after cortico-steroid therapy for smoke-inhalation injury. J Avian Med Surg 2005;19(2):138–41.
63. Graat EA, Ploeger HW, Henken AM, et al. *Eimeria acervulina*: influence of corticosterone-induced immunosuppression on oocyst shedding and production characteristics in broilers, and correlation with a computer simulation model. Vet Parisitol 1997;70:47–59.
64. Latour JG, Prejean JB, Margaret W. Corticosteroids and generalized Shwartzman reaction. Mechanisms of sensitization in rabbit. Am J Pathol 1971;65(1):189–202.
65. Antinoff N, Williams BH. Neoplasia. 3rd edition. St Louis (MO): Elsevier Saunders; 2012.
66. Palladia [Package insert]. Kalamazoo, MI: Zoetis. 2015.
67. Thompson KA, Patterson J, Fitzgerald S, et al. Treatment of renal carcinoma in a binturong (*Arctictis binturong*) with nephrectomy and a tyrosine kinase inhibitor. J Zoo Wildl Med, in press.
68. Piroxicam [package insert]. Sellersville, PA: Teva Pharmaceuticals USA. 2015.

Principles and Applications of Surgical Oncology in Exotic Animals

Michele A. Steffey, DVM, DACVS-SA

KEYWORDS

- Cancer • Oncology • Surgery • Surgical oncology • Interventional oncology
- Veterinary

KEY POINTS

- Optimal outcomes in the surgical removal of cancer are attained by a holistic approach to the disease, including knowledge of the biologic behavior of the tumor and appropriate staging.
- Treatment goals, whether curative intent or palliative intent, should be identified before surgery.
- Curative intent treatment plans may involve surgery alone, or multimodal therapies.
- Margin marking techniques are simple, inexpensive, and very useful for improved communication of information about microscopic disease.

INTRODUCTION

Treatment of cancer in exotic species is becoming increasingly prevalent, although formal research in this area remains sparse. A retrospective report on the prevalence of neoplasia in reptiles demonstrated that cancer was identified in 10% of the biopsy or necropsy submissions for reptile species, with individual groupings as follows: snakes (15%), lizards (8.5%), chelonians (2.7%), and crocodilians.[1] A recent online literature search by the author of the past 10 years of the *Journal of Avian Medicine and Surgery* and the *Journal of Zoo and Wildlife Medicine* revealed a total of 38 case reports of neoplasia; most of these reports occurred between 2011 and 2015, suggesting that treatment of cancer in exotic species is increasing in frequency. This is an exciting time for the exotic species practitioner, with shifting paradigms in client perceptions of cancer and increasing availability of advanced therapies. Although a number of therapeutic options exist for the treatment of neoplasia, surgical excision remains an important mainstay in the treatment of solid tumors. Aggressive

The author has nothing to disclose.
Surgical Oncology, University of California-Davis, School of Veterinary Medicine, 1 Shields Avenue, Davis, CA 95616, USA
E-mail address: masteffey@ucdavis.edu

Vet Clin Exot Anim 20 (2017) 235–254
http://dx.doi.org/10.1016/j.cvex.2016.07.010

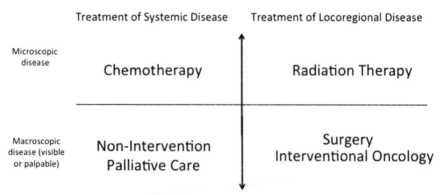

Fig. 1. Generalized schematic of the application of treatment modalities for cancer.

and well-planned surgical removal of localized solid neoplasms cures more veterinary patients than any other form of treatment.[2,3]

Surgical oncology is not just the physical act of cutting out a mass lesion, it emphasizes oncologic knowledge and a state of mind, with a goal to create the most effective treatment plan tailored to the disease, the patient comorbidities and quality of life, and the overarching goals of the client. To practice good surgical oncology, more than just surgical skills are needed, including an understanding of tumor biology and pathophysiology, an understanding of how other oncologic treatment options interact and complement each other (**Fig. 1**), and an understanding how preoperative, intraoperative, and postoperative decision making can impact patient outcome. Approaching the problem holistically, with the idea that the whole is more than the sum of its parts, generally improves patient outcomes and client satisfaction.

Surgical approaches to cancer generally work best in cases in which the disease is locoregional, or limited to a specific area (eg, a solitary mass, or a solitary mass and local lymph node metastasis but without systemic metastasis) (**Box 1**). It can be difficult to know where to start in surgical planning, but a clear differential diagnosis list based on an understanding of the types of tumors common to the species being treated is important. Optimizing a plan incorporates the understood biologic behavior for each of these differential diagnoses, the disease location, the disease extent, patient lifestyle and comorbidities, treatment alternatives, and expected prognosis. Depending on the differential diagnoses identified and their prioritization, workup may start with either imaging or tissue sampling.

Box 1
General principles for treatment of locoregional disease

1. Cancer is confined to an organ or area. If disseminated disease exists, regional therapy may still be indicated if it provides palliative relief for specific clinical signs (eg, cessation of hemorrhage, relief of obstruction), but in this case, veterinarians should be clear in the overall treatment goal.

2. There must be a therapeutic advantage of locoregional therapy over less invasive systemic therapy. There is likely no benefit to locoregional treatments if systemic therapy is efficacious and well tolerated (eg, lymphoma).

3. The proposed treatment should be technically feasible with minimal complications and/or acceptable risks.

IMAGING FOR SURGICAL PLANNING

Imaging for surgical planning should generally be performed before any sampling procedures to avoid artifact (eg, hemorrhage, gas introduced into the tissues) that may inhibit interpretation of results. Advanced imaging modalities, such as computed tomography (CT) and MRI, often provide improved diagnosis and characterization of small-volume disease and offer assistance in surgical planning, especially in anatomically challenging locations. After planning imaging, image-guided sampling can be performed (**Fig. 2**).

PREOPERATIVE SAMPLING

To optimize decisions about an overall treatment plan, including surgical dose, it is important to understand what fundamental tissue type is present so as to estimate biologic behavior of a mass, as the type or extent of treatment is generally determined by tumor type. The least invasive method of obtaining this information is often by cytologic evaluation. Samples of cells for staining and cytology often are obtained by fine-needle aspiration, or by impression smears. Sampling in this manner has few direct patient risks, although risks of needle tract contamination with neoplastic cells are possible,[4] and the direction from which the mass is sampled should ideally allow for en bloc resection of the tract along with the primary mass. As minimally invasive methods, such as fine-needle aspiration or impression smears, may result in samples of low cellularity, clients should be warned that samples may be nondiagnostic, that other factors including that processing artifacts may limit diagnosis, and that information that may impact future recommendations, such as tumor grade, is not estimable by cytologic evaluation. However, when a diagnostic sample can be attained, overall sensitivity and specificity of cytology for differentiating among inflammatory, benign

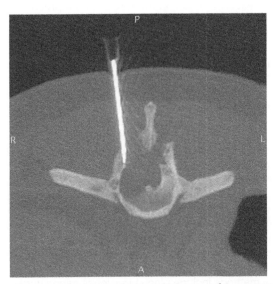

Fig. 2. Transverse maximum intensity projection CT image of an aggressive lesion of the thoracic spine of a dog ultimately diagnosed with metastatic pulmonary carcinoma. A needle was placed into the region of bone lysis with CT guidance to obtain a tissue sample for cytology. (*Courtesy of* Dr Allison Zwingenberger, University of California-Davis.)

neoplastic, and malignant neoplastic lesions is high,[5-7] and often identifies the class of tumor (epithelial vs mesenchymal), if not the specific tumor type.

Alternatively, if sufficient information to inform an overall treatment plan cannot be obtained from cytologic analysis, preoperative biopsy may be indicated. This is important for types of tumors in which identification of tumor grade impacts recommendations for staging diagnostics or extent of surgery. Additionally, if the client's willingness to consider expensive or potentially complicated surgery may be affected by the diagnosis, the prognosis associated with different tumor types, or the likelihood of aggressive biologic behavior within a given tumor type as estimated by tumor grade, then preoperative biopsy may be important.

When considering preoperative biopsy, practitioners must decide between an incisional or excisional biopsy. Excisional biopsy, in which all of the bulky disease is resected, may offer the potential for both diagnosis and cure depending on whether the lesion ultimately is determined to be benign or malignant in origin, and factors involved in the decision often include the size and location of the mass. But if histologic results are ultimately not what were expected, it is important to be aware that a poorly planned surgical approach associated with an excisional biopsy may negatively impact follow-up treatment. Once an excision has been performed, the local anatomy is significantly altered, and surgical invasion without sufficient surgical margins may provide the opportunity for residual tumor cells left behind to extend deeper and wider into tissues.[2] Although on first glance, an excisional biopsy may seem most straightforward, unless the tumor type is known at the time of the surgical procedure, the success of the excision and the long-term outcome of the patient may be compromised by doing too little or too much surgery.[2] If the tumor type is not known, large margins would be likely to cause patient morbidity, or excisional biopsy is likely to compromise future treatment, it is recommended to start with an incisional biopsy.

When an incisional biopsy procedure is planned, it is recommended to perform any imaging before excision. It is important to plan the procedure and ensure that the biopsy tract may be removed at a future surgery if necessary (eg, biopsy of oral masses should be performed via the oral cavity and not by an approach through the skin, as the definitive surgical approach will most likely occur from an oral approach). Practitioners should ensure that the biopsy incision orientation would not prohibit wound closure, or prevent future surgery or radiation therapy if indicated. Techniques to avoid nondiagnostic pathology should be emphasized, including obtaining sufficient sample volume, submitting all samples obtained, ensuring appropriate sample fixation, and minimizing pathologic artifact associated with trauma to the sample (eg, caused by instrument crush, electrocautery, or inappropriate tissue handling). A biopsy procedure in advance of a definitive surgical procedure may be contraindicated if the biopsy procedure itself is excessively difficult, dangerous, or requires essentially the same approach as the definitive procedure. For example, biopsy of a lung mass often requires an approach to the chest or is dangerous from a percutaneous/image-guided approach due to the proximity of neurovascular structures or risk of pneumothorax. So, in the case of a pulmonary mass lesion, if aspiration cytology is impractical, unsafe, or nondiagnostic, it is generally recommended to proceed directly to a definitive surgical excision rather than a biopsy procedure.

Incisional biopsy methods include pinch biopsies obtained under camera guidance (flexible or rigid endoscopy), percutaneous methods under image guidance (ultrasound, fluoroscopic, or CT-guided sampling using percutaneous biopsy instruments) (**Fig. 3**), punch biopsy (**Fig. 4**), wedge biopsy, or bone biopsy instruments (eg,

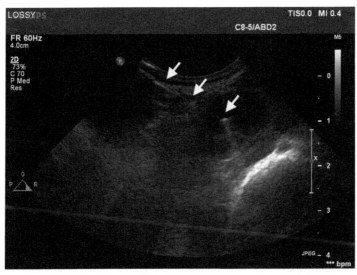

Fig. 3. Percutaneous ultrasound-guided biopsy using a commercial biopsy instrument. White arrows show the linear biopsy instrument placed to obtain a tissue sample for histopathology. (*Courtesy of* Dr Rachel Pollard, University of California-Davis.)

Jamshidi needle for smaller patients, or Michelle trephine for larger patients). In general, the instrument/method chosen should be tailored to each patient based on lesion location, patient size, and sample desired.

If a smaller biopsy instrument is chosen, it is generally recommended to obtain multiple biopsy samples from the lesion so as to obtain the greatest likelihood of obtaining a representative sample. It is recommended to avoid excessively soft/necrotic areas, which are likely to be nondiagnostic; at the same time, it is important to ensure that

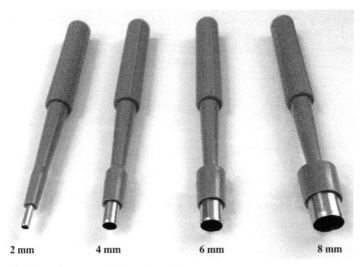

| 2 mm | 4 mm | 6 mm | 8 mm |

Fig. 4. Punch biopsy instruments in various sizes.

sampling is done deep enough that more than just the fibrous pseudocapsule is obtained. In general, for soft tissue biopsy samples, samples that include tissue near the palpable margin of the mass are useful to provide information on the microscopic margin where the neoplastic cells interact with normal tissues, although practitioners should take care not to extend dissection into uninvolved tissues that may allow seeding/extension of tumor cells. For bone biopsy, as a reactive zone of bone often exists at the periphery of most neoplastic bone lesions, biopsy techniques that include tissue from the center of the lesion are recommended to increase the likelihood that a diagnostic sample is obtained.[2]

SURGICAL DOSE

Like other oncologic treatments, surgery as a treatment for cancer also can be conceptualized as being applied in different doses. Surgical dose is optimally decided by incorporating information on tumor type, tumor grade, and tumor stage, and should be carefully evaluated and chosen before initiation of a definitive surgical procedure. Surgical dose is commonly described as curative intent (either wide excision in which a cuff of normal-appearing tissue is excised en bloc with the tumor and the pseudocapsule or reactive zone is not visualized, or radical excision in which the entire anatomic compartment in which the tumor is located is removed) or cytoreductive excision (sometimes described as marginal excision, which can lead to confusion, in which dissection is performed very close to the tumor pseudocapsule) and depends on the overall treatment plan for the patient.

DETERMINING THE ROLE OF SURGERY FOR A GIVEN PATIENT
Palliative Treatment Plans

If the determined overall treatment plan is palliative, when determining if there is a role for surgery, consider whether cytoreductive surgery would benefit the patient (**Box 2**). Would a surgical procedure improve function or reduce discomfort? As a general rule, palliative treatment plans do not impact systemic disease progression. Primary goals of palliative surgical procedures are to improve the patient's quality of life, and careful evaluation of the morbidity and/or complications of the procedure relative to the existing pain/dysfunction of the disease and the anticipated duration of relief expected from the procedure should be considered. Palliative surgery may be directed at the tumor itself, or as a bypass for functional problems. Although palliative procedures may be of real benefit to the patient, it is important that the intended goals and outcomes of the procedure are clearly communicated to the client.

Box 2
Examples of palliative procedures

- Amputation of a limb for an osteosarcoma lesion in which adjuvant chemotherapy is not planned: In this instance, although amputation alone will not greatly prolong the progression of systemic spread of this tumor and overall life span; management of focal pain and improved quality of life is provided by removal of the limb.

- Surgical debulking of a tumor causing hypercalcemia of malignancy in which complete lesion excision is not possible: In this instance, although it is anticipated that tumor recurrence and progression will occur, morbidity and management challenges associated with the secondary effects of the hypercalcemia are reduced.

- Nodulectomy combined with partial pancreatectomy for treatment of insulinoma in ferrets: This approach has demonstrated improved survival over nodulectomy alone.[43] Although surgical cure is unlikely in this scenario, as removal of the entire pancreas is not a realistic option, it is likely that the more aggressive surgical approach of partial pancreatectomy is removing undiagnosed low volume disease, and because this undiagnosed disease has a functional impact (insulin secretion), further reduction of disease burden results in improved disease-free intervals and survivals.

- Placement of a gastrointestinal feeding tube to bypass an obstructive upper gastrointestinal mass: The growth or spread of the primary disease is not impacted, but quality of life is improved by the ability to provide nutrition.

- Placement of a stent to alleviate pressure from an obstructive mass and restore luminal patency in neoplasms impacting major vessels or the gastrointestinal, urinary, or respiratory tracts (**Fig. 5**).

- Placement of a subcutaneous pleural port (**Fig. 6**) to allow for removal of recurrent malignant effusions that may be inhibiting normal physiologic function and quality of life. Subcutaneous port systems are available commercially[44] or may be customized using commonly available components.[45]

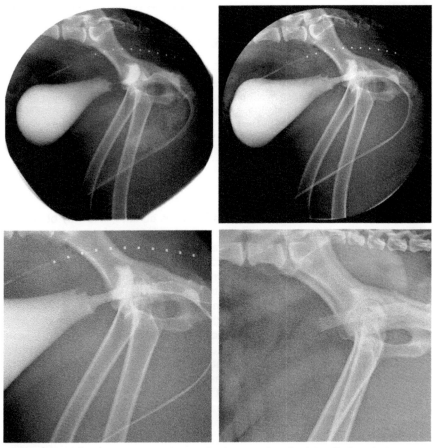

Fig. 5. Radiographic appearance of a urethral stent placed minimally invasively so as to palliate nearly complete urethral obstruction associated with lower urinary tract transitional cell carcinoma.

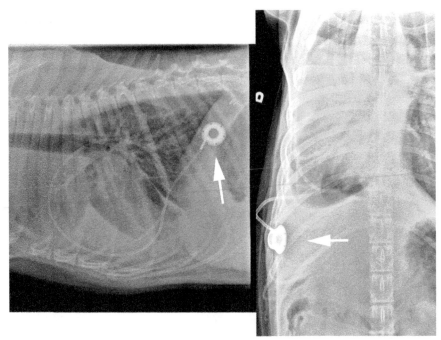

Fig. 6. Radiographic (lateral and dorso-ventral projections) appearance of a pleural port placed to allow long-term management of a malignant effusion. A soft fenestrated catheter allows increased surface area for drainage within the chest and connects to a subcutaneous port (*white arrow*). Special Huber needles always must be used to access the subcutaneous port to avoid damaging the silicone diaphragm, and sterile preparation of the skin is important to minimize risk of introducing infectious organisms into the implants.

Curative Intent Treatment Plans

If overall plan for treatment of a focal mass lesion is curative, this may be accomplished by a curative intent surgical procedure alone, or for some tumors, by a combination of cytoreductive surgery and adjuvant treatment, such as radiation. However, veterinarians should be clear on their surgical goals before taking the patient to surgery, as a well-planned cytoreductive surgery and adjuvant therapy combination has much more likelihood of optimizing patient outcome than a poorly planned excisional biopsy in which adjuvant therapy is applied as an afterthought.

In general, the goal of curative intent surgical excision is to attempt cure of the disease by surgery alone. The tumor is excised "en bloc" with a margin of normal tissue around it (see **Fig. 8**). Dissection near, and even visualization of, a tumor pseudocapsule is avoided. In general, if it is thought that curative intent surgical excision is possible, it is usually the first choice for management of focal mass lesions. It is important to avoid "peeling off" or "shelling out" tumors if the plan is for curative intent surgery.

Determining the appropriate operative margin for a given tumor remains a challenge in veterinary medicine. Given the variability in biologic behavior of various neoplasms, patient anatomic differences, and patient size differences, it is difficult to make "one-size-fits-all" recommendations for an operative surgical margin. Objective data on surgical margins and outcome to allow for informed, evidence-based recommendations is currently lacking for most neoplasms in most exotic species. As a rule of thumb, benign tumors or malignant tumor types that tend to be more microscopically localized and circumscribed (eg, carcinomas) generally do not require surgical margins as extensive as tumor types that tend to exhibit characteristics of microscopic local invasion (eg, sarcomas, mast cell tumors). Although the exact measurements for the desired margins may vary, the concepts of en bloc excisions and fascial planes as barriers to local tumor invasion are important principles of surgical oncology.

In the case of an aggressive treatment plan that encompasses cytoreductive surgery and adjuvant therapy, such as radiation, the surgical goal is to remove bulky disease and maximize the response to adjuvant therapies (chemotherapy, radiation therapy) that work best on microscopic disease while minimizing side effects that might limit those therapies. In general, cytoreductive surgery is chosen when (1) results, complications, or patient morbidities of a curative intent surgical procedure are likely to be unacceptable; (2) adjuvant therapies are available, and (3) adjuvant therapies are likely to have positive therapeutic impacts on the type of tumor being treated. No matter how well intentioned, a cytoreductive surgery plus adjuvant therapy plan would obviously not be optimal in situations in which the adjuvant therapy is not available, or if it is unlikely to be efficacious on the specific neoplasm, and it is important to have clear conversations about goals, plans for follow-up therapies, and anticipated outcomes with clients before the procedure. If adjuvant therapy is not an option because of client factors, it might be better overall to start with a different surgical or nonsurgical plan.

The first attempt at curative intent surgery usually has the best chance of success.[8] The surgical procedure is often easier for the surgeon, as the surgical anatomy is more normal, tissue planes are undisrupted, and less fibrous scar tissue is likely to be encountered. Conceptually, the tumor has less time to metastasize if all tumor is removed at the first surgery than if residual disease is left behind. Additionally, the center of a larger tumor may be a more hypoxic environment, less metabolically active, and more likely to be necrotic. The cells at the leading edge of a mass are more likely to be better vascularized and actively growing, and it is these cells that remain with a marginal excision. In general, surgical technique for a curative intent surgery should include planning of margins in advance with exact margin dimensions based on the best level of knowledge available regarding the tumor biology of the lesion in question. Margin planning should ensure that any previous biopsy tracts may be excised en bloc with the tumor and adhesions should be removed if present.[2] Good surgical technique, including early vascular ligation, gentle tissue handling, and minimization of seroma/hematoma formation is important. Sharp dissection is preferred over blunt dissection, as this will decrease the risk of straying from the planned margin and potentially leaving neoplastic cells in the patient.[2] The use of drains should be carefully considered. On one hand, it is better not to place drains if dead space can be adequately reconstructed by other means; however, if drain placement is unavoidable, ensure the drain tract location does not compromise further treatment (adjuvant radiation therapy or reexcision of scar if histopathology indicates incomplete margins). It is recommended to use new surgical instruments and change to clean gloves between tumor excision and wound closure and for each tumor site (if multiple separate excisions are planned). Inability to fully close the surgical wound in the case of larger masses and/or difficult locations should not be a blanket impediment to considering curative intent surgery, as depending on the tumor biology, the surgical wound may be allowed to heal by second intention, and as long as adequate margins have been achieved, long-term outcome can be good.[9] In general, it is better to manage a wound and/or consider delayed primary closure or a graft than to leave disease behind[10]; however, careful preoperative discussion with the owner is recommended for this approach.

DEFINING OPERATIVE MARGINS AT SURGERY

The topic of operative surgical margins is a difficult one to quantitate, and is an area that our physician counterparts struggle with as well. Overall surgical margin recommendations are based on retrospective analysis of operative margins and patient outcomes in historical populations, and these data are seriously lacking for most exotics. How best to apply this historical population data to an individual tumor resection is an evolving question in all species receiving surgical treatment of mass lesions, including humans. In general, tumors with a higher risk of microscopic local extension (eg, many soft tissue sarcomas, grade II or grade III mast cell tumors) require a more extensive surgical margin and a successful deep resection is usually accomplished by taking one fascial plane under the tumor. Tumors with less risk of microscopic local extension (eg, many carcinomas) generally do not require as extensive a resection margin. Although the resection margin is not as extensive, en bloc removal of some normal tissue surrounding the mass is still recommended and dissection at the mass pseudocapsule itself should be avoided. Overall, en bloc excisions should include as much tissue as needed to remove all cancer so as to prevent local recurrence; the problem rests in how to make this judgment at surgery. General rules of thumb inform current practice, but there is much debate about how these "rules" should be adapted for particularly small patients, or unclear anatomic barriers in which a tissue type changes from one compartment to another without a clear fascial plane. In general, in dogs, a 2-cm to 3-cm lateral margin and one fascial plane deep margin is generally recommended for tumors with higher risk of microscopic local extension (**Fig. 7**), and a 1-cm margin is generally recommended for tumors with lower risk of microscopic local extension.[9,11–14] Alternatively, a modified proportional margins approach has been proposed in which lateral tumor margins are equivalent to the largest diameter of the tumor.[15] Tumor grade and histologic margin status are important factors in making follow-up recommendations to clients, as lower grade tumors often have a much lower rate of local recurrence than higher-grade tumors, even with incomplete or close

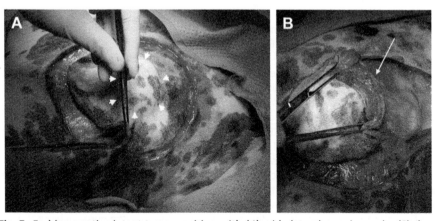

Fig. 7. En bloc curative intent tumor excision with (*A*) wide lateral margins and a (*B*) deep margin that includes a fascial or muscular plane (*arrow*). Arrowheads identify the palpable tumor margin. Notice that the tumor surface/pseudocapsule is never actually visualized during dissection.

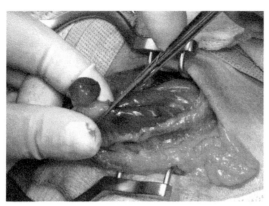

Fig. 8. Gastric leiomyoma resection in a guinea pig. Although ideal operative margins are not known for this tumor in this species, because a mesenchymal tumor was suspected, a full-thickness gastric resection was elected with 1-cm lateral margins.

histologic margins.[16,17] On the other hand, there is good evidence that even larger margins may be needed to obtain local control of certain tumors with very aggressive biologic behavior and a high risk of microscopic local extension, such as injection-site sarcomas in cats.[18] Therefore, if smaller surgical margins are elected due to anatomic

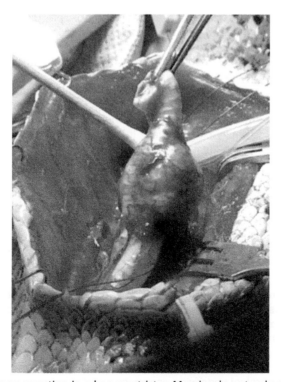

Fig. 9. Tracheal mass resection in a boa constrictor. Margins do not only apply to skin and subcutaneous masses. In tubular structures (gastrointestinal, respiratory, urinary tracts), margins along the length of the organ should be considered.

or other factors for tumor types that are prone to local extension, it becomes especially important to discuss the potential impacts with clients in advance, and to execute a surgical plan that will not preclude follow-up therapy if desired. It is for this reason that preoperative biopsy can be quite important in optimizing a surgical plan. The concepts of surgical margins also apply to neoplasms in locations other than the skin (**Figs. 8** and **9**). A survey of cases of squamous cell carcinoma in birds reported an odds ratio of 7.48 for complete or partial response to therapy if that patient received a complete surgical excision, and no other treatment category had a significant odds ratio, indicating the importance of complete surgical excision for this disease.[19] Although complete excision is clearly important, overall, there are few data regarding the specifics of recommended margins for successful local tumor excisions in a range of tumor types and grades in exotic species, and much work remains to be done in this area.

RECONSTRUCTION

Other important aspects of surgical planning for curative intent surgical procedures, or cytoreductive surgical procedures in which adjuvant treatment is planned, include plans for reconstruction. Curative intent surgical resections can be quite extensive and leave a large, difficult to reconstruct defect. In general, if the operating surgeon believes that a surgical cure is possible, it is better to be more aggressive and manage a wound than to leave cancer behind. However, the need for wound management in this eventuality should be discussed with the client in advance, and the treatment plan modified in the event that this is not feasible. When possible, direct appositional primary closure of the wound bed is often simplest and most desirable. Vascularized skin flaps may be desirable in areas of high tension, motion, or where adjuvant radiation therapy is planned. It is important to communicate clearly with any medical and radiation oncologists who may be collaborating on a patient's care regarding the use and timing of skin flaps. If surgical cure is possible but good options for vascularized flaps do not exist, and adjuvant radiation therapy is not a treatment option, the resection site may be managed as an open wound and allowed to heal by second intention or delayed primary closure later.[9] It is important to minimize the chance of transfer of neoplastic cells during wound reconstruction, and changing gloves and/ or using new instruments for wound closure than were used for mass resection may be recommended.

Primary reconstruction is preferred when possible, especially when adjuvant treatment is planned, as delays in healing may delay onset of adjuvant therapy, allowing tumor regrowth to occur. Once tumor regrowth is visible or palpable, adjuvant treatment is less efficacious. Minimizing dead space and avoiding seroma formation is important in this context; conversely, placement of a drain in a tumor excision bed may not be optimal and pros and cons of this decision should be weighed. Drains always should be exited through the subcutaneous tissue and skin such that the drain tract may be included in a surgical reexcision or radiation field if necessary. Considering tension lines may facilitate wound closure after large mass excisions; however, if postoperative radiation therapy is being considered, it is important to communicate with a radiation oncologist about how a radiation plan might impact surgical incisions. For example, a vertically oriented surgical scar over the thoracic wall may be easier to close with less tension, but this orientation may preclude an optimized radiation plan due to the need to protect underlying viscera, such as the lungs. In some cases, a horizontally oriented scar may be more useful. Similarly, a proximo-distally longitudinally oriented incision on an extremity is likely to be more amenable to postoperative radiation than an incision that is more oblique or circumferentially oriented around the limb due to the need to exclude some skin from the radiation margins so as to preserve adequate lymphatic drainage. The use of hemoclips is useful to differentiate visible scars associated with the tumor resection site from scars associated with mobilization of a skin flap, and helps to minimize radiation field planning.[20]

MARGIN MARKING AND COMMUNICATING WITH YOUR PATHOLOGIST

In general, no matter what the tumor type, communication with the evaluating pathologist about the histologic evaluation of surgical margins is important information.[11,21,22] This may be facilitated by tumor marking systems so as to communicate information about where a cut edge was located at the time of excision, or relative tissue depths. Although a number of methods may be used, the Davidson Marking System (IMEB Inc, San Diego, CA), which is sold as a set of formalin-stable inks in 5 to 7 colors, is an inexpensive and simple method that provides clear delineation of a cut edge (**Fig. 10**). However, without attention it is also easy to ink inappropriate tissues that do not convey margin information, which can be confusing to the interpreting pathologist and can impact the results received, so care should be taken when applying inks and subsequently handling the sample. Black, blue, and yellow are reported to be the best colors to use.[23] If margins are incomplete or close, based on histopathological evaluation, additional local excision

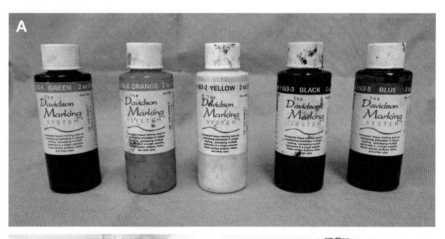

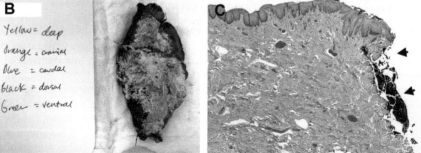

Fig. 10. (*A*) Davidson Marking System inks. (*B*) Tissue specimen with margins marked. (*C*) Histologic image demonstrating the microscopic appearance of a formalin-stable ink at the tumor resection margin (*arrowheads*). (Part [C] *Courtesy of* Dr Verena Affolter, University of California-Davis.)

with either primary tumor site/scar reexcision or radiation therapy has been shown to improve local control and overall survival.[24,25]

It is important to place tissue samples in fixative as soon as possible to prevent drying and artifact. If margin inking is to be done, this should be performed before placement of the sample in fixative. If this cannot be accomplished immediately (eg, the surgeon must focus first on closing the surgical incision), the sample should be wrapped in moist gauze and carefully preserved. Buffered formalin (10%) is commonly used in veterinary medicine as a fixative, and a biopsy should be placed in a 1:10 volume of fixative (tissue volume:fluid volume).[2]

One challenge in surgical planning and subsequent interpretation of histologic margins is that significant shrinkage of tissue has been documented after excision in specimens from dogs and cats.[26–30] However similar species-specific data are lacking in avian, reptile, and other exotic species. Canine skin-muscle-fascia specimens significantly decrease in size from gross preexcision dimensions after removal.[27] Suturing the specimen during surgery before excision will significantly improve alignment of tissue planes without creating distortion of the sample, but may alter the length, width, and lateral margins of the specimen.[27] As a result of tissue shrinkage, the surgeon should be aware that histologic margins read out by the interpreting pathologist will be very different from those measured and physically executed by the surgeon at the operating table, and this will need to be taken into consideration when interpreting results. Histologic margins are commonly reported as complete (often colloquially described as "clean") in which no tumor is seen at a margin cut edge; narrow (or "close"), which are still technically complete, but with tumor very near the cut edge (often only a few micrometers or a few cell layers away); or incomplete (often colloquially described as "dirty") in which tumor cells are seen at the margin cut edge. Further complicating interpretation, depending on the type of tumor, "close" or narrow margins may raise the concern that if the mass were sampled by the pathologist for sectioning in a slightly different location in the gross tissue specimen, microscopic margin assessment might have been positive. It is usually helpful to request a numerical measurement of distance of tumor from the cut edge of a histologic margin from the pathologist in making further treatment decisions. Other important information from a histopathology report used in making decisions about the need for further therapy and interpreting the potential biologic behavior, includes tumor type or subtype, tumor grade, presence of lymphatic or vascular invasion, and mitotic index.

TUMOR BED MARKING

Once an understanding of histologic margins has been obtained, this can be better translated to future therapeutic decision making if the tumor bed is also marked within the patient. This can be achieved, easily, inexpensively, and with low morbidity by placement of stainless steel surgical clips (**Fig. 11**) at the time of tumor resection.[20] It is important to place hemoclips in a manner such that the 3-dimensional extent of the tumor bed will be demonstrated even after closure; take care not to place clips such that, as the tissues are drawn together during wound reconstruction, the clips end up in a straight line at the wound center. In a prior study in dogs, there was a significant difference in radiation treatment field size when planned using information regarding the subcutaneous location of hemoclips in conjunction with the dermal surgical scar compared with radiation treatment field planning based on the dermal surgical scar alone.[20] This was most important in regions of looser skin (head, neck, trunk, perineum) compared with distal extremity tumors.[20]

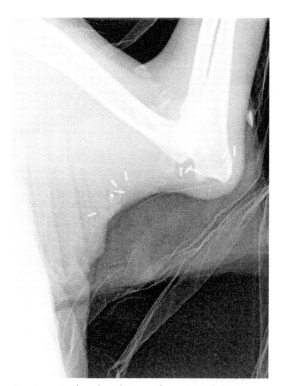

Fig. 11. Radiation treatment planning image demonstrating appearance of hemoclips placed to mark the site of tumor resection in anticipation of radiation planning. The tumor resection was primarily located in the axilla; however, hemoclips demonstrate to the radiation oncologist that the radiation field extends distal to the elbow. (*Courtesy of* Dr Katherine Hansen, University of California-Davis.)

PATIENT STAGING

Patient stage describes the spread of the tumor within the body (**Box 3**). Staging diagnostics may vary, including both imaging and sampling procedures, and may be done preoperatively or postoperatively relative to the primary tumor resection, depending on the anticipated biologic behavior of the tumor. Thoracic radiographs, and at times abdominal/coelomic ultrasound procedures, are commonly recommended, and identified lesions should be sampled with aspiration cytology or biopsy. Most commonly, the TNM system is used to describe the clinical extent of disease, and systemic and lymphatic tumor spread are differentiated. TNM descriptions differ for different types of tumor and are discussed elsewhere in greater detail for dogs and cats.[31–33] The lymphatic system is an important pathway for metastatic behavior of tumors with predisposition for spread, and should be carefully evaluated. Regional lymph nodes are the initial site of metastasis for many solid tumors. In canine oncology, in disease processes in which lymphatic metastasis is common (eg, carcinomas, oral melanomas, mast cell tumors), obtaining histopathology of the relevant lymph nodes may be prognostic and help to direct future therapeutic recommendations. Relevant disease and species-specific data in this area are lacking for most exotic patients, and species-specific differences in anatomy are important to consider: birds and reptiles do not have lymphatic tissue organized in the same way

---

Box 3
TNM system: general concepts

Primary Tumor

Tumor is assigned a numerical stage of T0, T1, T2, and so forth, related to a variety of tumor-specific factors (eg, size, level of clinical infiltration, evidence of local invasion).

Lymph Node

Patient is assigned a numerical stage of N0, N1, N2, or N3 related to level of tumor involvement in regional lymph nodes.

Systemic Metastasis

Patient is assigned a numerical stage of M0 (no evidence of metastasis), M1 (metastasis to one organ system), or M2 (metastasis to more than one organ system).

---

as mammalian species. Neoplastic masses in fish, including those that exhibit phenotypic characteristics of malignancy and might be more expected to metastasize, rarely exhibit metastatic behavior, and this may be associated with a variety of factors, including anatomic and physiologic differences in the lymphatic system.[34] However, in exotic mammals, the principles of lymphatic metastasis are likely to remain the same, and veterinarians should take the potential for lymphatic metastasis into account where relevant. Historically, lymphatic sampling has often been limited to lymph nodes that are visibly or palpably enlarged; however, this is highly inaccurate for prediction of metastasis.[35]

Patient staging assessments made by imaging or aspiration cytology are frequently known as "clinical stage," whereas those made on the basis of biopsy of lymph nodes or remote tissues and subsequent histopathology results are termed "pathologic stage." Surgical lymph node sampling can be very useful; however, lymphatic drainage from a tumor can be highly unpredictable and it can be difficult to be certain that the correct lymph node is assessed.[36] A technique of identifying the first lymph node receiving afferent lymphatics from a tumor margin (the sentinel lymph node) is used with increasing frequency in human and veterinary oncology. In people, this most commonly involves the use of lymphoscintigraphy in combination with visible blue dyes; however, lymphoscintigraphy is not widely available in veterinary medicine due to costs and regulatory challenges of working with radioactive injectable tracers. Other methods of sentinel lymph node identification are being studied in veterinary patients and it is likely that validated alternatives for this technique will be more widely available to veterinarians in the near future.

INTERVENTIONAL ONCOLOGY

Interventional oncologic procedures are a heterogeneous group of minimally invasive treatments that are performed under some form of imaging guidance, either through natural orifices or percutaneously through small incisions (**Box 4**). Very little outcome information is available on the use of these treatments for cancer in exotic species at this time, although a few case reports on the use of interventional techniques in exotic species exist.[37–42] In general, surgery almost always remains the optimal choice for treatment of local disease, but in cases in which surgery is not be possible, or the anticipated morbidity of the procedure may be too high, interventional procedures may provide options for improving duration and/or quality of life. At this time,

---

Box 4
Interventional oncology

- Transarterial bland embolization (TAE)
  - Occlusion of the arterial blood supply to a tumor by highly selective arterial catheterization and injection of small particles
- Intra-arterial chemotherapy
  - Direct delivery of a chemotherapeutic agent by highly selective arterial catheterization
- Transarterial chemoembolization (TACE)
  - Combination of particle embolization and arterial chemotherapy
- Palliative stenting of a malignant obstruction
  - Biliary tract
  - Gastrointestinal tract
  - Respiratory tract
  - Urinary tract (see **Fig. 5**)
  - Vascular obstructions
- Percutaneous thermal tumor ablation
  - Radiofrequency ablation
  - Microwave ablation
  - High-intensity focused ultrasound
  - Cryoablation (**Fig. 12**)
- Percutaneous drainage catheter placement in the management of malignant effusions[46]

---

interventional procedures remain mostly palliative, but they may provide benefit in ameliorating clinical signs. As with surgery, the costs, risks, and benefits of each interventional procedure should be weighed against the anticipated course of the disease, patient systemic health, client goals, and finances.

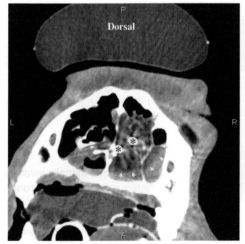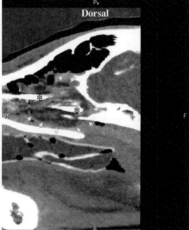

Fig. 12. CT-guided transnare cryoablation in a dog with a nasal tumor. Transverse slice and longitudinally reconstructed view of the skull. The 2 cryoprobes are indicated with a red asterisk. The extent of the iceball may be seen as hypodense relative to surrounding tissues (*yellow arrowheads*) and the treatment field can be monitored during the procedure.

SUMMARY

A wide variety of options exist for today's veterinary practitioner in the treatment of cancer, and this area continues to evolve rapidly. Surgical excision remains pivotal in cancer treatment, although optimal outcomes are achieved when the disease is approached with a thorough diagnostic and therapeutic plan. Treatment goals, whether curative intent or palliative intent, should be identified before surgery, and important oncologic surgical principles should be adhered to so as to attain the best outcome.

REFERENCES

1. Garner MM, Hernandez-Diver SM, Raymond JT. Reptile neoplasia: a retrospective study of case submissions to a specialty diagnostic service. Vet Clin North Am Exot Anim Pract 2004;7:653–71.
2. Ehrhart N, Culp WTN. Principles of surgical oncology. In: Kudnig ST, Seguin B, editors. Veterinary surgical oncology. Ames (IA): Wiley-Blackwell; 2012. p. 3–13.
3. Gilson SD, Stone EA. Management of the surgical oncology patient. Compend Contin Educ Pract Vet 1990;12:1047–105.
4. Nyland TG, Wallack ST, Wisner ER. Needle tract implantation following US-guided fine needle aspiration biopsy of transitional cell carcinoma of the bladder, urethra, and prostate. Vet Radiol Ultrasound 2002;43:50–3.
5. Eich CS, Whitehair JG, Moroff SD, et al. The accuracy of intraoperative cytopathological diagnosis compared with conventional histopathological diagnosis. J Am Anim Hosp Assoc 2000;36:16–8.
6. Cohen M, Bohling MW, Wright JC, et al. Evaluation of sensitivity and specificity of cytologic examination: 269 cases (1999-2000). J Am Vet Med Assoc 2003;222: 964–7.
7. Ghisleni G, Roccabianca P, Ceruti R, et al. Correlation between fine needle aspiration cytology and histopathology in the evaluation of cutaneous and subcutaneous masses from dogs and cats. Vet Clin Pathol 2006;35:24–30.
8. Vail D, Withrow S. Tumors of the skin and subcutaneous tissues. In: Withrow S, Vail D, editors. Small animal clinical oncology. 4th edition. St Louis (MO): Saunders; 2007. p. 375–401.
9. Prpich CY, Santamaria AC, Simcock JO, et al. Second intention healing after wide local excision of soft tissue sarcomas in the distal aspects of the limbs in dogs: 31 cases (2005-2012). J Am Vet Med Assoc 2014;244(2):187–94.
10. Withrow SJ. Surgical oncology: old and new ideas. Semin Vet Med Surg (small Anim) 1986;1:17–20.
11. Scarpa F, Sabattini S, Marconato L, et al. Use of hisotologic margin to predict recurrence of cutaneous malignant tumors in dogs and cats after surgical excision. J Am Vet Med Assoc 2012;240(10):1181–7.
12. Kuntz CA, Dernell WS, Powers BE, et al. Prognostic factors for surgical treatment of soft-tissue sarcomas in dogs: 75 cases (1986-1996). J Am Vet Med Assoc 1997;211(9):1147–51.
13. Fulcher RP, Ludwig LL, Bergman PJ, et al. Evaluation of a two-centimeter lateral surgical margin for excision of grade I and grade II cutaneous mast cell tumors in dogs. J Am Vet Med Assoc 2006;228(2):210–5.
14. Simpson AM, Ludwig LL, Newman SJ, et al. Evaluation of surgical margins required for complete excision of cutaneous mast cell tumors in dogs. J Am Vet Med Assoc 2004;224(2):236–40.

15. Pratschke KM, Atherton MJ, Sillito JA, et al. Evaluation of a modified proportional margins approach for surgical resection of mast cell tumors in dogs: 40 cases (2008-2012). J Am Vet Med Assoc 2013;243(10):1436–41.

16. Stefanello D, Morello E, Roccabianca P, et al. Marginal excision of low-grade spindle cell sarcoma of canine extremities: 35 dogs (1996-2006). Vet Surg 2008;37(5):461–5.

17. Schultheiss PC, Gardiner DW, Sangeeta Rao, et al. Association of histologic tumor characteristics and size of surgical margins with clinical outcome after surgical removal of cutaneous mast cell tumors in dogs. J Am Vet Med Assoc 2011; 238(11):1464–9.

18. Phelps HA, Kuntz CA, Milner RJ, et al. Radical excision with five-centimeter margins for treatment of feline injection-site sarcomas: 91 cases (1998-2002). J Am Vet Med Assoc 2011;239(1):97–106.

19. Zehnder A, Swift L, Sundaram A, et al. Multi-institutional survey of squamous cell carcinoma in birds. New Orleans: Proc Assoc Avian Vet; 2014. p. 3.

20. McEntee MC, Steffey MA, Dykes NL. Use of surgical hemoclips in radiation treatment planning. Vet Radiol Ultrasound 2008;49(4):395–9.

21. Donnelly L, Mullin C, Balko J, et al. Evaluation of histological grade and histologically tumour-free margins as predictors of local recurrence in completely excised canine mast cell tumours. Vet Comp Oncol 2015;13(1):70–6.

22. McSporran KD. Histologic grade predicts recurrence for marginally excised canine subcutaneous soft tissue sarcomas. Vet Pathol 2009;46(5):928–33.

23. Seitz SE, Foley GL, Maretta SM. Evaluation of marking materials for cutaneous surgical margins. Am J Vet Res 1995;56:826–33.

24. Kryl KL, Boston SE. Additional local therapy with primary re-excision or radiation therapy improves survival and local control after incomplete or close surgical excision of mast cell tumors in dogs. Vet Surg 2014;43(2):182–9.

25. Bacon NJ, Dernell WS, Ehrhart N, et al. Evaluaiton of primary re-excision after recent inadequate resection of soft tissue sarcomas in dogs: 41 cases (1999-2004). J Am Vet Med Assoc 2007;230(4):548–54.

26. RIsselada M, Matthews KG, Griffith E. Surgically planned versus histologically measured lateral tumor margins for resection of cutaneous and subcutaneous mast cell tumors in dogs: 46 cases (2010-2013). J Am Vet Med Assoc 2015; 247(2):184–9.

27. Risselada M, Matthews KG, Griffith E. The effect of specimen preparation on post-excision and post-fixation dimensions, translation, and distortion of canine cadaver skin-muscle-fascia specimen [early view]. Vet Surg 2016;45(5):563–70.

28. Sakthilia J, Smith AN, Schleis SE, et al. Effect of histologic processing on dimensions of skin samples obtained from cat cadavers. Am J Vet Res 2015;76(11): 939–45.

29. Miller JL, Dark MJ. Evaluation of the effect of formalin fixation on skin specimens in dogs and cats. Peer J 2014;2:e307.

30. Upchurch DA, Malenfant RC, Wignall JR, et al. Effects of sample site and size, skin tension lines, surgeon, and formalin fixation on shrinkage of skin samples excised from canine cadavers. Am J Vet Res 2014;75(11):1004–9.

31. Ryan S, Wouters EGH, van Nimwegan S, et al. Skin and subcutaneous tumors. In: Kudnig ST, Seguin B, editors. Veterinary surgical oncology. Ames (IA): Wiley-Blackwell; 2012. p. 55–85.

32. Liptak JM, Lascelles BDX. Oral tumors. In: Kudnig ST, Seguin B, editors. Veterinary surgical oncology. Ames (IA): Wiley-Blackwell; 2012. p. 119–77.

33. Martano M, Boston S, Morello E, et al. Respiratory tract and thorax. In: Kudnig ST, Seguin B, editors. Veterinary surgical oncology. Ames (IA): Wiley-Blackwell; 2012. p. 273–328.
34. Groff JM. Neoplasia in fishes. Vet Clini North Am Exot Anim Pract 2004;7:705–56.
35. Williams LE, Packer RA. Association between lymph node size and metastasis in dogs with oral malignant melanoma: 100 cases (1987-2001). J Am Vet Med Assoc 2003;222:1234–6.
36. Worley DR. Incorporation of sentinel lymph node mapping in dogs with mast cell tumors: 20 consecutive procedures. Vet Comp Oncol 2014;12(3):215–26.
37. Mejia-Fava J, Holmes SP, Radlinsky M, et al. Use of a nitinol wire stent for management of severe tracheal stenosis in an eclectus parrot (Eclectus roratus). J Avian Med Surg 2015;29(3):238–49.
38. Delk KW, Wack RF, Burgdorf-Moisuk A, et al. Percutaneous ureteral stent placement for the treatment of a benign ureteral obstruction in a Sumatran tiger (Panthera tigris sumatrae). Zoo Biol 2015;34(2):193–7.
39. Dallwig RK, Langan JN, Hatch DA, et al. Bilateral hydronephrosis secondary to endometriosis managed by endoscopic ureteral stent placement in a captive Guinea baboon (Papio papio). J Zoo Wildl Med 2011;42(4):747–50.
40. Wojick KB, Berent AC, Weisse CW, et al. Extracorporeal shock wave lithotripsy and endoscopic ureteral stent placement in an Asian small-clowed otter (Aonyx cinerea) with nephrolithiasis. J Zoo Wildl Med 2015;46(2):345–9.
41. Ferrel ST, Marlar AB, Garner M, et al. Intralesional cisplatin chemotherapy and topical cryotherapy for the control of choanal squamous cell carcinoma in an African penguin (Spheniscus demersus). J Zoo Wildl Med 2006;37(4):539–41.
42. Weiss C. Cryosurgery of the ferret adrenal gland. Exot DVM 1999;1(5):27–8.
43. Weiss CA, Williams BH, Scott MV. Insulinoma in the ferret: clinical findings and treatment comparison of 66 cases. J Am Anim Hosp Assoc 1998;34(6):471–5.
44. Brooks AC, Hardie RJ. Use of the PleuralPort device for management of pleural effusion in six dogs and four cats. Vet Surg 2011;40(8):935–41.
45. Cahalane AK, Flanders JA, Steffey MA, et al. Use of vascular access ports with intrathoracic drains for treatment of pleural effusion in three dogs. J Am Vet Med Assoc 2007;230(4):527–31.
46. Valtolina C, Adamantos S. Evaluation of small-bore wire-guided chest drains for management of pleural space disease. J Small Anim Pract 2009;59(6):290–7.

Principles and Applications of Radiation Therapy in Exotic Animals

Michael S. Kent, MAS, DVM, DACVIM (Oncology), DACVR (Radiation Oncology)

KEYWORDS

- Radiation therapy • Radiotherapy • Avian • Rabbit • Reptile • Oncology
- Small mammal

KEY POINTS

- Radiation therapy is increasingly available and being used to treat cancer in exotic animals using both external beam radiotherapy and strontium-90.
- Conventional dosing and fractionation schemes used to treat birds based on mammalian data may be insufficient to get treatment responses.
- Thymoma in the rabbit is very responsive to radiation therapy as a sole therapy with rapid clinical response, robust tumor responses, and long reported survival times.

INTRODUCTION

Radiation therapy is an increasingly used tool in managing the veterinary patients with cancer.[1] Knowledge of outcomes and side effects in dogs and cats treated with radiation therapy has grown substantially over the past decades, but there is still very little published on the use of radiation as a treatment modality in exotic animals. What is not known about the use of radiation to treat cancer across this large range of species is more than is known. There are also particular challenges that clinicians face when treating exotic animals, including the need for repeated anesthetic episodes; accurately and precisely positioning the animals at each treatment; and treating what are often very small patients and using small field sizes, which can make dose calculation difficult and in some cases limits the ability to treat an individual animal.

Radiation can be used as a definitive therapy if the goal is to cure the patient, or can be used in a palliative setting if the goal is decrease clinical signs by shrinking a tumor or by directly controlling pain. When talking with owners it is important to make sure

Disclosure: The author has nothing to disclose.
Department of Surgical and Radiological Sciences, School of Veterinary Medicine, University of California, Davis, 2112 Tupper Hall, 1 Shields Avenue, Davis, CA 95616, USA
E-mail address: mskent@ucdavis.edu

that they understand what is being attempted. The goal of therapy affects the dosing and number of treatments (fractions) used in prescribing a dose (**Box 1**).

Radiation therapy works by damaging the DNA, causing cells to die when they try to divide or in some cases through apoptosis. This process means that gross tumors may not decrease in size right away and that even acute side effects can occur after finishing a course of radiotherapy.

Radiation is most commonly used as a localized therapy, although wide field irradiation has been used in multiple species for hematopoietic tumors. It is also a therapy that works best in the setting of microscopic disease, meaning that it is often used as an adjuvant therapy to surgery when there is an incomplete surgical margin. In cases in which a tumor is not resectable or when using it to treat very radioresponsive tumors that are small, it is sometimes used as a sole modality. Radiation is also used as a palliative treatment in the gross disease setting when a tumor has already metastasized, when a tumor is not resectable, when surgery is not practical or feasible, or if the owner declines surgery. Radiation therapy can also be used along with chemotherapy. Chemotherapy can either be given systemically or by intralesional injection. The goals of combining radiation with chemotherapy are to increase chances of local control and also to treat known or suspected metastasis.

Radiation dose is quantified as units of energy delivered per mass of tissue. The SI unit for radiation dose is the Gray (Gy), which is equal to 1 J/kg. An older term for dose is the rad, which is equal to 1 cGy. Radiation doses are often, except for plesiotherapy, fractionated, meaning that the dose is broken up into multiple sessions. Total dose and fractionation schedules depend on the goals of therapy, the tolerance of the normal tissues that are also irradiated, and to some degree the radiotherapy technique used.

This dose can be delivered in a single or multiple fractions, depending on the type of radiation being used and the goals of therapy. For linear accelerator–based radiotherapy, curative intent radiotherapy is usually fractionated into 12 to 20 fractions of 2.5 to 4 Gy/fraction in veterinary medicine. By using a lower dose per fraction a higher total dose can be delivered while decreasing the risk of late side effects. The exception to this is stereotactic radiosurgery, in which, in veterinary medicine, patients are often treated in 1 to 5 fractions of 8 to 15 Gy/fraction. Palliative protocols vary widely in total dose and fractionation scheme and the ideal fractionation is not known. Usually a smaller number of fractions, between 4 and 6, are given using higher doses of radiation (6–9 Gy/fraction) in each treatment. This approach increases the risk of late side effects, but, in patients unlikely to live more than 6 months because of their tumor or concurrent disease, it can be a very good option.

Before calculating a dose of radiation the clinician must decide on the volume of tissue to irradiate. In radiation therapy, several volumes have been defined. The gross

---

Box 1
Components of a radiation prescription

- Type/source of radiation
- Total dose
- Dose per fraction (treatment)
- Frequency of fractions (eg, daily, Monday-Wednesday-Friday, weekly)
- Volume of tissue to be irradiated

target volume (GTV) is the area of gross disease or area of manipulated tissue in the case of postoperative therapy. The clinical target volume (CTV) is the GTV plus the volume added to account for microscopic extension of disease, which requires an educated guess and is often based on the tumor type and anticipated behavior. The planning target volume (PTV) is the volume to which a radiation dose is prescribed and encompasses the CTV plus a margin in place for patient setup, treatment, and machine uncertainties.

There are several types of radiation therapy treatments available for use in veterinary medicine: teletherapy, plesiotherapy, brachytherapy, and systemic radiotherapy using radionucleotides. Teletherapy is radiation therapy delivered at a distance, usually using a linear accelerator, although in the past orthovoltage and cobalt-60 machines were used. Plesiotherapy is a type of radiotherapy in which a radioactive source is placed on the tumor, whereas in brachytherapy a radioactive source is either implanted into a tumor permanently by using seeds or temporarily using catheters and an afterloader device. Systemic radiotherapy involves a radiopharmaceutical being given to the patient with the idea that the tumor can be targeted. The most commonly used forms of radiotherapy to treat malignant tumors are teletherapy and plesiotherapy.

Linear accelerators work by accelerating electrons and directing them at a target to create photons. The photons in turn interact with the tissue they are directed at to create electrons, which cause ionization in the tumor. The photon beam can be shaped by using blocks and newer designed units have multileaf collimators that allow finer shaping of the beam. In general, the volume to be irradiated is placed at the isocenter of the machine, which is the point in space on which the radiation beam centers as the linear accelerator rotates around, allowing the tumor to be targeted from multiple angles. By dividing the dose into multiple beams that intersect at 1 point the dose to surrounding normal tissue can be decreased and a more homogeneous dose placed into the treatment volume.

Dose calculation can either be done by hand, in which in general a single point in the tumor is picked and the dose calculated, or, in cases in which there is normal tissue that needs to be spared or the shape to be treated is complex, computerized treatment planning can be done. In this case a computed tomography (CT) scan of the patient taken in the position to be treated can be imported into the software and a treatment plan developed. Other imaging modalities, such as MRI or PET, can then be merged onto the CT scan to allow better tumor delineation. CT scans are generally used to calculate dose because they allow the different densities of tissue in a patient to be accounted for in the dose calculation; this is called tissue heterogeneity correction. CT is also known to have better spatial resolution than MRI or PET scans. The dose is then displayed on the patient images and the plan can be optimized to deliver the maximum dose to the tumor while minimizing dose to the surrounding tissues. The software can also produce a dose-volume histogram, which shows the doses of radiation received by varying volumes of tumor and normal tissues (**Fig. 1**). Although this can be of great value in helping plan a treatment, the additional advanced imaging required adds expense for the owner.

Achieving the same position for each treatment that the patient was imaged in for treatment planning is necessary to deliver the planned dose. There are 2 main elements to ensure this. First, by using patient positioning devices that are custom made for each patient at the time of imaging, and second by the use of on-board imaging at the time of treatment. Multiple patient positioning devices have been described in veterinary medicine, including the use of moldable cushions, vacuum-locked bags, orthoplastic molds, and bite block systems.[2–6] Although these have

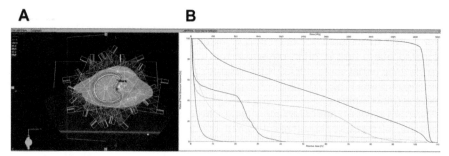

Fig. 1. (A) Intensity modulated radiotherapy plan from a rabbit diagnosed with a thymoma. (B) Dose-volume graph showing the volume of normal tissue receiving the prescribed dose (*red line*) and doses being received by normal tissues (*purple, gold, blue, teal,* and *brown lines*). (*Courtesy of* Radiation oncology and CAPE services, Veterinary Medical Teach Hospital, Davis, CA.)

been designed for use in the dog and the cat, many can also be used in exotic animal patients (**Fig. 2**). By combining the use of positioning devices and imaging, a high level of accuracy and precision can be achieved, which helps limit the amount of margin that must be used in the PTV, which in turns spares more normal tissue.

ELECTRON RADIOTHERAPY

Most newer linear accelerators are able to treat with electrons as well as photons. These electrons are created in a linear accelerator by scattering the accelerated electrons instead of having them hit a target in the machine. Linear accelerators offer a variety of different energies, allowing different depths of penetration. The depth of tissue to which a dose is delivered depends on the energy of the electrons used. Electrons are charged particles that have the advantage compared with photons of being able to largely control the depth of penetration of the radiation delivered, thereby sparing normal tissues beyond the area intended to be irradiated (**Fig. 3**). For example, a 6-MeV electron beam has about 2 cm of tissue dosed effectively, with very little dose

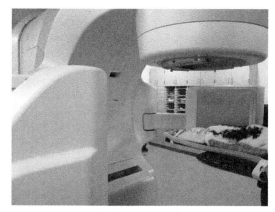

Fig. 2. Rabbit in a thermoplastic mask with a moldable cushion used for patient positioning to allow precise and accurate dose delivery. (*Courtesy of* Radiation oncology and CAPE services, Veterinary Medical Teach Hospital, Davis, CA.)

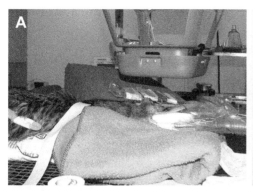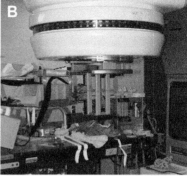

Fig. 3. (*A*) A mallard duck positioned under an electron cone for treatment of a melanoma on the bill. (*B*) A bird with a squamous cell carcinoma of the uropygial gland positioned under a linear accelerator for treatment with electrons. (*Courtesy of* Radiation oncology and CAPE services, Veterinary Medical Teach Hospital, Davis, CA.)

reaching beyond 3 cm of depth. This property can be very useful for treating tumors such as thoracic wall tumors.

INTENSITY MODULATED RADIOTHERAPY

Intensity modulated radiotherapy (IMRT) is a radiotherapy technique that allows better shaping of the dose in 3 dimensions onto a tumor, by changing the fluence of the beam as it is delivered. With this technique, a high dose gradient at the edges of the treatment field can be achieved, meaning that the dose decreases very rapidly. Although this can be beneficial in sparing normal tissue abutting a tumor, if positioning is not exact there is the potential to miss the tumor volume and put the high-dose area in normal tissue. IMRT treatments are accomplished by using advanced imaging, computerized treatment planning, multileaf collimators in the head of the linear accelerator, and on-board imaging to allow the precise patient setup needed to deliver the treatment. Although this type of treatment requires specialized equipment and increased time to deliver, it does allow better sparing of surrounding normal tissues and has the potential to decrease side effects and increase the dose delivered to the tumor.[7]

STEREOTACTIC RADIOSURGERY

Stereotactic radiosurgery is another specialized type of radiotherapy that is done using a linear accelerator. The linear accelerators have to be specifically equipped for this type of treatment and need to have some type of on-board imaging to allow the precise and accurate patient setups needed. With stereotactic radiosurgery, very small tissue margins are used and generally treatments with high doses per fraction are used to attempt to ablate the tumors (**Fig. 4**). Stereotactic radiosurgery is still a new treatment modality in veterinary medicine, with only a few published reports.[8–12]

STRONTUIM-90 PLESIOTHERAPY

Strontium-90 (^{90}Sr) is a radioactive element that can be placed on the surface of a tumor to deliver radiation. ^{90}Sr is a beta emitter, meaning that an electron is produced by nuclear decay of a neutron. ^{90}Sr has a half-life of approximately 29 years and emits an

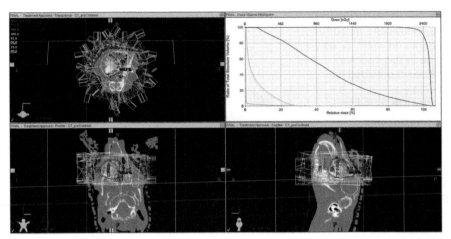

Fig. 4. A stereotactic radiosurgery plan for a rabbit diagnosed with a maxillary osteosarcoma. (*Courtesy of* Radiation oncology and CAPE services, Veterinary Medical Teach Hospital, Davis, CA.)

electron with an energy of 2.27 MeV. With this energy the maximal dose is delivered at the surface and decreases rapidly, with only about 10% of the delivered dose reaching a depth of 3 mm. This property has both advantages and disadvantages; delivering the dose superficially means that it is not effective for deep-seated tumors, but it has the advantage of limiting the dose to deeper, normal tissues, meaning that a high dose can be given in a single or several fractions without damage to normal underlying tissue. This property also means that the treatment can be repeated if needed. The active area of the probe is less than 1 cm in diameter, which means that larger lesions are treated with overlapping circles. The probe is generally held in a device during treatment to minimize exposure to personnel (**Fig. 5**). Although the dose rate is determined by the age of the individual probe, most treatments can be done in 3 to 5 minutes per application. In veterinary medicine there are published reports of using ^{90}Sr in cats with oral and nasal planum squamous cell carcinoma and cutaneous mast cell

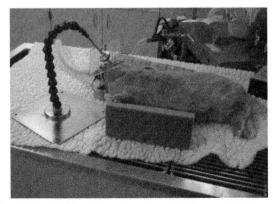

Fig. 5. Rabbit being treated with a strontium-90 probe for an eyelid plasmacytoma. (*Courtesy of* Radiation oncology and CAPE services, Veterinary Medical Teach Hospital, Davis, CA.)

tumors.[13–16] In dogs and horses it has been reported for the treatment of conjunctival squamous cell carcinoma.[17] There is also a case report of a lingual plasmacytoma in a dog treated with ^{90}Sr as well as the treatment of limbal melanoma and hemangiosarcoma in this species.[18–20] More specific information regarding ^{90}Sr in exotic animal species is provided later.

RADIATION SIDE EFFECTS: GENERAL CONSIDERATIONS

Side effects from radiation therapy are generally broken down into acute effects and late effects. A grading system for mammalian veterinary patients has been developed.[21] Acute effects occur toward the end of therapy or soon after the conclusion of therapy and are caused by damage to the rapidly dividing normal tissues in the radiation field. These effects include mucositis and moist and dry desquamation. Fatigue has also been reported in people as an acute side effect. Late or chronic effects of radiation therapy occur months to years after treatment. These effects can be life threatening and are more likely to affect quality of life. These side effects include fibrosis, ulceration, necrosis, and second tumor formation. In most cases, acute effects resolve within several weeks of finishing therapy.

FISH

Although clinically radiation therapy has been anecdotally used in fish there are no published reports and a single conference proceeding describes the use of electron radiotherapy that was unsuccessfully used to treat a goldfish (*Carassius auratus*) with a myxoma on the face. This treatment was attempted after failing intralesional bleomycin. In this case, 2 single fractions approximately 1 month apart of 8 Gy using 6-MeV electrons were used in an attempt at palliative care. The fish was euthanized 23 days after the second dose because of progressive disease.[22]

REPTILES

There are a few case reports in the literature of using radiation therapy to treat cancer in reptiles. A female Madagascar ground boa (*Boa madagascariensis*) was treated with a linear accelerator for a pharyngeal squamous cell carcinoma with a planned dose of 30 Gy delivered in 3 once-weekly treatments of 10 Gy. Five days after receiving the second dose the boa had open-mouthed breathing and dysecdysis and was euthanized. The mass had increased in size during the course of treatment.[23] A male bearded dragon (*Pogona vitticeps*) was treated with a linear accelerator for a squamous cell carcinoma of the upper eyelid that had recurred after surgical debulking. Radiation was delivered using 6-MeV electrons from a linear accelerator to a total dose of 48 Gy delivered in 10 fractions given 3 times per week. No acute effects from the radiation treatment were noted. At a 3-month recheck the mass had largely regressed, with the remaining tissue presumed to be granulation tissue.[24] Given the lack of information in reptiles, more work needs to be done in these animals before the efficacy of radiation therapy can be known.

BIRDS

There is very limited knowledge when it comes to irradiating birds. Most clinical information is in the form of case reports, with many lacking complete follow-up. The effectiveness of radiation therapy in birds also has not yet been well defined and more work needs to be done to determine an effective dosing and fractionation scheme for this species.

There are several case reports in the literature regarding the use of teletherapy with linear accelerators, cobalt-60 units, orthovoltage machines, and a cesium irradiator. A presumed female umbrella cockatoo was treated with orthovoltage radiotherapy after having a debulking surgery for an orbital osteosarcoma. She received a total dose of 68 Gy given in 17 fractions on Mondays, Wednesdays, and Fridays over a 6-week period. Although the bird remained well during the course of radiotherapy she died 2 months after finishing treatment with neurologic signs. Because the owners declined necropsy examination it is not known whether this represented tumor progression or was secondary to radiation effects on the brain.[25] In another case, a male budgerigar (*Melopsittacus undulatus*) was treated with a ^{137}cesium unit for a metacarpal region mass diagnosed as a hemangiosarcoma. He was treated to a total dose of 40 Gy in ten 4-Gy fractions given on Mondays, Wednesdays, and Fridays. The mass responded completely, but there was a suspected new lesion noted outside the radiation field 4 weeks later. Eight weeks after that the bird developed ataxia, lethargy, and anorexia and was euthanized. On necropsy, multiple lesions were identified and found to be hemangiosarcoma.[26] A macaroni penguin (*Eudyptes chrysolophus*) was treated with radiation therapy for a malignant melanoma in the subcutaneous tissues near the right nares. This bird was treated with a total of 36 Gy in alternating-day 6-Gy fractions. There was a complete response noted by 15 weeks, although the penguin developed a new lesion outside the radiation field 29 months later and a survival time of 39 months was reported. Although details of this individual bird were not presented in this case series, the authors stated that there was metastasis at the time of death.[27] A case of a male thick-billed parrot (*Rhynchopsitta pachyrhyncha*) that was treated with electron radiotherapy using a linear accelerator for a melanoma located along the mandibular beak has also been reported. He received a total dose of 50 Gy in twenty 2.5-Gy fractions on a Monday-through-Friday schedule. A good clinical local response to radiotherapy was noted, with the only side effect noted from treatment being some feather loss in the radiation field. The bird died approximately 11.5 weeks after starting therapy from complications associated with systemic metastasis, which was confirmed on necropsy.[28] Another case of a mandibular beak tumor, this time a squamous cell carcinoma, in a Buffon's macaw (*Ara ambigua*) treated with a cobalt-60 unit has been reported. He received a total dose of 48 Gy delivered in 12 fractions on Mondays, Wednesdays, and Fridays over 4 weeks. After finishing the course, a biopsy revealed active tumor and an additional 8-Gy boost was delivered. This treatment was complicated by a continued and concurrent infection. Another biopsy was taken and showed little tumor response to the prescribed radiation dose. Intralesional cisplatin was then attempted. The bird died 1 week later after aspirating. Necropsy confirmed the diagnosis and did not show signs of metastasis.[29] A female American flamingo (*Phoenicopterus ruber*) diagnosed with a digital squamous cell carcinoma was treated with radiotherapy using a cobalt-60 unit. Initially she received a total dose of 30 Gy in three 10-Gy fractions on days 0, 7, and 21. As the tumor continued to grow, 2 additional fractions of 10 Gy once weekly were given 1 month later. Because there was no response, the toe was amputated.[30]

There is a single case reported of intralesional cisplatin combined with radiation to treat a female blue and gold macaw (*Ara ararauna*) diagnosed with a fibrosarcoma on the wing. She received a total dose of 40 Gy delivered in ten 4-Gy fractions on Mondays, Wednesdays, and Fridays. In addition, her tumor was injected with cisplatin (0.3 mg/cm^3) 10 minutes before the first, third, and eighth treatments. A complete response was achieved by 2 months after finishing treatment. The bird died 15 months later of respiratory disease. Because no necropsy was done it is not known whether there was pulmonary metastasis or not.[31]

There is also limited information in the published literature for the use of ^{90}Sr in birds, but there a case series presented in abstract form describing its use. A male budgerigar (*M undulatus*) with a uropygial gland carcinoma, a female budgerigar (*M undulatus*) with a uropygial squamous cell carcinoma, and a female cockatiel (*Nymphicus hollandicus*) with a uropygial gland papillary adenoma were all treated with 100 Gy of radiation using ^{90}Sr. All had good responses with lack of recurrence in the first 2 at 9 and 8 months and regression of the tumor at last recheck at 8 weeks after therapy, with none of the cases having adverse radiation reactions.[32] In another abstract, a single case of a female African gray parrot (*Psittacus erithacus*) that was treated with ^{90}Sr using 2 fractions of 100 Gy 1 week apart after surgical debulking of an uropygial gland carcinoma has been reported. In this case there were no reported side effects and the site remained tumor free at 6-month follow-up.[33]

There is also a single report of whole-body low-dose irradiation in a male black swan (*Cygnus atratus*) for the treatment of a T-cell chronic lymphocytic leukemia after a poor response to various chemotherapeutics. He received a total dose of 2 Gy delivered in ten 20-cGy fractions twice weekly. The total white blood cell count decreased but was still markedly increased. One-hundred and eighteen days after finishing radiotherapy the bird began showing tremors and died 6 days later. Necropsy did not reveal the cause of the tremors, although hyperviscosity syndrome was suspected.

Overall the data indicate a variable response to radiotherapy and that it may be that birds require an increased total dose to have the same effect on their tumors as mammalian species. Although this is not an established fact, there are some clues in the literature that indicate that normal tissues in birds are more resistant to the effects of radiation, which in turn could indicate that their tumors are more resistant as well. In total body radiation experiments the $LD_{50/60}$ (lethal dose for 50% of cases at 60 days) for chickens was 9 Gy, which is more than twice the lethal dose for humans, dogs, and many other species.[34] Japanese quail were found to have an $LD_{50/30}$ of 22.5 Gy, which is higher than that reported for any mammalian species.[34] Perhaps more relevant to radiotherapy for the treatment of cancer, Barron and colleagues irradiated 3 ring-necked parakeets to 48, 60, or 72 Gy in 4-Gy fractions delivered on Mondays, Wednesdays, and Fridays. They also had a nonirradiated control group. The birds were observed for visible skin effects, and body weight and food intake were measured. None of the birds in any of the groups showed any radiation side effects. Biopsies taken at the end of treatment were compared with biopsies taken from the control group. No histologic changes were found in the epidermis in the 48-Gy or 60-Gy groups, and there were only mild changes, including mild, multifocal anisokaryosis of keratinocytes in the epidermis and mild to moderate dermatitis and folliculitis, in the 72-Gy group. No ill effects were noted at 6-month and 9-month reevaluation in any of the birds. The investigators went on to report that 4 Gy delivered in 18 fractions to a total dose of 72 Gy was delivered clinically to 3 psittacines treated with different skin tumors with good results, but no further description was given.[35]

In a recent study of whether the dose calculated using a computerized treatment planning software program was actually delivered in a group of military macaws that had their choana regions experimentally irradiated, the delivered dose was 1.2% to 8.6% less than planned. It is hard to say what accounted for these differences because some of this may have been inherent in their experimental design, but the investigators hypothesized that this may in part be caused by the complex anatomy with multiple air-filled cavities and the skin and subcutaneous thickness. Both of these things could lead to inadequate dose buildup, which in turn could account for delivering a decreased dose of radiation compared with the planned dose.[36]

These data taken in conjunction with the lack of clinical responses in dosing schemes based on mammalian species mean that more work needs to be done in determining ideal dosing and fractionation schemes for the treatment of avian neoplasia. In a 2010 survey of radiation facilities in the United States, Canada, and Europe, 6 of the 24 responding facilities reported treating birds.[1] If clinicians are to advance the field and learn how to appropriately treat birds with various neoplastic conditions using radiation therapy, a concerted effort will be needed.

RODENTS

To the author's knowledge there are no clinical reports of using radiotherapy in rodent species to treat cancer. It is reasonable to consider treating appropriate cases using information gained from other mammal species, given that there has been experimental cancer research done in rats and mice in many studies.

RABBITS

There is perhaps more known about irradiating rabbits than other exotic animals. There are several case series published on the treatment of thymomas in rabbits. The first study, from 2006, describes a course of palliative radiotherapy using a linear accelerator. Each rabbit received a total dose of 24 Gy delivered in three 8-Gy fractions over a 4-week period. All 3 rabbits had an improved quality of life and a reduction in clinical signs. Two of the rabbits were still clinically doing well at 6 months but were then lost to follow-up. The third case was reported to be in remission at 24 months after therapy. No adverse radiation affects were reported.[37] A multi-institutional retrospective study of 19 rabbits treated with a variety of different machines and dosing schemes found a median survival of 313 days. If the 3 rabbits that died during the course of therapy are excluded from analysis, the median survival time was 727 days. The only prognostic factor found for survival was that the rabbits that had a body weight lower than the mean (1.57 kg) were more likely to have a shorter survival time. In 7 of the rabbits the time to resolution of clinical signs was available and ranged from 4 to 42 days. Six of these rabbits had a second CT scan done during the course of therapy, showing a decrease in tumor mass of between 30% and 86.6%, indicating that these tumors are very responsive to radiation therapy.[38] This finding also means that repeat imaging during the course of therapy should be considered to avoid overdosing normal tissues that may move into the originally planned tumor volume as the tumor shrinks. An acute case of radiation pneumonitis was noted 3 months after treatment, 1 case of myocardial failure was confirmed on necropsy 12 months after completing radiotherapy, and 1 case of alopecia in the radiation field was noted. In a recently published prospective study in which 15 rabbits were treated with an IMRT arc radiotherapy plan using a linear accelerator at a single institution, median survival was not reached. Two rabbits died during the study period, at 677 and 777 days, and three were lost to follow-up. The mean follow-up time was 801.3 days. These rabbits were treated to a total dose of 40 Gy in six 6.67-Gy fractions every other day. Fourteen of the rabbits had a complete response on a 40-day recheck CT scan. The final rabbit also achieved a complete response but not until 6 months after treatment. This study used adaptive planning with the rabbits undergoing additional diagnostic CT scans on days 5 and 9 of treatment, showing a reduction in mean volume of more than 50%, again showing the need for careful imaging and radiotherapy replanning during the course of treatment.[8] No acute or late radiation side effects were reported in this study.

There is also a published case report of a female spayed Netherland dwarf rabbit that was diagnosed with a nasal adenocarcinoma that was treated with an orthovoltage unit after surgical debulking of the mass, although there was gross disease left behind. A total dose of 48 Gy was given in 6 once-weekly 8-Gy fractions. Repeat CT scans up to 1 year after treatment showed no tumor recurrence and the rabbit was alive at more than 3 years after treatment. The investigators did report bilateral cataracts and altered color and texture of the hair as radiation-induced side effects.[39] In another case report, a female New Zealand white mixed-breed rabbit diagnosed with an amelanotic melanoma was treated with surgical debulking and 150 Gy of radiation using ^{90}Sr to the tumor bed intraoperatively. The rabbit was reported to have died approximately 6 months later, with no evidence of local recurrence. Because no necropsy examination was done it is not known whether or not the tumor had metastasized or there was another cause of death.[40] An intact male rabbit was treated with radiotherapy after surgical debulking of a maxillary acanthomatous ameloblastoma. The type of machine and radiation were not indicated. The rabbit received a total dose of 38 Gy delivered in twelve 3.17-Gy fractions. These fractions were initially given 3 times weekly but then switched to twice weekly when anorexia developed in the third week of therapy. No recurrence was noted at 1 year. No mention of side effects secondary to the radiation therapy were mentioned.[41]

Besides the clinical data from published reports and clinical series of rabbits that were irradiated, there are data in the literature on radiation side effects from experimentally irradiated rabbits. These data suggest that rabbits respond similarly to other species in terms of acute and late side effects.[42–44] In the case of skin, rabbits can acutely have alopecia with either dry or moist desquamation. This condition generally resolves within several weeks and over time the hair grows back, although it is likely to be coarser and the color dilute (**Fig. 6**).

FERRETS

Although radiotherapy is generally not a component traditionally used in the most commonly reported tumors that occur in ferrets (endocrine tumors and lymphoma), there are several reports in the literature of using radiotherapy clinically to treat neoplasia in ferrets. A female European ferret (*Mustela putorius furo*) that had been

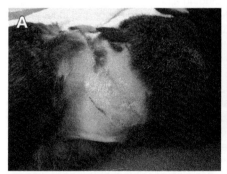
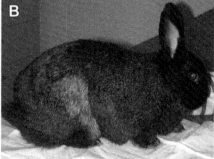

Fig. 6. (*A*) Rabbit on last day of radiotherapy after receiving 48 Gy of electron radiotherapy using a linear accelerator for an incompletely excised myxofibrosarcoma. Note areas of alopecia and dry desquamation. (*B*) Same rabbit 3 months after treatment showing hair regrowth with leukotrichia. (*Courtesy of* Radiation oncology and CAPE services, Veterinary Medical Teach Hospital, Davis, CA.)

diagnosed with lymphoma and failed a COP-based chemotherapy protocol was treated with a single dose of doxorubicin and an orthovoltage unit as a salvage therapy. Clinically the disease was confined to a single lymph node, although the animal was not completely staged, which is why radiation was attempted. She received a total dose of 40 Gy delivered in eight 5-Gy fractions twice weekly. She achieved a complete response. The ferret relapsed 4 months after completion of the course of radiation and went on to receive further chemotherapy. In total the ferret lived 23 months after initial diagnosis.[45]

A female ferret was diagnosed with a perianal apocrine gland tumor. The mass was not surgically resectable and the area was treated using a cobalt-60 unit to a total dose of 48 Gy in twelve 4-Gy fractions on Mondays, Wednesdays, and Fridays. By the end of treatment there was a complete clinical response. Nodal metastasis was noted 2 months later. The ferret became clinical approximately 3 months later and the enlarged sublumbar lymph nodes were treated with an additional course of radiotherapy consisting of three 8-Gy doses on days 0, 7, and 21 to a total dose of 24 Gy. There was a good clinical response, although again this was short lived and the ferret was euthanized approximately 1 month later.[46]

In another case report, a male castrated ferret presented with recurrence of a perianal mass. Biopsy revealed an apocrine gland adenocarcinoma that was thought to be of anal sac origin. Because the 2 masses were invasive into the underlying tissues, surgery was not deemed possible and the ferret was treated with orthovoltage radiation therapy. The planned total dose was to be 48 Gy delivered in twice-weekly 4-Gy fractions. After the sixth fraction the mass was no longer palpable but the ferret developed anorexia, dyspnea, and coughing. There was pleural effusion present, which was cytologically examined and revealed a mesothelioma. The ferret died at home shortly after that.[47]

There are several reports in the literature describing preputial tumors in ferrets. In one report a male castrated ferret was treated with a cobalt-60 unit to a total dose of 40 Gy in eight 5-Gy treatments twice weekly for an adenocarcinoma. This treatment was done after 2 previous surgeries with recurrence in the gross disease setting. There was a complete response by the end of therapy but recurrence in the field at 4 months and an additional new lesion developed outside the radiation field. A second course of radiotherapy using a larger field was then used after gross resection of the new tumor to a total dose of 25 Gy delivered in five 5-Gy fractions over 13 days. There was local recurrence approximately 2 months later, including a new lesion along the spine, and the ferret was euthanized. The skin side effects reported were minor and included erythema and dry desquamation, which resolved.[48] In a separate report regarding a preputial mass, a preputial adenocarcinoma that was treated with surgery with 1-cm margins had no reported recurrence at 23 months when it represented for an insulinoma and adrenal tumor. The other ferret was treated with surgery and despite reported clean margins for its carcinoma had local recurrence at 3 months. After a second surgical procedure, which was pathologically read again as having a clean margin, the ferret received radiotherapy. Full details of the radiation treatments were not provided, but the ferret was given 36 Gy in total in twelve 3-Gy fractions over a 4-week period. There was local recurrence reported soon after, further therapy was not attempted, and the ferret was euthanized 3 months later.[49] Although it is possible that the tumor was inherently radioresistant, it is also possible that the dose was not sufficient to kill all of the tumor.

A male castrated ferret diagnosed with a retrobulbar adenocarcinoma was initially treated with incomplete surgical debulking, including exenteration of the eye. He was treated with postoperative radiotherapy using a cobalt-60 unit to a total dose of 32 Gy in 4 once-weekly 8-Gy fractions. The only noted acute side effect was erythema in the radiation field, which resolved with a late effect of a hair coat color and texture change in that area. At 200 days the ferret was clinically normal.[50]

A male castrated ferret was treated with radiation therapy using a linear accelerator and electrons 2 months after undergoing a partial maxillectomy for an oral squamous cell carcinoma. It was thought that tumor extended to the surgical margin, although the tissue was cauterized, so this was difficult for the pathologist to assess. The ferret was treated to a total dose of 54 Gy in eighteen 3-Gy fractions delivered once daily on Monday through Thursday and twice on Fridays to the primary tumor resection site and to a total dose of 45 Gy in fifteen 3-Gy fractions given Monday through Friday to the mandibular lymph node. The investigators reported some alopecia and erythema in the irradiated tissues, which resolved by 2 months. At the time of the report the ferret was clinically free of disease at 3 months after therapy.[51]

There have also been many studies done using ferrets as an experimental model of radiation-induced nausea and vomiting. From these studies and those reviewed earlier, clinically reported side effects seem similar to those of other mammals.

Radiation has proved to be an effective tool in managing dogs and cats for many types of tumors. As more experience is gained in exotic animal medicine in treating tumors, radiation also promises to be a valuable tool. However, clinicians must determine the optimal methods, dosing, and treatment schedules for these unique patients if they are to take full advantage of its promise.

REFERENCES

1. Farrelly J, McEntee MC. A survey of veterinary radiation facilities in 2010. Vet Radiol Ultrasound 2014;55(6):638–43.
2. Charney SC, Lutz WR, Klein MK, et al. Evaluation of a head-repositioner and Z-plate system for improved accuracy of dose delivery. Vet Radiol Ultrasound 2009;50(3):323–9.
3. Dieterich S, Zwingenberger A, Hansen K, et al. Inter- and intrafraction motion for stereotactic radiosurgery in dogs and cats using a modified Brainlab frameless stereotactic mask system. Vet Radiol Ultrasound 2015;56(5):563–9.
4. Kent MS, Gordon IK, Benavides I, et al. Assessment of the accuracy and precision of a patient immobilization device for radiation therapy in canine head and neck tumors. Vet Radiol Ultrasound 2009;50(5):550–4.
5. Kippenes H, Gavin PR, Sande RD, et al. Comparison of the accuracy of positioning devices for radiation therapy of canine and feline head tumors. Vet Radiol Ultrasound 2000;41(4):371–6.
6. Hansen KS, Theon AP, Dieterich S, et al. Validation of an indexed radiotherapy head positioning device for use in dogs and cats. Vet Radiol Ultrasound 2015; 56(4):448–55.
7. Lawrence JA, Forrest LJ. Intensity-modulated radiation therapy and helical tomotherapy: its origin, benefits, and potential applications in veterinary medicine. Vet Clin North Am Small Anim Pract 2007;37(6):1151–65, vii–iii.
8. Dolera M, Malfassi L, Mazza G, et al. Feasibility for using hypofractionated stereotactic volumetric modulated arc radiotherapy (Vmat) with adaptive planning for treatment of thymoma in rabbits: 15 cases. Vet Radiol Ultrasound 2016;57(3): 313–20.
9. Farese JP, Milner R, Thompson MS, et al. Stereotactic radiosurgery for treatment of osteosarcomas involving the distal portions of the limbs in dogs. J Am Vet Med Assoc 2004;225(10):1567–72, 1548.

10. Glasser SA, Charney S, Dervisis NG, et al. Use of an image-guided robotic radio-surgery system for the treatment of canine nonlymphomatous nasal tumors. J Am Anim Hosp Assoc 2014;50(2):96–104.

11. Kubicek L, Milner R, An Q, et al. Outcomes and prognostic factors associated with canine sinonasal tumors treated with curative intent cone-based stereotactic radiosurgery (1999-2013). Vet Radiol Ultrasound 2016;57(3):331–40.

12. Nolan MW, Griffin LR, Custis JT, et al. Stereotactic body radiation therapy for treatment of injection-site sarcomas in cats: 11 cases (2008-2012). J Am Vet Med Assoc 2013;243(4):526–31.

13. Goodfellow M, Hayes A, Murphy S, et al. A retrospective study of (90)Strontium plesiotherapy for feline squamous cell carcinoma of the nasal planum. J Feline Med Surg 2006;8(3):169–76.

14. Hammond GM, Gordon IK, Theon AP, et al. Evaluation of strontium Sr 90 for the treatment of superficial squamous cell carcinoma of the nasal planum in cats: 49 cases (1990-2006). J Am Vet Med Assoc 2007;231(5):736–41.

15. Turrel JM, Farrelly J, Page RL, et al. Evaluation of strontium 90 irradiation in treatment of cutaneous mast cell tumors in cats: 35 cases (1992–2002). J Am Vet Med Assoc 2006;228(6):898–901.

16. Nagata K, Selting KA, Cook CR, et al. 90Sr therapy for oral squamous cell carcinoma in two cats. Vet Radiol Ultrasound 2011;52(1):114–7.

17. Nevile JC, Hurn SD, Turner AG, et al. Management of canine corneal squamous cell carcinoma with lamellar keratectomy and strontium 90 plesiotherapy: 3 cases. Vet Ophthalmol 2015;18(3):254–60.

18. Ware K, Gieger T. Use of strontium-90 plesiotherapy for the treatment of a lingual plasmacytoma in a dog. J Small Anim Pract 2011;52(4):220–3.

19. Donaldson D, Sansom J, Adams V. Canine limbal melanoma: 30 cases (1992-2004). Part 2. Treatment with lamellar resection and adjunctive strontium-90beta plesiotherapy–efficacy and morbidity. Vet Ophthalmol 2006;9(3):179–85.

20. Donaldson D, Sansom J, Murphy S, et al. Multiple limbal haemangiosarcomas in a border collie dog: management by lamellar keratectomy/sclerectomy and strontium-90 beta plesiotherapy. J Small Anim Pract 2006;47(9):545–9.

21. Ladue T, Klein MK, Veterinary Radiation Therapy Oncology Group. Toxicity criteria of the veterinary radiation therapy oncology group. Vet Radiol Ultrasound 2001;42(5):475–6.

22. Stevens B, Vergneau-Grosset C, Rodriguez C, et al. Treatment of a facial myxoma in a goldfish (*Carassius auratus*) with intralesional bleomycin chemotherapy and radiation therapy. Paper presented at: International Association for Aquatic Animal Medicine. Virginia Beach (VA), May 21–26, 2016.

23. Steeil JC, Schumacher J, Hecht S, et al. Diagnosis and treatment of a pharyngeal squamous cell carcinoma in a Madagascar ground boa (*Boa madagascariensis*). J Zoo Wildl Med 2013;44(1):144–51.

24. Bishop T, Cumming B. Treatment of a squamous cell carcinoma in a bearded dragon (*Pogona vitticeps*) using radiation therapy. Paper presented at: Association of Avian Veterinarians, Australasian Committee and Unusual Pets and Avian Veterinarians. Cairns (Australia), April 22–25, 2014.

25. Fordham M, Rosenthal K, Durham A, et al. Intraocular osteosarcoma in an umbrella cockatoo (*Cacatua alba*). Vet Ophthalmol 2010;13(Suppl):103–8.

26. Freeman KP, Hahn KA, Adams WH, et al. Radiation therapy for hemangiosarcoma in a budgerigar. J Avian Med Surg 1999;13:40–4.

27. Duncan AE, Smedley R, Anthony S, et al. Malignant melanoma in the penguin: characterization of the clinical, histologic, and immunohistochemical features of

malignant melanoma in 10 individuals from three species of penguin. J Zoo Wildl Med 2014;45(3):534–49.

28. Guthrie AL, Gonzalez-Angulo C, Wigle WL, et al. Radiation therapy of a malignant melanoma in a thick-billed parrot (*Rhynchopsitta pachyrhyncha*). J Avian Med Surg 2010;24(4):299–307.

29. Manucy TK, Bennett RA, Greenacre CB, et al. Squamous cell carcinoma of the mandibular beak in a Buffon's macaw (*Ara ambigua*). J Avian Med Surg 1998; 12(3):158–66.

30. Abu J, Wunschmann A, Redig PT, et al. Management of a cutaneous squamous cell carcinoma in an American flamingo (*Phoenicopterus ruber*). J Avian Med Surg 2009;23(1):44–8.

31. Lamberski N, Théon AP. Concurrent irradiation and intratumoral chemotherapy with cisplatin for treatment of a fibrosarcoma in a blue and gold macaw (*Ara ararauna*). J Avian Med Surg 2002;16(3):234–8.

32. Nemetz L, Broome M. Strontium-90 therapy for uropygial neoplasia. Paper presented at: Proc Annu Conf Assoc Avian Vet. New Orleans (LA), August 16–20, 2004.

33. Pignon C, Azuma C, Mayer J. Radiation therapy of uropygial gland carcinoma in psittacine species. Paper presented at: Association of avian veterinarians. Seattle, Washington, August 6–12, 2011.

34. Zallinger C, Tempel K. The physiologic response of domestic animals to ionizing radiation: a review. Vet Radiol Ultrasound 1998;39(6):495–503.

35. Barron HW, Roberts RE, Latimer KS, et al. Tolerance doses of cutaneous and mucosal tissues in ring-necked parakeets (*Psittacula krameri*) for external beam megavoltage radiation. J Avian Med Surg 2009;23(1):6–9.

36. Cutler D, Shiomitsu K, Liu C, et al. comparison of calculated radiation delivery versus actual radiation delivery in military macaws (*Ara militaris*). J Avian Med Surg 2016;30(1):1–7.

37. Guzman Sanchez-Migallon D, Mayer J, Gould J, et al. Radiation therapy for the treatment of thymoma in rabbits (*Oryctolagus cuniculi*). J Exot Pet Med 2006; 15:138–44.

38. Andres KM, Kent M, Siedlecki CT, et al. The use of megavoltage radiation therapy in the treatment of thymomas in rabbits: 19 cases. Vet Comp Oncol 2012;10(2): 82–94.

39. Nakata M, Yasutsugu M, Tsuboi M, et al. Surgical and localized radiation therapy for an intranasal adenocarcinoma in a rabbit. J Vet Med Sci 2014;76(12):1659.

40. Brandão J, Blair R, Kelly A, et al. Amelanotic melanoma in the rabbit: a case report with an overview of immunohistochemical characterization. J Exot Pet Med 2015;24(2):193–200.

41. Huynh M, Desprez I, Volait L, et al. Acanthomatous ameloblastoma in a rabbit treated by surgery and radiation therapy. Paper presented at: Association of Exotic Mammal Veterinarians. Orlando (FL), 2014.

42. Du Z-Z, Ren H, Song J-F, et al. Rabbit model of radiation-induced lung injury. Asian Pac J Trop Med 2013;6(3):237–41.

43. Meirelles RP, Hochman B, Helene Junior A, et al. Experimental model of cutaneous radiation injury in rabbits. Acta Cirurgica Brasileira 2013;28(11):751–5.

44. Lin Z, Wu VW, Ju W, et al. Radiation-induced changes in peripheral nerve by stereotactic radiosurgery: a study on the sciatic nerve of rabbit. J Neurooncol 2011; 102(2):179–85.

45. Hutson CA, Kopit MJ, Walder EJ. Combination doxorubicin and orthovoltage radiation therapy, single-agent doxorubicin, and high-dose vincristine for salvage therapy of ferret lymphosarcoma. J Am Anim Hosp Assoc 1992;28(4):365–8.

46. Graham JE, Roberts RE, Wilson GH, et al. Perianal apocrine gland adenocarcinoma in a ferret. Compendium on Continuing Education for the Practising Veterinarian North American Edition 2001;23(4):359–62.
47. Nakata M, Miwa Y, Nakayama H, et al. Localised radiotherapy for a ferret with possible anal sac apocrine adenocarcinoma. J Small Anim Pract 2008;49(9):476–8.
48. Miller TA, Denman DL, Lewis GC Jr. Recurrent adenocarcinoma in a ferret. J Am Vet Med Assoc 1985;187(8):839–41.
49. van Zeeland YR, Lennox A, Quinton JF, et al. Prepuce and partial penile amputation for treatment of preputial gland neoplasia in two ferrets. J Small Anim Pract 2014;55(11):593–6.
50. McBride M, Mosunic CB, Barron GHW, et al. Successful treatment of a retrobulbar adenocarcinoma in a ferret (*Mustela putorius furo*). Vet Rec 2009;165(7):206–8.
51. Graham J, Fidel J, Mison M. Rostral maxillectomy and radiation therapy to manage squamous cell carcinoma in a ferret. Veterinary Clin North Am Exot Anim Pract 2006;9(3):701–6.

Index

Note: Page numbers of article titles are in **boldface** type.

A

Ablation, percutaneous thermal tumor, 251
ACOPA protocol, for chemotherapeutics, in ferret oncology, 230
ACTH stimulation test, for guinea pigs, 116
Actin, smooth muscle, as rabbit tumor marker, 143
Adenitis, sebaceous, in rabbits, 165
Adenocarcinomas, chemotherapeutics for, 216
 in avians, gastrointestinal, 76
  respiratory, 75
  urogenital, 76–77, 79
 in chinchilla, 119
 in ferrets, endocrine, 192
  integumentary, 188
  oral, 193
  perianal, 266
  preputial gland, 186, 202–203, 266
  reproductive tract, 185–186
  retrobulbar, 266–267
 in fish, 23, 25–26, 30
  vent, 31, 34
 in gerbils, 122
  uterine, 123
 in hamsters, gastrointestinal, 122
  uterine, 120
 in invertebrates, 6
 in rabbits, 139–140
  respiratory, 115
  testicular, 149, 159, 161
  uterine, 148–149, 158–159
 in reptiles, 89–93, 95, 99
 renal, chemotherapeutics for, 211–212
 salivary gland, chemotherapeutics for, 216
Adenomas, in chinchilla, 119
 in ferrets, integumentary, 188
 in fish, 23
 in gerbils, 122, 124
 in guinea pigs, 112
  pulmonary, 117
 in invertebrates, 5–7
 in mice, 126
 in rabbits, bile duct, 148
  uterine, 149, 158

Vet Clin Exot Anim 20 (2017) 271–306
http://dx.doi.org/10.1016/S1094-9194(16)30063-9
1094-9194/17

Moving?

Make sure your subscription moves with you!

To notify us of your new address, find your **Clinics Account Number** (located on your mailing label above your name), and contact customer service at:

Email: journalscustomerservice-usa@elsevier.com

800-654-2452 (subscribers in the U.S. & Canada)
314-447-8871 (subscribers outside of the U.S. & Canada)

Fax number: 314-447-8029

Elsevier Health Sciences Division
Subscription Customer Service
3251 Riverport Lane
Maryland Heights, MO 63043

Printed and bound by CPI Group (UK) Ltd, Croydon, CR0 4YY

07/10/2024

01040503-0006